Recent Progress in Hepatic Surgery

Recent Progress in Hepatic Surgery

Edited by **Amelia Foster**

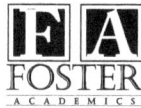

FOSTER
A C A D E M I C S

New Jersey

Published by Foster Academics,
61 Van Reypen Street,
Jersey City, NJ 07306, USA
www.fosteracademics.com

Recent Progress in Hepatic Surgery
Edited by Amelia Foster

International Standard Book Number: 978-1-63242-350-4 (Hardback)

Contents

Preface

This book has been an outcome of determined endeavour from a group of educationists in the field. The primary objective was to involve a broad spectrum of professionals from diverse cultural background involved in the field for developing new researches. The book not only targets students but also scholars pursuing higher research for further enhancement of the theoretical and practical applications of the subject.

The book integrates recent advancements made in the field of hepatic surgery. The liver was referred to as a hostile organ by Longmire since it welcomes sepsis and malignant cells so warmly, bleeds so freely, and is usually the first organ to get injured in blunt abdominal trauma. To balance these negative factors, it has an excellent characteristic: its capability to regenerate after a great loss of substance. This book highlights a great range of topics including secondary liver tumors, liver tumors in infants and children, hepatobiliary trauma, hepatic trauma and portal hypertension. It would serve as an important source of reference for students, researchers and physicians.

It was an honour to edit such a profound book and also a challenging task to compile and examine all the relevant data for accuracy and originality. I wish to acknowledge the efforts of the contributors for submitting such brilliant and diverse chapters in the field and for endlessly working for the completion of the book. Last, but not the least; I thank my family for being a constant source of support in all my research endeavours.

Editor

Secondary Liver Tumors

Hesham Abdeldayem, Amr Helmy, Hisham Gad,
Essam Salah, Amr Sadek, Tarek Ibrahim,
Elsayed Soliman, Khaled Abuelella, Maher Osman,
Amr Aziz, Hosam Soliman, Sherif Saleh,
Osama Hegazy, Hany Shoreem, Taha Yasen,
Emad Salem, Mohamed Taha, Hazem Zakaria,
Islam Ayoub and Ahmed Sherif

Additional information is available at the end of the chapter

1. Introduction

The liver is a common site of metastases. The most relevant metastatic tumor of the liver to the surgeon is colorectal cancer because of the well-documented potential for long-term survival after complete resection. However, a large number of other tumors commonly metastasize to the liver, including cancers of the upper gastrointestinal system (stomach, pancreas, biliary), genitourinary system (renal, prostate), neuroendocrine system, breast, eye (melanoma), skin (melanoma), soft tissue (retroperitoneal sarcoma), and gynecologic system (ovarian, endometrial, cervix). [1]

The high frequency of liver metastases is caused by: [2]

1. The liver's vast blood supply, which originates from portal and systemic systems.

2. The fenestrations of the hepatic sinusoidal endothelium may facilitate penetration of malignant cells into the hepatic parenchyma.

3. Humoral factors that promote cell growth and cellular factors, such as adhesion molecules, favor metastatic spread to the liver.

4. The liver's geographic proximity to other intra-abdominal organs may allow malignant infiltration by direct extension.

Not so long ago, oncologists were so pessimistic about the appearance of hepatic metasta-ses that "no treatment" was often the recommendation. Advancing technology and im-proved surgical techniques now offer potential therapeutic options for patients with such lesions. Patient selection is the most important aspect of surgical therapy for metastatic disease in the liver and clinical follow-up of resected patients has identified those most and least likely to benefit. Therefore, realistic expectations and honest patient education is an important aspect of treatment. [1]

1.1. Clinical presentation

The clinical presentation of patients with liver metastases is variable and subtle. Most pa-tients are asymptomatic; a minority may report abdominal pain, jaundice, or pruritus. Hep-atic metastases from gastrointestinal carcinoid tumors are associated with release of vasoactive peptides and serotonin into the systemic circulation. Symptoms of the carcinoid syndrome, specifically flushing, sweats, and diarrhea, frequently occur in this setting. Liver metastases from neuroendocrine tumors can lead to significant symptoms caused by the production of functioning hormones. [1]

Physical examination may reveal hepatomegaly, a friction rub over hepatic metastases, or ascites caused by hepatic venous obstruction or peritoneal carcinomatosis. [2]

1.2. Histopathology

The histologic appearances of metastatic deposits in the liver may resemble those of the pri-mary tumors; however, there can be marked differences. These differences exist because metastatic foci are derived from a select subpopulation of tumor cells. Cells that are capable of successful metastasis are believed to have specific characteristics, such as high motility, resistance to immune-mediated destruction, and a high concentration of matrix receptors or matrix-degrading enzymes.

Because the metastatic cell population may not be representative of the primary tumor, it can be difficult to determine the site of origin based on the histologic appearance of the metastases alone.

The initial light-microscopic findings can be used to categorize the tissue into one of three groups:

1.   poorly differentiated carcinoma or adenocarcinoma,

2.   well-differentiated adenocarcinoma, and

3.   squamous carcinoma.

In most cases, immunohistochemical studies further differentiate these metastases. (Table 1) [3]

Tumor	Antigens
Colonic adenocarcinoma	CEA
Pancreatic carcinoma	CEA, pancreatic carcinoma-associated antigen
Lung carcinoma	CEA, cytokeratin, neuron-specific enolase
Breast carcinoma	CEA, milk-fat globulin, hCG
Thyroid carcinoma	Thyroglobulin
Prostate carcinoma	Prostate-specific acid phosphatase, PSA
Melanoma	S-100, vimentin, neuron-specific enolase
Carcinoid	Chromogranin, neuron-specific enolase
Lymphoma and leukemia	CLA
Sarcoma	
Smooth muscle	Type IV collagen, vimentin, desmin
Skeletal muscle	Myoglobin, vimentin, desmin
Neurogenic	S-100, myelin basic protein
Cartilage	S-100, vimentin
Bone	Vimentin
Germ cell tumors	α-fetoprotien, α1-antitrypsin
Trophoblastic tumors	hCG, α-Fetoprotein

Table 1. Immunohistochemical antigens for the identification of primary tumors.

Abbreviations: CEA, carcinoembryonic antigen; CLA, common leukocyte antigen; hCG, human chorionic gonadotropin; PSA, prostate-specific antigen.

1.3. Biochemical Laboratory Tests

The laboratory tests that are available for liver function assessment are not very sensitive. CEA remains the most sensitive test for metastatic colon cancer, but even this test can be normal in the presence of liver metastases, especially with minimal hepatic disease.

1.4. Imaging Techniques

The choice among the various techniques, and the sequence with which they are used, should be guided primarily by the clinical indication, taking into account the primary type and the different possible treatments, which also depend on the general status of clinical history of the patient. Dedicated liver imaging is not needed in patients diagnosed with disseminated, inoperable disease. [4]

1.4.1. Ultrasonography

1.4.1.1. Transabdominal ultrasonography (US)

US presents several advantages, including low cost, absence of irradiation, wide availability, and portability. Transabdominal ultrasound generally has a lower sensitivity for tumor detection than does CT scan or MR imaging, especially for lesions less than 2 cm in size. US is most commonly used for screening for metastases because of its wide availability. Hepatic metastases may be hypoechoic, hyperechoic, cystic, or of mixed echogenicity on ultrasound. Hyperechoic masses are observed more commonly in vascular tumors, such as renal cell and islet cell tumors. Hypovascular lesions, such as lymphoma, appear as hypoechoic masses. [5]

1.4.1.2. Contrast-enhanced US

Contrast-enhanced US, using intravascular microbubble contrast agents, has shown similar accuracy compared to CT and MR. An advantage of contrast-enhanced US is the potential for characterization of liver lesions based on morphologic evaluation as well as temporal vascular enhancement pattern. During the portal venous phase, benign lesions typically enhance more than the liver, whereas malignant lesions enhance less. [6]

1.4.1.3. Endoscopic ultrasound (EUS)

EUS is a well-established tool for diagnosing and staging various gastrointestinal tumors, especially pancreatic cancer; however, it is not used often for hepatic imaging. A few reports in the literature address the use of EUS in the evaluation of hepatic metastases. EUS can detect lesions that are not seen on conventional CT scanning and allows for tissue sampling using fine-needle aspiration. [4]

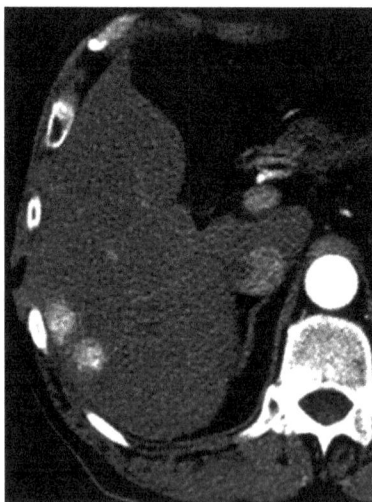

Figure 1. Computed tomography of hypervascular liver metastases from a renal primary tumor at the arterial phase.

1.4.1.4. Intraoperative US (IOUS)

IOUS involves a direct scan of the liver, allowing the use of higher-frequency transducers with higher resolution. IOUS can also be useful at detecting small, deep hepatic metastases not palpable. IOUS is more accurate than conventional CT scanning or MR imaging for delineating liver lesions and is regarded as an important tool in determining resectability and prognosis. [7]

1.4.2. Computed Tomography

1.4.2.1. Noncontrast Computed Tomography

Contrast CT is sometimes not possible because of contrast allergic reactions or renal impairment. Although the sensitivity and specificity of noncontrast CT is far reduced as compared to contrast CT, it may help in identifying hypervascular metastases (especially carcinoid tumors, islet cell tumors, and renal cell carcinomas) or visualizing calcifications or hemorrhage. Noncontrast CT often fails to distinguish hypovascular tumors from the liver parenchyma. Nonenhanced blood vessels may also appear as low-attenuation masses and be confused with metastases. [4]

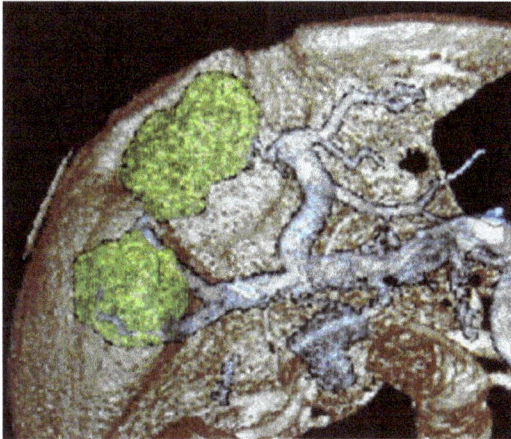

Figure 2. Computed tomography 3-D reconstruction before surgical showing liver metastases (http://c2i2.digithala-mus.com/winter2003/Imaging%20update%20in%20metastatic%20liver%20disease.asp).

1.4.2.2. Contrast Computed Tomography

The CT appearance of liver metastases varies according to the pathologic type of the primary tumor. Most lesions are seen best in the portal venous phase, and some lesions are best seen in delayed venous and occasionally arterial phases. Metastases from melanomas, sarcomas, neuroendocrine tumors, and renal cell carcinomas (fig. 1) are hypervascular and there-

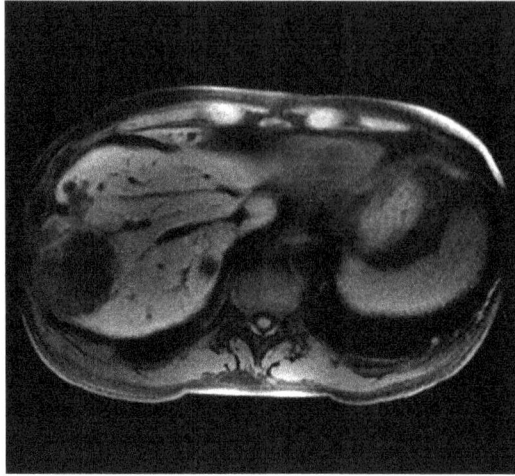

Figure 3. Liver metastases after Mn DPPD or mangafodipir injection.

fore better visualized during the hepatic arterial phase. Metastases from colorectal cancer are hypovascular and therefore better visualized during the portal venous phase. [8]

1.4.3. Magnetic Resonance Imaging (MRI)

T1-weighted images generally show hepatic metastases as low-intensity lesions, whereas T2-weighted images show these lesions to be areas of increased signal intensity. Dynamic, breath-hold MR imaging with a gadolinium-based contrast material is considered to be the most sensitive MR technique for detection of hepatic metastases (fig. 3). Similar to CT, MR angiography can be used as a noninvasive method to evaluate hepatic vasculature. Novel MR contrast agents have the potential for improving detection of liver metastases. [8, 9]

1.4.4. Positron Emission Tomography (PET)

PET, in which a radioactively labeled tracer is administered to the patient and the scanner collects the emitted positron radioactivity to generate an image, allows imaging of cellular processes (such as cellular proliferation (18F-labeled thymidine), hypoxia (18F-labeled Miso), and blood flow ([15O]water) to be visualized. The majority of clinical experience relies on the uptake and use of glucose in human cells. 18F-Fluorodeoxyglucose 18FDG, the most commonly used marker in PET imaging, is an analogue of glucose in which a carbon atom is replaced by a radioactive fluorine isotope. 18FDG is transported into cells, where it accumulates to create an intense signal on PET imaging. Malignant lesions typically have increased 18FDG uptake because of the increased expression of glucose transporter proteins and elevated levels of glycolysis. [10, 11]

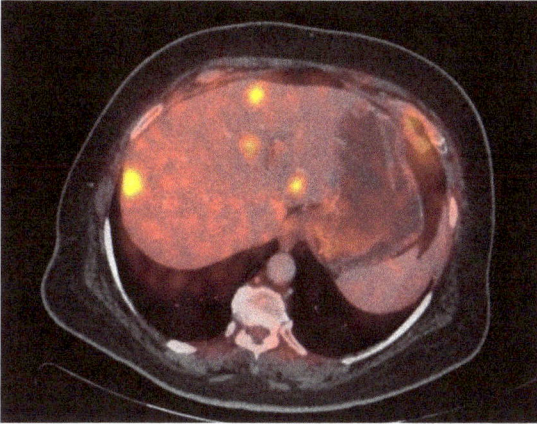

Figure 4. PET/CT Cancer pancreas with liver metastases (http://www.radrounds.com/photo/petct--2context).

1.4.5. PET/CT (fig. 4)

Despite excellent clinical results with FDG PET, the technique is intrinsically limited by the lack of precise and reliable anatomic information. Foci of increased uptake that are clearly located in the liver parenchyma are readily identified and usually correspond to metastases, but the bowel uptake is highly variable and may be focally increased in regions close to the liver, and therefore be mistaken with peripheral liver lesions. Combined PET/CT scanners allow the precise localization of the abnormal areas of uptake. Modern PET/CT devices are equipped with high-end CT scanners, fully capable of performing full diagnostic CT studies. [11]

2. Colorectal Liver Metastases (CLM)

The liver is the most common site for hematogenous metastasis from colorectal cancers (CRC). A quarter of patients with primary colorectal carcinoma are found to have synchronous hepatic metastasis. Nearly half of patients who undergo resection of the colorectal primary eventually develop metachronous liver metastasis. [2]

CRC principally spreads through two mechanisms:

1. Via portal venous drainage.

2. To regional lymph nodes and then through central lymphatics into the systemic circulation or

2.1. Prognostic Variables and Staging Systems

All patients with colorectal metastases by definition are grouped as stage IV in the TNM staging system, but considerable diversity exists within this group. The prognosis of a pa-

tient with a solitary liver metastasis found years after resection of a node-negative right colon cancer is different from the prognosis of a patient with synchronously discovered diffuse
bilateral liver metastases at the time of operation for a perforated node- positive colon cancer. A classification system that can discriminate between these patients and provide meaningful prognostic information is essential. This classification system must enable the
comparison of patients from diverse publications and facilitate patient selection for adjuvant
therapy or clinical trials. [2, 12]

2.1.1. Independent predictors of prognosis include [2]

1. the presence of extrahepatic disease,

2. a positive resection margin,

3. nodal metastases from primary cancer,

4. a short disease-free interval,

5. largest tumor greater than 5 cm,

6. more than one liver metastasis, and

7. CEA greater than 200 ng/mL.

- The first two parameters are data that are determined intraoperatively only because preoperative evidence of extrahepatic disease and inability to obtain negative margins would be
relative contraindications to surgery. There is no role for surgical debulking in this setting.

- Using the last five criteria, a preoperative clinical risk score (CRS) system was created
with each positive criterion counting as 1 point.

- This CRS is a simple, easily remembered staging system for classifying patients with liv-
er-exclusive metastatic colorectal cancer

2.1.2. Prognostic Scoring System for Hepatic Colorectal Metastases: Clinical risk score (CRS)

- Node-positive primary tumor

- Disease-free interval <12 mo between colon resection and appearance of metastases

- Size of largest lesion >5 cm

- >1 tumor

- CEA >200 ng/dL

Sum of points with 1 point assigned for each positive criterion

- The presence of any one of these characteristics still was associated with a 5-year survival.

- No single criterion can be considered a contraindication to resection.

- The total score out of 5 is highly predictive of outcome.

- A score of 2 or less places a patient in a good prognostic group, for whom resection is ideal.

- For scores of 3 or 4, outcome is less favorable, and patients should be considered for aggressive trials of adjuvant therapy.

- For a score of 5, long-term disease-free survivors rarely are encountered, and resections in this high-risk group should be accompanied by trials of adjuvant therapy.

- This CRS proved useful in selection of patients for neoadjuvant therapy and ablative therapies and in stratification of patients enrolled in clinical trials

- A high CRS has been associated with sufficiently high incidence of occult metastatic disease that fluorodeoxyglucose positron emission tomography (FDG PET) can be justified as a preoperative test

- The yield from laparoscopy in the preoperative staging of patients with hepatic colorectal metastases also has been correlated with the CRS.

- For patients with a high CRS, a laparoscopy can save patients with disseminated disease from having a laparotomy, minimizing morbidity and hospital stay, whereas patients with a low CRS can avoid the added anesthesia and operating room time associated with a negative laparoscopy. [2, 12]

2.1.3. Molecular Determinants of Outcome

There are reports that molecular characteristics that predict response to chemotherapy, such as tumor thymidylate synthase levels or levels of the transcription factor E2F-1, are important in predicting the outcome It is likely that these and other molecular determinants will be incorporated into postoperative prognostic scales in the future. [2]

2.2. Medical Treatment

Over the past 3 decades, the most widely used chemotherapeutic agent in the treatment of metastatic CRC has been 5-fluorouracil (5-FU), used either alone or in combination with other chemotherapies. [13]

Now, the most commonly used regimens are: FOLFOX, FOLFIRI, and FOLFOXIRI.

2.2.1. FOLFOX is a made up of the drugs

- FOL – Folinic acid (leucovorin), a vitamin B derivative used as a "rescue" drug for high doses of the drug methotrexate and that modulates/potentiates/reduces the side effects of fluorouracil;

- F – Fluorouracil (5-FU) fluorouracil (5-FU), a pyrimidine analog and antimetabolite which incorporates into the DNA molecule and stops synthesis; and

- OX – Oxaliplatin (Eloxatin) A platinum-based drug, usually classified as alkylating agents, although it is not actually alkylating groups (functions by a similar mechanism)

This regimen is recommended for 12 cycles, every 2 weeks. The recommended dose schedule given every two weeks is as follows:

- Day 1: Oxaliplatin 85 mg/m² IV infusion in 250-500 mL D5W and leucovorin 200 mg/m² IV infusion in D5W both given over 120 minutes at the same time in separate bags using a Y-line, followed by 5-FU 400 mg/m² IV bolus given over 2-4 minutes, followed by 5-FU 600 mg/m² IV infusion in 500 mL D5W (recommended) as a 22-hour continuous infusion.

- Day 2: Leucovorin 200 mg/m² IV infusion over 120 minutes, followed by 5-FU 400 mg/m² IV bolus given over 2-4 minutes, followed by 5-FU 600 mg/m² IV infusion in 500 mL D5W (recommended) as a 22-hour continuous infusion.FOLFOX4 regime.

Premedication with antiemetics, including 5-HT3 blockers with or without dexamethasone, is recommended.

FOLFOX4				
drug	dose	administration	time	term
Oxaliplatin	85 mg/m²	IV infusion	2 h	day 1
Folinic acid	200 mg/m²	IV infusion	2 h	day 1 + 2
Fluorouracil	400 mg/m²	IV bolus	2 min	day 1 + 2
Fluorouracil	600 mg/m²	IV infusion	22 h	day 1 + 2

Table 2.

2.2.2. FOLFIRI is is made up of the following drugs:

- FOL – folinic acid (leucovorin).

- F – fluorouracil (5-FU); and

- IRI – irinotecan (Camptosar), a topoisomerase inhibitor, which prevents DNA from uncoiling and duplicating.

The dosage consists of: Irinotecan (180 mg/m² IV over 90 minutes) concurrently with folinic acid (400 mg/m² [or 2 x 250 mg/m²] IV over 120 minutes).

Followed by fluorouracil (400-500 mg/m² IV bolus) then fluorouracil (2400-3000 mg/m² intravenous infusion over 46 hours).

This cycle is typically repeated every two weeks. The dosages shown above may vary from cycle to cycle.

FOLFOX and FOLFIRI are widely considered to be equivalent in the metastatic setting and are generally selected according to the toxicity profile. The FOLFOX regimen is characterized by a higher rate of grade 3 and 4 neurotoxicity and neutropenia. The FOLFIRI is associated with more nasuea and vomiting, mucositis, and alopecia.

2.2.3. Folfoxiri

- irinotecan, oxaliplatin, fluorouracil, and folinate

FOLFOXIRI has been shown to have better results than FOLFIRI and FOLFOX in several studies.

2.2.4. Cetuximab (Erbitux) and panitumumab (Vectibix)

Both are monoclonal antibodies against the epidermal growth factor receptor (EGFR) and are now an important part of the treatment algorithm for unresectable colorectal metastases. Cetuximab is a chimeric monoclonal antibody approved for treatment of metastatic CRC in combination with irinotecan in patients with disease refractory to irinotecan or as a single agent in patients who cannot tolerate irinotecan or oxaliplatin. Panitumumab is a fully humanized monoclonal antibody and therefore appears to have a lower rate of serious infusion reactions compared with cetuximab. Like cetuximab, panitumumab is approved for single-agent therapy in patients who have progressed on standard chemotherapy. [2]

2.3. Regional treatment for metastatic colorectal cancer

The rationale for a regional approach to what normally would be thought of as a systemic process is based on the concept that tumor cells from gastrointestinal malignancies, especially colorectal cancer, spread hematogenously via the portal circulation, making the liver the first site of metastasis in most patients. This stepwise spread of cancer from primary site to liver and from there to other organs provides an opportunity to prevent dissemination of tumor to other sites by direct treatment of hepatic metastases. In this way, metastatic colorectal cancer differs from most other metastatic malignancies. In addition, the remarkable ability of the liver to regenerate after hepatic resection has enabled aggressive surgical options for hepatic metastases. There is no doubt that surgery alone can cure a subset of patients. [14]

Liver resection has become the standard treatment for metastatic lesions from colorectal primaries. With many series reporting long-term survival for these patients, even before the era of modern chemotherapy, 5-year, 10-year, and 20-year survivals with hepatic resection can be expected to reach 40%, 25%, and 20%. [2]

2.3.1. Preoperative evaluation

All patients with CLM benefit from evaluation by a multidisciplinary team comprising physicians (surgeons, medical oncologists, radiologists, pathologists), nurses, social workers, and research coordinators. The central tenets in the preoperative evaluation of patients for potential surgical resection of CLM are:

1. establishing the diagnosis,
2. anatomically defining the liver lesion for diagnosis and surgical planning, and
3. staging to rule out extrahepatic disease.
4. evaluation of the patient's fitness for operation;

5. estimation of an individual's tumor biology.

Preoperative biopsy of CLM is rarely indicated or beneficial for assessment of CLM, and has been associated with tumor dissemination and decreased survival. Preoperative biopsy may have usefulness for confirmation of extrahepatic disease when a change in therapy is planned based on the biopsy results. [1]

2.3.1.1. Evaluation of Fitness for Operation

A careful evaluation of a patient's physiologic capability to tolerate hepatic resection is necessary to ensure favorable outcomes after hepatectomy. History, physical examination, and routine laboratory studies (complete blood count, liver function testing, and coagulation studies) are relied on to screen for underlying liver dysfunction.The criteria for patient operability are similar to the criteria considered for any major laparotomy. A history of cardiac and pulmonary disease must be investigated because these patients are at significant risk for perioperative complications. Any previous liver disease that might have impaired hepatic function should be evaluated because this determines the volume of liver than can be resected safely. [2, 14]

2.3.1.2. Anatomic and Functional parameters

Determination of resectability is primarily based on preoperative imaging. High-quality cross-sectional imaging is critical for gauging the extent of disease, response to preoperative therapy, and for operative planning (The role of preoperative imaging was discussed above). [14]

Patients should be routinely reimaged after any course of systemic therapy; preferably within 4 weeks of planned resection. Meticulous preoperative attention to the relationships of CLM to arterioportal inflow, biliary drainage, and hepatic venous outflow is necessary and allows for an informed and efficient hepatectomy. Preoperative imaging may also help to identify the presence of concomitant parenchymal disease (eg, fibrosis/cirrhosis, portal hypertension, steatohepatitis) or extrahepatic disease. [2]

Resectability of CLM has been well defined by the American Hepato-Pancreato-Biliary Association (AHPBA)/Society of Surgery of the Alimentary Tract (SSAT)/Society of Surgical Oncology (SSO) in a 2006 consensus statement as an expected margin-negative (R-0) resection resulting in preservation of at least 2 contiguous hepatic segments with adequate inflow, outflow, and biliary drainage with a functional liver remnant (FLR) volume of more than 20% (for healthy liver). [1, 14]

2.3.1.3. Tumor biology

Careful evaluation of all patients in a multidisciplinary setting allows for better identification of those patients most likely to benefit from surgical resection as opposed to those who would benefit more from nonoperative therapies, given their particularly aggressive disease. Consideration of this question is far from an exact science, but valuable information can be gleaned from factors such as [1]

1. the stage of primary disease,

2.   number and distribution of CLM,

3.   tumor histology,

4.   response to chemotherapy,

5.   rate of growth of CLM on serial imaging,

6.   rate of increase in serum carcinoembryonic antigen (CEA).

2.3.1.4. Diagnostic laparoscopy

Diagnostic laparoscopy has a role in staging those patients in whom preoperative imaging or high-risk scores suggest a high likelihood for finding intra-abdominal extrahepatic disease or for patients with indeterminate intrahepatic lesions that may be best characterized by IOUS. Laparoscopy is useful at identifying peritoneal disease or the involvement of periportal lymph nodes not apparent on preoperative imaging. When laparoscopy is employed, laparotomy can be avoided in patients with unresectable disease. [1, 2]

2.3.2. Operative technique

The goal should be a safe R-0 hepatectomy allowing for preservation of adequate FLR volume to avoid hepatic insufficiency. Given the significant decrease in survival between R-0 and R-1/2 resections, the ability to achieve R-0 resection, is paramount. The optimal width of resection margin is unclear, with no clear minimum margin established. A predicted margin width of less than 1 cm should not be used as an exclusion to resection. The extent of resection depends on the number and location of metastases relative to the portal triads and hepatic veins. Anatomic resections, which are facilitated by intraoperative ultrasound, are preferred to wedge resections. Anatomic resections permit excision of parenchymal areas distal to the tumor, where vascular micrometastases tend to occur, and, most importantly they are less likely to have positive margins. [14, 15]

The principles of hepatic resection are no different for colorectal metastases than for any other hepatic surgery. Technical details of liver mobilization and various anatomic hepatectomies have been well described elsewhere in this book. Most procedures can be divided into distinct stages: [1, 2, 14, 15]

1.   exploration,

2.   liver mobilization,

3.   intraoperative ultrasonography,

4.   inflow control,

5.   outflow control,

6.   parenchymal transection, and

7.   hemo- and biliostasis.

The abdomen must be explored thoroughly for evidence of extrahepatic metastases. In particular, the celiac axis and portocaval and hilar lymph nodes must be palpated, and any suspicious nodes should be removed and examined by frozen section.

Most surgeons routinely use intraoperative ultrasound after mobilization of the liver. IOUS can delineate better the interior anatomy of the liver, including intrahepatic vessels, and hepatic resection can be performed more safely and in a more anatomically oriented fashion. In addition to the initial planning, the operation can be monitored by the repeated use of IOUS because the resection line is displayed in relation to the lesion and blood vessels. [14, 15]

2.3.3. Follow-up

Patients after hepatic resection usually are monitored in an attempt to identify early recurrence that may be amenable to further resection. Currently, most patients undergo serial physical examination, serum CEA level, annual chest x-ray, and CT of the abdomen and pelvis every 3 to 4 months for the first 2 years and then every 6 months for the next 5 years. [16]

2.3.3.1. Adjuvant Chemotherapy

1- Adjuvant Systemic Chemotherapy

Although the use of oxaliplatin-based or irinotecan-based chemotherapies in this setting is common, there are no clear data from comparative studies supporting such practice. [17]

2- Adjuvant Hepatic Arterial Infusion Chemotherapy

Regional chemotherapy, via the hepatic artery, is a theoretically attractive mode of adjuvant therapy, because the liver is the most common site for tumor recurrence after liver resection and is the sole site of recurrence in 40% of patients.

The rationale for HAI of chemotherapy is based on the concept that most metastatic liver tumors preferentially derive their blood supply from the hepatic artery, whereas normal hepatic tissue relies on the portal venous blood supply.

The ability of the hepatic parenchyma to extract and metabolize chemotherapy drugs to nontoxic metabolites offers a unique opportunity to administer highly toxic drug levels to tumor cells, while minimizing systemic toxicity. The most extensively studied agent is 5-fluorouracil-2-deoxyuridine (FUDR), an analogue of 5-FU that can be concentrated 100-fold to 400-fold in the liver because of a 95% hepatic extraction ratio. [17, 18, 19, 20]

2.4. Controversial issues

2.4.1. Downstaging of unresectable tumor and neoadjuvant chemotherapy.

Potential benefits of prehepatectomy chemotherapy include [2, 20]

1. the potential to render formerly unresectable patients resectable i.e. the possibility for downstaging liver metastases,

2. in vivo testing of chemotherapeutic efficacy,

3. identification of occult intra- or extrahepatic metastases, and

4. early exposure of subclinical microscopic metastases to systemic therapy.

5. with prudent monitoring and attention to comorbidities, allows for improved patient selection

Patients with tumor progression during preoperative chemotherapy have a significantly worse outcome CLM. Potential downsides of preoperative chemotherapy are largely related to hepatic toxicities that may be clinically relevant. Oxaliplatin has been linked to steatohepatitis and sinusoidal obstruction; irinotecan has been associated with steatohepatitis and periportal inflammation. A preoperatively treated liver is more fibrotic, often with perivascular adhesions. The planes of resection are difficult to dissect, making the procedure more challenging overall. Despite the operative complexity, the perioperative morbidity and mortality in the trials of resection after neoadjuvant chemotherapy do not seem to be higher than series of de novo hepatic resection. [1, 2]

One controversial issue is the treatment of a patient with a *complete clinical response* to neoadjuvant chemotherapy. When there is no visible tumor left to resect, should a blind resection, based on the site of previous metastasis, be undertaken? Suggested practice is to use intraoperative ultrasound to attempt to identify the lesion, and if this is not possible a hepatic resection of the area previously involved with tumor is performed. This is not, however, a universally accepted practice. [1, 2, 20]

Patients who present with liver lesions that are potentially resectable for cure should be offered a surgical resection because there are no definite data supporting a neoadjuvant chemotherapeutic approach.

2.4.2. Repeated resection for recurrent tumor

In the absence of extrahepatic disease and in a patient with a good performance status and adequate hepatic reserve, a repeat hepatectomy may be considered. Approximately one third of recurrence is amenable to further resection The presence of adhesions and the altered anatomy of the liver, particularly the position of the vasculature and biliary system, make this technically challenging.

There is a higher likelihood of further recurrence, however, and the study of adjuvant therapy should be encouraged in these patients. [21]

2.4.3. Synchronous Metastases

Synchronous CLM are noted in 20% to 30% of patients at the time of initial colorectal cancer diagnosis. Surgical management of this group of early metastases has been debated in terms of disease biology, operative approach (staged vs. simultaneous colorectal and liver resection), the order of resection, and timing of chemotherapy. [2, 22]

Some suggests that synchronous diagnosis of metastases portends a worse prognosis, perhaps as a result of a failure to detect micrometastatic foci in the liver. Delaying hepatic resection may increase survival in the surgically resected group by selecting out the patients with aggressive tumor biology who would be unlikely to derive a survival benefit from resection. Although delayed resection does not seem to impair survival, it does increase the volume of resected liver, a factor that is predictive of postoperative complications. [22]

Potential benefits of simultaneous CLM resection include [2]

1.   avoidance of morbidity of a second laparotomy and anesthesia, and

2.   decreased time to initiation of chemotherapy.

Risks of simultaneous resection are related to the magnitude and complexity of the combined operation.

A selective approach to synchronous CLM should be based on careful consideration of the technical complexity and risks for the colorectal and liver resections, as well as judicious intraoperative decision making. Good judgment is required in selection of patients for a simultaneous or a staged resection in close coordination with medical oncologists and collaborating surgeons. [1]

2.4.4. Bilobar Metastases

Bilobar metastases are no longer an absolute contraindication to resection. Possible options include:

1.   Extended hepatectomy,

2.   2-stage hepatectomy,

3.   Combined hepatic resection and ablation.

4.   For patients with insufficient FLR, portal vein embolization (PVE) may be a useful adjunct to increase the size of the FLR and allow for safe extended hepatectomy.

Two-stage hepatectomy for patients with bilobar metastases involves an initial hepatectomy with contralateral portal vein ligation or postoperative PVE, followed by chemotherapy. After restaging, a second hepatectomy is performed based on response to PVE/chemotherapy and ability to achieve resection with an adequate FLR. A proportion of patients will not be eligible for second hepatectomy because of disease progression, inadequate FLR, or perioperative or chemotherapy-associated complications. [23, 24]

2.4.5. Extrahepatic Colorectal Metastases

In the past, extrahepatic disease has been labeled an absolute contraindication to resection of CLM. However, with the advent of more effective systemic therapies, a growing body of literature supports R-0 resection of CLM and extrahepatic metastases. [25]

- An assessment of tumor biology is critical to selecting patients for resection of CLM as well as extrahepatic metastases. For patients found to have extrahepatic metastases preoperatively, a short course of preoperative chemotherapy followed by reimaging is prudent to better define the disease biology.

- Intraoperative decision for previously unrecognized intra-abdominal extrahepatic metastases is difficult. The following should be considered:

1. the complexity and extent of the R-0 hepatic resection,

2. the complexity of resection of the R-0 extrahepatic metastases,

3. the physiologic age of the patient,

4. availability of postoperative chemotherapeutic options, and

5. the patient's risk of rapid progression with the additional finding of extrahepatic metastases.

3. Neuroendocrine Liver Metastases (NLMs)

The liver is the most common site of metastatic disease for neuroendocrine tumors. Nonoperative therapies for advanced neuroendocrine malignancies are associated with minimal response rates, short durations of disease stability, and no clear survival benefit. [26]

3.1. Pathology and Classification

Most NLMs are of gastrointestinal or pancreatic origin, or so-called gastroenteropancreatic (GEP) tumors GEP neuroendocrine tumors historically are divided into two broad types: carcinoid and noncarcinoid. Either type may or may not be associated with hormone production causing a clinical endocrinopathy (functional or nonfunctional). [26, 27]

Traditionally, gastrointestinal carcinoids have been classified by their site of origin—foregut (lung, thymus, stomach, duodenum, pancreas, bile duct, gallbladder, and liver), midgut (small intestine, appendix, and proximal colon), and hindgut (distal colon and rectum)—because of the various biologic and biochemical features shown within these groups. Pancreatic neuroendocrine tumors have been classified by whether they are functional or not. [26, 28]

Regardless of origin, neuroendocrine tumors are similar histopathologically. Many histologic and morphologic features may be shared by benign and malignant tumors. Histologically, neuroendocrine tumors typically are well differentiated, and atypia and mitoses are rare.

Neuroendocrine tumors stain positive for chromogranin A, neuron-specific enolase, and synaptophysin, which confirms neuroendocrine cell origin. Neuroendocrine tumors also stain positively for one or more endocrine hormones immunohistochemically. [27]

Morphologically, neuroendocrine tumors can be solitary or multiple and solid or cystic. Tumor size alone is not a reliable indicator of malignancy. Neuroendocrine tumors greater than 2 cm throughout the GEP tract have a greater probability of malignant behavior, however, than tumors less than 2 cm. Gross or microscopic vascular invasion may occur for any GEP neuroendocrine tumors, although major vascular invasion is most typical of pancreatic NECs. Only the confirmed presence of metastases confers an unequivocal diagnosis of malignancy. [28]

Regardless of whether NECs are classified as carcinoid or noncarcinoid, the natural history of patients with unresected or unresectable hepatic metastases generally has been similar. Overall, patients with unresected hepatic metastases from NEC have an approximately 30% 5-year survival The presence of liver metastases alone is the most significant factor adversely affecting outcome Five-year survival with and without liver metastases from NECs is approximately 30% to 40% and 90% to 100%. [26]

3.2. Treatment of NLMs

3.2.1. Liver resection

The treatment of hepatic metastases from NECs is aimed at reduction of the mass of malignant tissue (cytoreduction) chiefly for two reasons. [29]

First, metastatic gastrointestinal neuroendocrine tumors are usually indolent and slow growing because most are low-grade malignancies (WHO classification). Chemotherapeutic and radiotherapeutic regimens targeted at rapidly dividing cells are relatively ineffective, targeting only a paucity of the total population of malignant cells.

Second, symptoms secondary to expression and secretion of biologically active peptides by these tumors are directly related to overall mass of tumor, although production of peptides may be heterogeneous among individual metastases. Similarly, pain and debilitating decrease in performance status may have a negative impact on quality of life for nonfunctional NECs metastatic to the liver. Cytoreduction of the tumor is the most direct and immediately effective method to provide symptomatic relief.

These reasons, coupled with improved safety for hepatic resection, have prompted hepatic resection as a primary therapeutic option for patients with functional and nonfunctional metastatic GEP NECs. Currently, hepatic resection of NLMs is recommended if the primary tumor and regional disease are resectable or resected, and greater than 90% of hepatic metastases are resectable or ablatable.

The concept of hepatic resection for NLMs has grown because of several clinical observations: [30]

1.   the protracted natural history of NECs compared with other gastrointestinal tract cancers,

2. the often prolonged duration of intrahepatic disease before evidence of extrahepatic progression,

3. the clinical impression that the severity of clinical endocrinopathies correlates with the intrahepatic volume of metastatic disease,

4. the frequent resectability of the primary and regional neuroendocrine tumors despite metastatic disease, and

5. the rarity of underlying concomitant hepatic disease (fibrosis or cirrhosis).

3.2.1.1. Debulking strategy

When complete resection of gross liver disease is not feasible or in the presence of unresectable extrahepatic disease, resection as a tumor debulking strategy should be considered in patients with extreme hormonal symptoms refractory to other treatments or with tumors in locations that would affect short-term quality of life, such as large lesions abutting the hepatic hilum (resulting in biliary obstruction) or the colon/duodenum (resulting in gastrointestinal obstruction). [31, 32]

3.2.1.2. Subsequent plan for treatment of recurrence. [26, 33]

1. For solitary recurrences, either resection or ablation is appropriate. Percutaneous ablative approaches often are preferable.

2. Repeat hepatic resection is advised for lesions in sites that preclude safe radiofrequency ablation (RFA) (i.e., surface metastases adjacent to bowel, near bile ducts, or near diaphragm).

3. Sequential ablation or resection is undertaken as recurrence is recognized until precluded by extent of recurrence within the liver.

4. Extensive recurrent intrahepatic metastases are treated by embolization or chemoembolization with or without systemic chemotherapy in the absence of extrahepatic disease and chemotherapy in the presence of extrahepatic disease.

3.2.2. Liver transplantation

Liver transplantation (OLT) has been employed increasingly to treat metastatic NEC. OLT may be indicated if the primary and regional NEC has been resected, and distal metastases have been excluded. While transplantation has the benefits of removing all hepatic disease burden, rapid disease recurrence is near universal. Long-term actuarial survival among patients transplanted for NLM is poor compared with overall patient and graft survival rates for all indications. At present, liver transplantation cannot be considered a viable option for unresectable NLM. OLT should be considered as an investigative treatment alternative in specialty centers. [34]

3.2.3. Radiofrequency Ablation

Radiofrequency ablation (RFA) can provide local control and short-term symptomatic relief from NLM when resection is not possible. Successful ablation typically occur in the treatment of small metastases (<5 cm). [35-38]

3.2.4. Ethanol Ablation

Percutaneous ethanol injection permits ablation of metastases located adjacent to structures at risk of damage by RFA. It can be performed on metastases located adjacent to vital structures (e.g., the hepatic flexure of the colon); adjacent to large vessels vulnerable to the heat-sink effect; and adjacent to central bile ducts, where subsequent biliary stricture may occur. [61]

3.2.4.1. Guidelines for Ablation

General guidelines in the ablation of liver metastases are analogous to the treatment of hepatocellular carcinoma and colorectal metastases. [35-38]

There are three clinical scenarios for ablation of neuroendocrine hepatic metastases:

1. adjunct to concurrent surgical resection of hepatic metastases,

2. treatment of limited hepatic metastases in patients unfit for operation, and

3. primary therapy when clinical expertise or intraoperative circumstances preclude safe resection.

3.2.5. Hepatic arterial therapy

Because neuroendocrine tumors usually are highly vascular lesions that predominantly derive blood supply from the hepatic artery (as opposed to the normal hepatic parenchyma that derive the majority of blood supply from the portal vein), opportunities exist for selected ischemia of NLM and/or delivery of directed chemotherapy via hepatic artery therapy. Hepatic arterial embolization with cyanoacrylate, gel foam particles, polyvinyl alcohol, and microspheres have all been used to achieve distal embolization without surgical ligation of the hepatic artery. Chemoembolization provides an intratumoral concentration of chemotherapy that is 10 to 20 times higher than systemic administration.

Complete response and long-term survival are not common after hepatic arterial therapy, as the periphery of the tumor is spared from ischemia or chemotherapy. Thus, embolization of lesions close to the hepatic hilum is generally unsuccessful, as the periphery of the tumor will still cause mass-effect associated symptoms. [39, 40]

The morbidity of embolization approaches include liver abscess, transient liver failure, pleural effusion, and postembolization syndrome, the latter consisting of fever, abdominal pain, leukocytosis, and a transient increase in liver enzymes and/or bilirubin. Multiple sessions of therapy are often needed with varying intervals between sessions. Contraindications to hepatic arterial therapy include hepatic failure, portal vein occlusion, uncorrectable coagulopathy, and renal failure. [40]

3.2.6. Medical treatment

A- Somatostatin Analogues

Short-acting somatostatin analogue therapy is used to prevent or to treat the carcinoid crisis periprocedurally for any intervention, including resection, transplantation, ablation, or embolization. Somatostatin analogue treatment generally is well tolerated. Steatorrhea, diarrhea, abdominal discomfort, and biliary sludge or gallstones can develop, but rarely preclude continued use. [41]

B- Chemotherapy

Systemic chemotherapy generally is reserved for patients with advanced or progressive disease in whom other treatment efforts have failed Streptozocin-based combinations with 5-FU and doxorubicin have resulted in objective responses. Carcinoid tumors may be less sensitive to cytotoxic agents because of the preponderance of low-grade malignant (well-differentiated) histology and low proliferation index. [24]

C- Interferon Alfa

Systemic interferon alfa may be used to treat advanced NEC. The mechanism of interferon alfa is mediated through direct inhibitors of the cell cycle (G1/S phase) and of protein and hormone production, through antiangiogenesis, and indirectly through increased immune stimulation. Adverse reactions to interferon alfa are common. Chronic fatigue and hematologic cytopenias are the most common side effects. [42]

3.3. Primary hepatic neuroendocrine tumors

NECs may arise primarily within the liver. The diagnosis presumes a thorough search and exclusion of an extrahepatic NEC. The cell of origin is unknown. Pancreatic heterotopia has been postulated as a source of these tumors. Some tumors may arise from intrahepatic biliary tract radicles because carcinoids of the extrahepatic biliary tract are more common. Primary hepatic neuroendocrine tumors may be metastases from an occult primary NEC or a primary NEC that had spontaneously regressed. [24]

4. Non-colorectal Non-neuroendocrine Liver Metastases (NCNNLM)

Except for gastrointestinal primaries, the liver is not the primary filter for venous blood. In other words, liver metastases from nongastrointestinal cancers indicate systemic tumor spread; this makes selection of patients a crucial factor to offer hepatic resection to patients who may benefit the most.

Tumor biologies among NCNNLM vary widely, and their treatment requires dedicated multidisciplinary teams with expertise in diverse areas including hepatic surgery, surgical oncology, medical oncology, radiation oncology, diagnostic imaging, and interventional radiology. Patient care must be individualized, especially in the absence of data to clearly guide therapy. [43]

4.1. Treatment options

4.1.1. Resectional treatment

The potential utility of surgery in NCNNLM relates to several factors:

1. advances in chemotherapy have led to effective control of extra hepatic disease for certain tumor types, supporting a rationale for surgical resection of LM in the presence of presumed or de facto systemic disease;

2. improvements in patient preparation for surgery, surgical technique and perioperative care have reduced the perioperative risk of hepatic resection, tipping the risk–benefit ratio in favor of surgical resection in selected cases;

3. the increased emphasis on multimodality treatment approaches has improved patient selection and strengthened the role of hepatic resection as a key component of integrated multidisciplinary care in selected patients with NCNNLM.

Although it might appear that patients with isolated liver metastases can benefit from hepatic resection, the proper selection of patients that may potentially benefit from treatment remains the most critical issue. Patient selection criteria depend on the primary tumor type. After selection based on patient performance status and evaluation of comorbidities, staging studies are required not only to assess the overall disease status of the patient but also to characterize liver lesions and their precise location relative to intrahepatic vascular structures. Assessment of the liver volume that will remain after resection is an equally important component of surgical planning for extensive hepatectomy. [43, 45]

Patient selection and oncologic outcome of metastasectomy depends fundamentally on complete resection of all disease. Preoperative studies are essential in defining both the extent and the limits of surgical resection. Hepatic volumetry to assess the planned future liver remnant (FLR) volume is a critical tool for the selection of patients who will undergo major hepatic resection If the future liver remnant is of inadequate volume, preoperative portal vein embolization can be used to induce hypertrophy of the future liver remnant to allow safe resection. Liver tumors are deemed resectable if preoperative evaluation shows that complete resection of the tumor-bearing liver leaves an adequate remnant volume with adequate vascular inflow, outflow, and biliary drainage. The treatment of each individual tumor type requires expertise in staging, systemic therapy, and hepatic surgery. [43, 45]

4.1.2. Nonresectional treatment

Percutaneous and intraoperative ablative techniques may play a role in the treatment of many types of liver tumors because the therapy

1. can be performed percutaneously or with minimally invasive approaches,

2.   is associated with low morbidity and mortality, and

3.   can help preserve liver parenchyma in selected patients.

The role of nonresectional ablative approaches for NCNNLM is not well defined. Data and experience are still accruing, and for now such treatment should be considered only in those centers that can provide the full spectrum of therapies for liver metastases. [43]

4.1.3. Hepatic arterial therapies

The utility of hepatic arterial therapies in the treatment of NCNNLM is not well understood. TACE, TAE, and hepatic artery infusion are not considered standard therapy for NCNNLM. For certain tumor subtypes, including unresectable soft tissue sarcomas (STS) and gastrointestinal stromal tumors (GIST), these approaches hold promise. [43, 45]

4.2. Specific tumor types

4.2.1. Gastrointestinal tumors

Overall reported survival rates for patients with NCNNLM from gastrointestinal tumors (esophageal, stomach, duodenum, pancreas, and small bowel) are worse than for those with nongastrointestinal LM.

4.2.1.1. Esophagus and stomach

Currently, there are no accepted indications for resection of esophageal cancer LM, either for palliation or cure. The justification for resection of gastric cancer liver metastases remains controversial. A few published series from Japan and Korea, where the incidence of gastric cancer is high, specifically address gastric cancer LM. Currently, hepatic resection for gastric adenocarcinoma cannot be recommended as standard of care. Data supporting hepatic resection in highly selected patients need confirmation by additional clinical studies. [43]

4.2.1.2. Small bowel

Metastases from small bowel adenocarcinoma are most often widespread and associated with a dismal outcome regardless of treatment. There currently are no data to support resection of small bowel LM except in highly selected cases. [43]

4.2.1.3. Anus

Liver metastases from anal adenocarcinoma are very uncommon, and a meaningful discussion of the indications for resection is difficult. [43]

4.2.2. Bile ducts and pancreas

4.2.2.1. Gallbladder, hilar bile ducts, and ampulla

There currently are no generally accepted indications for hepatic resection in patients with gallbladder cancer, cholangiocarcinoma, or ampullary carcinoma. Judicious recommendations should be made on a case-by-case basis. [43, 45]

4.2.2.2. Pancreas

Even for pancreatic carcinoma patients without LM, the overall survival is poor. LM from pancreatic adenocarcinoma occurs nearly always in the setting of disseminated systemic disease.. In the majority of cases, benefit cannot be expected from hepatic resection for this disease. [43, 45]

4.2.3. Breast

Although it has not been formally proven that liver resection prolongs survival for selected patients with liver metastases of breast cancer, recent studies suggest that with careful patient selection, resection of breast LM can produce long-term survival. Some authors also suggest that patients first should undergo systemic chemotherapy, and that only patients who do not progress should undergo liver resection. [45]

4.2.4. Genitourinary

4.2.4.1. Kidney

In patients with hepatic metastases of renal tumors in whom a complete resection seems possible, surgical exploration may be justified. The number of studies evaluating renal tumors including Wilms' tumors, renal cell adenocarcinomas, and nephroblastomas are few, and the cohorts of patients are small. [43, 45]

4.2.4.2. Testicle

Effective chemotherapeutic regimens are available for most reproductive tumors. Treatment with chemotherapy can lead to complete responses. Surgical resection is considered a necessary salvage treatment in the absence of complete radiographic response to systemic therapy, because residual teratomas have been known to degenerate into invasive carcinoma. [43]

"Salvage" hepatic resection may be considered because

1. resection is the only way to confirm a complete response in the residual liver masses,

2. teratomas may progress to malignant transformation in 30% of cases,

3. mortality and morbidity from hepatic resection is low, and

4. if feasible, concomitant resection of liver metastases and residual retroperitoneal disease is associated with favorable outcome.

Because of the small number of published cases, however, no general conclusions can be drawn.

4.2.4.3. Uterus and ovary

The concept of hepatic resection for LM from ovarian cancer has evolved from the fact that cytoreductive surgery can significantly alter the natural history of ovarian cancer metastatic to the peritoneum. Resection of ovarian LM may be considered in carefully selected patients that are candidates for complete cytoreduction after evaluation by a multidisciplinary team. [43]

4.2.5. Melanoma

Most patients with liver metastases of melanoma have unresectable disease owing to extrahepatic disease or disseminated hepatic metastases. Isolated liver metastasis from cutaneous melanoma is uncommon. Uveal melanoma is a distinct entity that seems to have a different tumor biology, and it commonly spreads to the liver.. Hepatic resection has been performed in both populations, although outcomes differ based on the primary site of origin. Hepatic resection for uveal or cutaneous melanoma should only be considered in a multidisciplinary setting and by experienced hepatic surgeons. [43, 45]

4.2.6. Adrenal

Hepatic resection can provide acceptable results in selected patients with limited adrenal metastases, particularly for palliation of symptoms in patients with secreting hepatic tumors. For patients with symptomatic disease who are not candidates for surgery, ablative therapy such as RFA may be an effective alternative therapy for symptom control. [43]

4.2.7. Soft tissue sarcoma and gastrointestinal stromal tumor

Hepatic resection for STS metastases is indicated for disease confined to the liver. Patients with retroperitoneal and intra-abdominal visceral STS and those with leiomyosarcomas are more likely to have liver-only metastatic disease than are patients with extra-abdominal STS.

The treatment strategy for patients with liver metastases from gastrointestinal stromal tumors has changed since the development of the targeted agent imatinib mesylate, which achieves dramatic tumor response rates. Imatinib is now the first-line treatment. Therapy with imatinib has revolutionized the treatment of patients with GIST and has been used alone and in conjunction with hepatic resection for GIST LM. "Complete" radiographic response assessed by CT or PET, including cystic changes after imatinib treatment of GIST, are not necessarily equivalent to complete pathologic response. Because hepatic lesions contain viable tumor in >85% of cases after chemotherapy and biologic therapy, the goal of surgical treatment is complete removal of all residual disease including small residual cystic lesions and "scars." [43, 45]

4.2.8. Squamous cell carcinoma

Because the dataset is so heterogeneous, standard recommendations cannot be made, except that careful patient selection for hepatic resection is mandatory. [43]

4.2.9. Lung cancer

Resection of liver metastases of lung cancer has been reported, and in selected patients long-term survival has been achieved. [43]

4.2.10. Unknown primary cancer

Patients presenting with liver metastases from an unknown primary tumor are a challenge to manage because median overall survival is approximately 5 months. The treatment plan for these patients should be individualized and discussed in a multidisciplinary team. [43, 45]

Author details

Hesham Abdeldayem*, Amr Helmy, Hisham Gad, Essam Salah, Amr Sadek, Tarek Ibrahim, Elsayed Soliman, Khaled Abuelella, Maher Osman, Amr Aziz, Hosam Soliman, Sherif Saleh, Osama Hegazy, Hany Shoreem, Taha Yasen, Emad Salem, Mohamed Taha, Hazem Zakaria, Islam Ayoub and Ahmed Sherif

*Address all correspondence to: habdeldayem64@hotmail.com

Department of Surgery, National Liver Institute, Egypt

References

[1] Kemeny, N., & Kemeny, M. L. (2008). Dawson Liver Metastases. *From: Abeloff: Abeloff's Clinical Oncology, 4th ed. / Chapter 59Liver Abeloff: Abeloff's Clinical Oncology, 4th ed.,* Copyright © 2008 Churchill Livingstone, An Imprint of Elsevier.

[2] Winter, J., & Auer, R. A. C. (2012). Metastatic malignant liver tumors Colorectal cancer Chapter 81A. *From: Jarnagin & Blumgart: Blumgart's Surgery of the Liver, Pancreas and Biliary Tract, 5th ed. / Chapter 81A- Metastatic malignant liver tumors,* Copyright © 2012 Saunders, An Imprint of Elsevier.

[3] Haskell, C. M., Cochran, A. J., Barsky, S. H., & Steckel, R. J. (2008). Metastasis of unknown origin. *Curr Probl Cancer,* 12, 5-58.

[4] Faingold, R., Albuquerque, P. A. B., & Carpineta, L. (2011). *Hepatobiliary Tumors Radiol Clin N Am,* 49-679, doi:10.1016/j.rcl.2011.05.002.

[5] Bipat, S., Leeuwen, M. V., Comans, E., et al. (2005). Colorectal liver metastases: CT, MR imaging, and PET for diagnosis-meta-analysis. *Radiology*, 237, 123-131.

[6] Krix, M., & Kiesslink, F. (2004). Low mechanical index contrast-enhanced ultrasound better reflects high arterial perfusion of liver metastases than arterial phase computed tomography. *Invest Radiol*, 39, 216-222.

[7] Rydzewski, B., Dehdashti, F., Gordon, B. A., et al. (2002). Usefulness of intraoperative sonography for revealing hepatic metastases from colorectal cancer in patients selected for surgery after undergoing FDG PET. *Am J Roentgenol*, 178, 353-358.

[8] Voroney, J. J., Brock, K. K., Eccles, C., et al. (2006). Prospective comparison of CT and MRI for liver cancer delineation using deformable image registration. *Int J Radiat Oncol Biol Phys*, 66, 780-791.

[9] Das, C. J., Dhingra, S., Gupta, A. K., et al. (2009). Imaging of paediatric liver tumors with pathological correlation. Clin Radiol the, 64, 1015-25.

[10] Takahashi, S., Kuroki, Y., Nasu, K., et al. (2006). Positron emission tomography with F-18 fluorodeoxyglucose in evaluating hepatic metastases down staged by chemotherapy. *Anticancer Res*, 26, 4705-4711.

[11] Hustinx, R., Witvrouw, N., & Tancredi, T. (2008). *Liver Metastases PET Clinics- 32-CopyrightSaunders*, An Imprint of Elsevier.

[12] Nordlinger, B., Guiguet, M., Vaillant, J. C., et al. (1996). Surgical resection of colorectal carcinoma metastases to the liver. A prognostic scoring system to improve case selection, based on 1568 patients. *Association Fran?aise de Chirurgie. Cancer*, 77, 1254-1262.

[13] Adam, R., Aloia, T., Figueras, J., et al. (2006). Liver Met Survey: analysis of clinicopathologic factors associated with the efficacy of preoperative chemotherapy in 2,122 patients with colorectal liver metastases. *In 2006 ASCO Annual Meeting. Atlanta, Georgia*, USA, Am Soc Clin Oncol.

[14] Hao, C. Y., & Ji, J. F. (2006). Surgical treatment of liver metastases of colorectal cancer: strategies and controversies in 2006. *Eur J Surg Oncol*, 32, 473-483.

[15] Abdalla, E. K., Vauthey, J. N., Ellis, L. M., et al. (2004). Recurrence and outcomes following hepatic resection, radiofrequency ablation, and combined resection/ablation for colorectal liver metastases. *Ann Surg*, 239, 818-827.

[16] Pozzo, C., Basso, M., Quirino, M., et al. (2006). Long-term followup of colorectal cancer (CRC) patients treated with neoadjuvant chemotherapy with irinotecan and fluorouracil plus folinic acid (5FU/FA) for unresectable liver metastases. *In: 2006 ASCO Annual Meeting. Atlanta, Georgia*, USA, American Society of Clinical Oncology, 3576.

[17] Huitzil-Melendez, F., Capanu, M., Haviland, D., & Kemeny, N. E. (2007). Evaluation of the impact of systemic (SYS) neoadjuvant chemotherapy (neoadj) in patients (pts) with resectable liver metastasis (mets) from colorectal carcinoma (CRC) treated with

adjuvant hepatic arterial infusion (HAI) and SYS chemotherapy. *In: 2007 Gastrointes-tinal Cancers Symposium. Orlando, Florida*, USA, American Society of Clinical Oncolo-gy, 14503.

[18] Mentha, G., Majno, P. E., Andres, A., et al. (2006). Neoadjuvant chemotherapy and resection of advanced synchronous liver metastases before treatment of the colorectal primary. *Br J Surg*, 93, 872-878.

[19] Kemeny, N. E., Jarnagin, W., Gonen, M., et al. (2005). Phase I trial of hepatic arterial infusion (HAI) with floxuridine (FUDR) and dexamethasone (DEX) in combination with systemic oxaliplatin (OXAL), fluorouracil (FU) + leucovorin (LV) after resection of hepatic metastases from colorectal cancer. *In: 2005 ASCO Annual Meeting. Orlando, Florida* , USA, American Society of Clinical Oncology.

[20] Adam, R., Delvart, V., Pascal, G., et al. (2004). Rescue surgery for unresectable color-ectal liver metastases downstaged by chemotherapy: a model to predict long-term survival. *Ann Surg*, 240, 644-658.

[21] Petrowsky, H., Gonen, M., Jarnagin, W., et al. (2002). Second liver resections are safe and effective treatment for recurrent hepatic metastases from colorectal cancer: a bi-institutional analysis. *Ann Surg*, 235, 863-871.

[22] Tanaka, K., Shimada, H., Matsuo, K., et al. (2004). Outcome after simultaneous color-ectal and hepatic resection for colorectal cancer with synchronous metastases. *Sur-gery*, 136, 650-659.

[23] Bolton, J. S., & Fuhrman, G. M. (2000). Survival after resection of multiple bilobar hepatic metastases from colorectal carcinoma. *Ann Surg*, 231, 743-751.

[24] Kornprat, P., Jarnagin, W. R., Gonen, M., et al. (2007). Outcome after hepatectomy for multiple (4 or more) colorectal metastases in the era of effective chemotherapy. *Ann Surg Oncol*, 14, 1151-1160.

[25] Headrick, J. R., Miller, D. L., Nagorney, D. M., et al. (2001). Surgical treatment of hep-atic and pulmonary metastases from colon cancer. *Ann Thorac Surg*, 71, 975-990.

[26] Khan, S., Nagorney, D. M., & Que, F. G. (2012). *Metastatic malignant liver tumors : Neu-roendocrine Chapter 81B- Jarnagin & Blumgart: Blumgart's Surgery of the Liver, Pancreas and Biliary Tract* (5th ed), Copyright © 2012 Saunders, An Imprint of Elsevier.

[27] Sutcliffe, R., Maguire, D., Ramage, J., et al. (2004). Management of neuroendocrine liver metastases. *Am J Surg 187*, 39-46.

[28] Clary, B. (2006). Treatment of isolated neuroendocrine liver metastases. *J Gastrointest Surg 10*, 332-334.

[29] Que, F., Sarmiento, J. M., & Nagorney, D. M. (2002). Hepatic surgery for metastatic gastrointestinal neuroendocrine tumors. *Cancer Control*, 9, 67-79.

[30] Guruswamy, K. S., Ramamoorthy, R., Sharma, D., et al. (2009). Liver resection versus other treatments for neuroendocrine tumours in patients with resectable liver metastases. Cochrane Database Syst Rev 2. CD007060.

[31] Touzios, J. G., Kiely, J. M., Pitt, S. C., et al. (2005). Neuroendocrine hepatic metastases: does aggressive management improve survival? *Ann Surg 241,* 776-785.

[32] Sarmiento, J. M., Heywood, G., Rubin, J., et al. (2003). Surgical treatment of neuroendocrine metastases to liver: a plea for resection to increase survival. *J Am Coll Surg 197,* 29-37.

[33] Sarmiento, J. M., & Que, F. G. (2003). Hepatic surgery for metastases from neuroendocrine tumors. *Surg Oncol Clin N Am 12,* 231-242.

[34] van Vilsteren, F. G. I., Baskin-Bey, E. S., Nagorney, D. M., et al. (2006). Liver transplantation for gastroenteropancreatic neuroendocrine cancers: defining selection criteria to improve survival. *Liver Transpl 12,* 448-456.

[35] Henn, A. R., Levine, E. A., Mc Nulty, W., & Zagoria, R. J. (2003). Percutaneous radiofrequency ablation of hepatic metastases for symptomatic relief of neuroendocrine syndromes. *Am J Roentgenol,* 181, 1005-1010.

[36] Wettstein, M., Vogt, C., Cohnen, M., et al. (2004). Serotonin release during percutaneous radiofrequency ablation in a patient with symptomatic liver metastases of a neuroendocrine tumor. *Hepatogastroenterology,* 51, 830-832.

[37] Gilliams, A., Cassoni, A., Conway, G., et al. (2005). Radiofrequency ablation of neuroendocrine liver metastases: the Middlesex experience. *Abdom Imaging,* 30, 435-441.

[38] Mazzaglia, P. J., Berber, E., Milas, M., et al. (2007). Laparoscopic radiofrequency ablation of neuroendocrine liver metastases: a 10year experience evaluating predictors of survival. *Surgery,* 142, 10-19.

[39] Osborne, D. A., Zervos, E. E., Strosberg, J., et al. (2006). Improved outcome with cytoreduction versus embolization for symptomatic hepatic metastases of carcinoid and neuroendocrine tumors. *Ann Surg Oncol,* 13, 572-581.

[40] Guruswamy, K. S., Pamecha, V., Sharma, D., et al. (2009). Palliative cytoreductive surgery versus other palliative treatments in patients with unresectable liver metastases from gastro-entero-pancreatic neuroendocrine tumours. Cochrane Database Syst Rev 1. CD007118.

[41] Pasieka, J. L., Mc Ewan, A. J. B., & Rorstad, O. (2004). The palliative role of 131I-MIBG and 111In-octreotide therapy in patients with metastatic progressive neuroendocrine neoplasms. *Surgery,* 136, 1218-1226.

[42] Faiss, S., Pape, U. F., Bohmig, M., et al. (2003). Prospective, randomized, multicenter trial on the antiproliferative effect of lanreotide, interferon alfa, and their combination for therapy of metastatic neuroendocrine gastroenteropancreatic tumors-the International Lanreotide and Interferon Alfa Study Group. *J Clin Oncol,* 21, 2689-2696.

[43] Jürgen, Weitz., Ronald, P., & De Matteo, . (2012). Noncolorectal nonneuroendocrine metastases Chapter 81C- Jarnagin & Blumgart: Blumgart's Surgery of the Liver, Pancreas and Biliary Tract, 5th ed. Copyright © 2012 Saunders, An Imprint of Elsevier.

[44] Adam, R., Chiche, L., Aloia, T., et al. (2006). Hepatic resection for noncolorectal nonendocrine liver metastases: analysis of 1,452 patients and development of a prognostic model. *Ann Surg*, 244, 524-535.

[45] Reddy, S. K., Barbas, A. S., Marroquin, C. E., et al. (2007). Resection of noncolorectal nonneuroendocrine liver metastases: a comparative analysis. *J Am Coll Surg*, 204, 372-382.

Chapter 2

Transplantation for Hepatocellular Carcinoma

Ahmad Madkhali, Murad Aljiffry and
Mazen Hassanain

Additional information is available at the end of the chapter

1. Introduction

Hepatocellular carcinoma (HCC) is the third leading cause of cancer mortality world-wide, accounting for more than 500,000 deaths annually. Major risk factors include chronic liver disease and liver cirrhosis due to hepatitis B and C viral infections, alcoholic liver disease and non-alcoholic steatohepatitis (NASH). Surgical resection and liver transplantation are the only potentially curable options for patients with HCC. While surgical resection is the treatment of choice in patients with good hepatic function, it is contraindicated in those with moderate to severe cirrhosis (Child class B or C), leaving these patients with liver transplantation as the only option. Moreover, transplantation is the optimal treatment even for small, otherwise resectable disease. This is a reflection of a number of factors. Liver transplantation will most likely result in a microscopically negative resection, which is the most effective oncologic treatment. Most HCCs are multifocal especially in the background of cirrhosis, though pre-neoplastic lesions may not be visible on periopera-tive evaluation; they are likely to continue to evolve into new primary HCCs. Further-more, transplantation eliminates cirrhosis and restores normal hepatic function. However, limited organ availability mandates the restriction of liver transplantation to patients with early stage tumors who are not candidates for resection.

2. Organ allocation

In an effort to prioritize liver transplant candidates according to the highest short-term risk of mortality from end stage cirrhosis, the model for end-stage liver disease (MELD) scoring system was implemented in 2002 (table 1). To impart more urgent access to liver transplan-tation for patients with small HCCs, additional points within the scoring system were allotted to these patients. This is done to equilibrate their risk of death in comparison with the mortality of end-stage cirrhosis. The original scoring exception included lesions smaller than 2 cm, which resulted in an over distribution of donor livers to patients with HCC (with many expected small tumors turning out not to be HCC on explanted pathology). Therefore, the scoring exception was modified later by reducing the upgrade for Stage II tumors and eliminating it for Stage I tumors. Using the American Liver Tumor Study Group Modified TNM staging system, current UNOS guidelines do not allow upgrading of candidates with Stage I disease, irrespective of biopsy confirmation; only candidates with Stage II HCC disease are upgraded on the waiting list to a MELD score of 22 (equivalent to a 15% probability of candidate death within 3 months) with the intent to shorten their waiting time. From 2002-2007 in UNOS database, patients with an "HCC MELD-exception" had similar survival to patients without HCC.

MELD score component, calculation and mortality prediction	
Serum bilirubin (mg/dL)	
Serum creatinine (mg/dL)	
INR	
MELD = 3.8[Ln serum bilirubin (mg/dL)] + 11.2[Ln INR] + 9.6[Ln serum creatinine (mg/dL)] + 6.4	
* If a patient has had 2 or more hemodialysis treatments or 24 hours of CVVHD in the week prior to the time of the scoring, Creatinine will be set to 4 mg/dL	
MELD score	Mortality in 3 months
- <9	1.9 %
- 10–19	6.0 %
- 20–29	19.6 %
- 30–39	52.6 %
- >40	71.3%

Table 1. MELD score component, calculation and mortality prediction

3. Criteria for transplantation

Retrospective study by *Mazzaferro* and colleagues established that favorable results could be achieved in patients with cirrhosis with either a solitary HCC ≤5 cm or with up to 3 nodules ≤3 cm, criteria that came to be called "the Milan criteria (Table3)." The 5-year survival of these early-stage patients exceeded 70%. Recipient age, gender, type of viral infection, or Child-Pugh score (table 2) did not affect survival after transplantation. In a multivariate analysis by *Marsh JW* and colleagues, found that independent predictors of tumor-free survival included lymph node status, depth of vascular invasion, greatest tumor dimension, lobar distribution, and tumor number.

The strict application of the Milan criteria by UNOS for MELD upgrades allocation disadvan-tages patients with HCC with tumor profiles exceeding the criteria's maximal size or multifoca

CHILD – PUGH SCORE			
Clinical and laboratory parameter	**Scores**		
	1	2	3
Encephalopathy (grade)	None	1-2	3-4
Ascites	None	Slight	Moderate
Albumin (g/dL)	> 3.5	2.8-3.5	< 2.8
Prothrombin time prolonged (sec)	1-4	4-6	6
Bilirubin (mg/dL)	< 2	2-3	> 3
· For primary biliary cirrhosis	< 4	4-10	> 10
Class A = 5–6 points; Class B = 7–9 points; Class C = 10–15 points. Class A: Good operative risk Class B: Moderate operative risk Class C: Poor operative risk			

Table 2. Child Pugh score

parameters but in whom favorable outcomes after liver transplantation have been demonstrated. There is an ongoing debate within the liver transplantation community regarding whether to expand indications for liver transplantation as primary therapy for HCC. For patients with HCC disease beyond Milan criteria in whom there is no macroscopic evidence of vascular invasion or extrahepatic spread, the survival rates after liver transplantation are generally comparable with patients transplanted for disease within the criteria. Most groups report a 5-year survival of more than 50% in patients transplanted for HCC beyond Milan, which many investigators have argued is the minimum acceptable survival rate. In 2001 *Yao* and colleagues at the University of California, San Francisco (UCSF) defined an expanded set of HCC criteria (solitary tumor ≤ 6.5 cm, or ≤ 3 nodules with the largest tumor ≤ 4.5 cm and total tumor diameter ≤ 8 cm)(table3) for which 1 and 5-year survival rates after LT were 90% and 75%, respectively. Retrospectively evaluating post- liver transplantation survival for patients with tumors beyond Milan criteria but within ''UCSF'' expanded criteria by pre-transplantation imaging and explant pathology, the group at the University of California, Los Angeles (UCLA) confirmed acceptable 1,3-, and 5-year survival rates of 82%, 65%, and 52%, respectively. Moreover, the difference in 5-year recurrence-free survival after liver transplantation for HCC in the UCLA study did not reach statistical significance between Milan criteria and UCSF expanded criteria tumor groups (74% vs 65%, P =.09). Liver transplantation in such candidates is controversial and widely adopted. The short-term outcomes are similar to those who are transplanted within the Milan criteria.

Group from Edmonton have study Total Tumor Volume (TTV) in patients with HCC who had liver transplant based on Milan or UCSF criteria in 3 centers and they found TTV < 115 cm^3 has lower recurrence rate than TTV > 115 cm^3. In same study they also found that patients beyond Milan but within TTV < 115 cm^3 had survivals similar to those of patients within Milan. On the contrary, patients with TTV >115 cm^3 demonstrated lower survival than those within TTV <115 cm^3 when pathology (5-year: 47% versus 79%, P < 0.001) and radiology staging (5-year: 53% versus 76%, P < 0.1) was used.

Milan criteria:
- Single lesion ≤ 5 cm or
- ≤3 nodules each ≤ 3 cm
Without vascular invasion.
"UCSF" expanded criteria:
- Single lesion ≤ 6.5 cm or
- ≤ 3 nodules with the largest tumor ≤ 4.5 cm and total tumor diameter ≤ 8 cm
Without vascular invasion.

Table 3. Criteria for liver transplantation

4. Pre-transplant treatment for HCC

The major limitation for liver transplantation as therapy for early-stage HCC is the insufficient number of donor livers. There is always a waiting period between candidate listing and transplantation. If the waiting period extends over a sufficient length of time, the tumor will grow and eventually hinders transplantation. In a study by *Yao* and colleagues of patients with HCC on the waiting list, a 6-month waiting period for liver transplantation was associated with a 7.2% cumulative dropout probability, increasing to 37.8% and 55.1% at 12 and 18 months, respectively. In this setting the treatment of HCC prior to liver transplantation has three potential goals: (a) controlling tumor growth and vascular invasion during the waiting time and therefore decrease dropouts from the waiting list; (b) carrying out neoadjuvant therapy to improve the post-transplant outcome by reducing the risk of postoperative recurrence, and (c) downstaging the HCC burden to make a patient eligible for transplantation.

Followups for patients on waiting list are required every three months by CT or MRI to ensure continued eligibility for liver transplantation.

5. Percutaneous ablation therapy

5.1. Bridging therapy

Bridge therapy is used to decrease tumor progression and the dropout rate from the liver transplantation waiting list. It is considered for patients who meet the transplant criteria. A number of studies have investigated the role of locoregional treatment as a bridge to liver transplantation in patients on a waiting list. These studies included radiofrequency ablation (RFA), transarterial chemoembolization (TACE), surgical resection, conformal radiation therapy, and sorafenib as "bridge" therapies.

5.1.1. TACE

The rationale for using TACE as a bridge therapy prior to OLT is to control tumor growth while the patient awaits an organ. In addition, TACE could cause significant tumor necrosis, which may reduce tumor dissemination, making it a potential neoadjuvant therapy. TACE can also be used to learn more about the natural history and behavior of a particular tumor prior to liver transplantation. *Decaens et al.* failed to demonstrate survival benefit in a retrospective case-control study comparing 100 patients who underwent TACE prior to liver transplantation (median 1 session/patient) versus 100 matched controls without prior treatment. Mean waiting time was 4.2 months, and 5-year post-LT survival rates were 69% versus 63% (p = ns); dropout was not analyzed. *Yao et al.* retrospectively studied 168 HCC patients who underwent liver transplantation, 88 of whom received TACE (in most cases immediately prior to LT). For patients with HCC within the Milan criteria, 5-year recurrence-free survival was 96% for the TACE group versus 87% for controls (p = 0.12), but for HCC beyond the Milan criteria the difference was statistically significant (86% vs. 51%, p = 0.05). *Roayaie et al.* reported a 46% dropout rate, but only advanced HCC (>5 cm) were included in this study. *Graziadei et al.* found no dropout from the waiting list in patients treated wit TACE meeting Milan criteria and the mean waiting time was only 178 days. Furthermore, the monitoring protocol of repeat staging and the criteria for dropout was not specified. In view of this study and others, the dropout rate ranged from 15 to 46%. The rate of dropout was related to the tumor state and to the duration in the waiting list, the higher rate (46%) being observed in more advanced HCC and when the mean waiting time was 340 days. A systematic review of bridging therapy with TACE by *Lesurtel et al.* concluded that there was insufficient good quality evidence to demonstrate that TACE either improved post-LT survival, altered post-LT complication rates, or impacted on waitlist drop out.

Although pre-liver transplantation TACE does not influence post-LT overall survival and disease-free survival, it remains indicated in context of clinical trial when the period on the waiting list is more than 6 months.

5.1.2. Percutaneous ablation therapy

Patients with small tumors can have ablation either by percutaneous ethanol injection, radiofrequency or any other technique. Pre-transplant RFA ablation for HCC as a strategy to reduce dropout has been addressed in view studies. More than 80% of patients were in the Milan criteria with approximately 1 year on the waiting list. The dropout rate ranged from 0 to 14%. In a nonrandomized series from Toronto of 74 patients bridged using ablation compared with 79 non-bridged patients, the analysis of dropout for tumor progression identified a difference (p < 0.005) that became apparent only with prolonged waiting time superior to 300 days.

The main concern with this approach is seeding due to tumor puncture as has been reported for diagnostic biopsy. However, puncture-related seeding is usually a case of poorly differentiated tumors and to peripheral tumors that cannot be approached through a rim of non-tumoral liver.

In conclusion, due to small size of these studies and the heterogeneous nature of the study populations, as well as the absence of randomized clinical trials evaluating the utility of bridge therapy for reducing the liver transplantation waiting list dropout rate, limit the conclusions that can be drawn. Therefore, if liver transplantation can be done without significant delay (i.e. within 6 month) would the optimum. However, in patients whose waiting time is predicted to be prolonged, an RCT of TACE and/or ablation as bridging therapy to decrease dropout of transplantation could be justified.

5.2. Liver resection

Advances in liver surgery have significantly improved the safety of resection. Resection can be used as a treatment for HCC prior to liver transplantation in three different settings. First, resection can be used as a primary therapy, and liver transplantation reserved as a "salvage" therapy for patients who develop recurrence or liver failure. A second justification for resection prior to transplantation is that it helps refine the selection process. Resection, indeed, gives access to detailed pathological examination of the tumor and the surrounding liver parenchyma. Important prognostic information can be obtained from the entire resected tumor, including differentiation (which proved to be heterogeneous within the tumor), satellite nodules, microvascular invasion, and capsular effraction. As a result, resection may help deny transplantation in patients with tumors apparently within the Milano criteria but with histological features of especially poor prognosis (undetected macrovascular invasion in particular). On the other hand, resection may help decide transplantation in patients with tumors slightly outside the Milano criteria but with histological features of good prognosis. Third, resection can be used as a "bridge" therapy for patients who have already been enlisted for liver transplantation. Resection as the first line treatment for patients with small HCC with preserved liver function, followed by salvage transplantation only for recurrence or liver failure is an attractive option. Initial resection with negative margins, gives rapid access to an effective therapy, without the need for a donor, and offers 5-year survival rates exceeding 50% with a good quality of life. The main obstacle to this strategy is the risk of "loss of chance" in case of rapid and extensive recurrence not amendable to salvage liver transplantation. At the time of recurrence, salvage liver transplantation is only applicable in patients with a tumor within the Milan criteria. Initial data showed that patients with HCV infection who developed recurrence after partial resection had multifocal tumors and/or vascular invasion at the time of recurrence.

Although limited resection appears to be sufficient in this setting, it is associated with increased risk of post resection liver failure and is only appropriate for patients with peripheral tumors and Child A cirrhosis and no portal hypertension. As disadvantage for this approach the subsequent liver transplantation would be more difficult due to increase operative time and blood loss.

The use of laparoscopic approaches for peripheral tumors may further contribute to expand this strategy by minimizing technical difficulties during the transplant procedure.

5.3. Tumor dowenstaging

The role of downstaging of tumors before liver transplantation has been explored. Downstaging is done using HCC directed therapy that aims at reducing the size and/or number of HCC lesions. *Graziadei et al.* achieved downstaging to within Milan using TACE in 15/36 patients (41%). Among those downstaged, four dropped out prior to LT, one remained waiting, and 10 underwent LT; there were six deaths including three HCC recurrences, and 4- year post-transplant survival of 41%. *Yao et al.* reports successful downstaging in 21/30 patients with HCC beyond UCSF using a multimodality approach including resection in four cases. There were two deaths related to downstaging treatment (one postresection). Among 16 patients transplanted there was one death and no recurrence, but follow-up was limited (median 16 months). Recent prospective studies have demonstrated that downstaging (prior to transplant) with percutaneous ethanol injection (PEI), RFA, TACE and transarterial radioembolization (TARE) with yttrium 90 microspheres improves disease-free survival following transplant. However, such studies have used different selection criteria for the downstaging therapy and different transplant criteria after successful downstaging. In some studies response to locoregional therapy has been associated with good outcomes after transplantation. Further validation is needed to define the end-points for successful downstaging prior to transplant.

6. Living donor transplantation

Efforts to address the large waiting list of liver transplantation candidates and to decrease the dropout rate have included several strategies such as living donor LT, domino LT, split LT, the use of extended criteria donors, and donors after cardiac death. Living donor LT appears to be an effective option for patients with HCC within the Milan criteria, essentially equivalent in terms of survival to OLT, and it is cost effective if waiting times exceed 7 months. There are few data to support the use of living donor LT for patients with HCC who exceed the Milan criteria, although its use for this purpose is becoming increasingly common.

7. Immunsupression

Immunsupresion is used post liver transplantation to reduce graft rejection but, especially in transplantation for HCC, is associated with a risk of tumor growth. While results of liver transplantation including survival and rates of rejection were dramatically improved in cyclosporine treated patients compared with "historical controls", a high incidence of neoplasm and its aggressive phenotype were found to be due to cyclosporine and its activation of transforming growth factor-beta (TGFβ). *Vivarelli* and colleagues reported an increase in 5-year recurrence free survival in patients treated with smaller cumulative doses of cyclosporine in the first year following liver transplantation for HCC. Furthermore, they observed a significantly higher mean cyclosporine level in patients with HCC recurrence. Tacrolimus, another calcineurin inhibitor was also found to promote cell cycle progression by an increase in cdk4 kinase activity and thus was linked to increased tumor recurrence.

On the other hand, the calcineurin-independent immunosuppressive agent sirolimus, a binder of mTOR, inhibits tumor growth in cell lines, and it inhibits primary and metastatic tumor growth *in vivo*. In a study by *Wang Z et al*, looking at HCC in mouse model of human HCC, they identify that sirolimus induces cell cycle arrest and blocke proliferation of an HCC cell line, also sirolimus found to prevent tumor growth and metastatic progression by down-regulating the mRNA expression of VEGF and HIF-1α.

Several retrospective reports suggest a lower risk of post-transplant tumor recurrence in patients with HCC with the use of sirolimus as compared to other types of immunosuppressive agents (such as the calcineurin inhibitors tacrolimus and cyclosporine). However, these reports are limited by small size and uncertainty as to whether the observed benefits were due to a specific antitumor effect or an impact on liver transplant in general.

8. Surveillance

There is no consensus as to the optimal approach for post-transplant surveillance. Guidelines from the National Comprehensive Cancer Network (NCCN) suggest the follow up after liver transplant with triphasic CT every 3-6 months for 2 years, then every 6-12 months. AFP levels every 3 months for 2 years, if initially elevated, then every 6-12 months.

9. Survival

There is a clear survival benefit and low recurrence rate after transplantation for hepatocellular carcinoma. When surgeons adhere to Milan criteria, 5-year survival rates after transplantation range from 70% to 80%, and tumor recurrence rates are approximately 10%. Since the initial report by Yao and colleagues that demonstrated acceptable survival rates using the UCSF criteria (90% 1-year survival rates and 75% 5-year survival rates) and showed no survival deference from Milan criteria in 1,3 and 5 years, long-term survival need to be further identified.

10. Recurrence

Tumor recurrence remains a main limitation to the long-term survival of patients following liver transplantation for HCC. While the majority of patients recur in the first two years after transplantation, late recurrence is not infrequent. Most common sites of recurrence are liver graft, lung, bone, abdominal lymph nodes, adrenal glands and peritoneum. The incidence of recurrent HCC following transplantation has been reported to vary, ranging from 6-56%. However, in cases in which the Milan selection criteria were adopted, risk of recurrence decreased to 10–15% at 5 years. While several recipient and tumor specific factors are prognostically important, primary tumor size, number of lesions, grade of tumor and presence of vascular invasion have been noted to be the most significan clinical risk factors for both recurrence and survival. De-novo tumor development from recurrent hepatitis and cirrhosis in the liver graft can occur, however presence of microscopic foci of disease in lymph nodes or distant organs at the time of transplantation, as well as hematogenous or peritoneal tumor dissemination during transplantation, are mechanisms attributed to disease recurrence. Recurrent disease following liver transplantation for HCC may involve an extrahepatic site in 10-43% of patients.

Successful surgical salvage has been reported for intrahepatic and/or confined extrahepatic HCC metastases. In a study by *Regalia et al*, involving several Italian centers, 7 out of 21 patients (30%) underwent salvage resection of recurrent HCC of the liver (2), lung (2), bone (1), skin or other sites (2). Surgical resection was associated with a survival of 15.5 months, which was better than the 5.5 months noted among patients treated with a non-surgical approach. *Schlitt et al.* reported on 39 patients with recurrent disease, 9 intrahepatic recurrences, 15 extrahepatic disease and 15 had both intra and extrahepatic recurrence. Eleven of these patients were able to undergo complete removal of the recurrent disease, including 5 patients with an intrahepatic recurrence; 7 (63%) were alive at 4.3 years of follow-up. As with HCC of the native liver, the utilization of resection versus ablation to treat recurrence in the allograft is dependent on surgical judgment, as well as the size and location of the tumor. While resection may be more applicable to more superficial and larger tumors, ablative techniques may be sufficient and appropriate in the setting of smaller and more deeply situated tumors. Although liver resection for intrahepatic HCC recurrence has been reported by several centers, most series are limited by a small sample size.

Reports of repeat liver transplantation as a treatment of recurrent intrahepatic HCC are limited to a few very select case series and is not the standard of care.

Another potential approach to intrahepatic HCC recurrence is the utilization with TACE and RFA. *Ko et al*, reported on 28 patients with recurrent HCC who underwent one or more cycles of TACE after transplantation (mean, 2.5 cycles). In this study, the targeted tumor reduced in size by ≥25% in 19 of the 28 study patients (68%). However, intrahepatic or extrahepatic metastasis occurred in 21 of the 28 patients (75%) during the 3-month follow-up period and mean survival was only 9 months.

Systemic therapeutic options for recurrent HCC are limited. While cytotoxic agents have traditionally had marginal effect in the treatment of HCC, systemic therapy with molecular targeted therapy has been shown to prolong survival in recent trials. Sorafenib, a multitargeted kinase inhibitor, demonstrated a significant overall survival benefit in patients with advanced or metastatic HCC when compared with placebo in two separate Phase 3 trials. These studies were carried out in patients who presented initially with advanced disease (mostly liver confined disease), and did not include patients who had previously undergone curative-intent therapy, such as surgical resection or liver transplantation. A number of retrospective studies have reported acceptable safety data for sorafenib in liver transplant patients, with very few unexpected toxicities or interaction with immunosuppressive medications. The numbers in these studies are small, and there is clearly a need for a prospective trial to fully assess the potential survival benefit of sorafenib in this setting.

Radiation therapy is another option for patients with recurrent unresectable HCC. Three dimensional conformal radiation, as well as stereotactic body radiation therapy and radioembolization, have been utilized in the treatment of primary unresectable HCC. In addition, radiation therapy is a treatment option for symptomatic palliation of extrahepatic disease. *Yamashi et al*, reported on 28 patients with metastatic HCC involving the portal and/or peripancreatic lymph nodes who were treated with radiation therapy. A total of 18 (64%) and five (18%) patients achieved partial responses and complete responses, respectively. The 1- and 2-year overall survival rates were 53% and 33%, respectively. In one study, *Seong et al.* investigated the effectiveness of palliative radiation therapy for HCC bone metastasis. In this study, 51 patients received radiation therapy for 77 bony metastatic lesions, with a median total dose of 30 Gy. There was pain relief in 56 lesions (73%), however, median and 1 year survival were only 5 months and 15%, respectively. In aggregate, these studies suggest that recurrent metastatic HCC may be sensitive to palliative radiation therapy. Therefore, radiation therapy should be considered for palliation of metastatic HCC lesions.

Abbreviation

HCC Hepatocellular carcinoma

HIF-1α Hypoxia-inducible factor 1, alpha

MELD Model for end-stage liver disease

RFA Radiofrequency ablation

PEI Percutaneous ethanol injection

TACE Transarterial chemoembolization

TGFβ Transforming growth factor-beta

TNM Classification of Malignant Tumors (Tumor, lymph Node, Metastasis)

VEGF Vascular endothelial growth factor

UNOS United Network for Organ Sharing

UCSF University of California, San Francisco

Author details

Ahmad Madkhali[1], Murad Aljiffry[2] and Mazen Hassanain[1,3]

1 Department of surgery, College of Medicine, King Saud University, Riyadh, Saudi Arabia

2 Department of surgery, College of Medicine, King Abdulaziz University, Jeddah, Saudi Arabia

3 College of Medicine, Liver Disease Research Centre, King Saud University, Riyadh, Saudi Arabia

References

[1] Jordi Bruix, and Morris Sherman. Management of Hepatocellular Carcinoma: An Update. HEPATOLOGY, Vol. 53, No. 3, 2011.

[2] Peter Abrams, J. Wallis Marsh. Current Approach to Hepatocellular Carcinoma.Surg Clin N Am 90 (2010) 803–816

[3] Mazzaferro V, Regalia E, Doci R et al. Liver transplantation for the treatment of small hepatocellular carcinomas in patients with cirrhosis. N Engl J Med 1996; 334: 693–699.

[4] Marsh JW, Dvorchik I, Bonham CA, et al. Is the pathologic TNM staging system for patients with hepatoma predictive of outcome? Cancer 2000; 88(3):538–43.

[5] Yao FY, Bass NM, Nikolai B, et al. A follow-up analysis of the pattern and predictors of dropout from the waiting list for liver transplantation in patients with hepatocellular carcinoma: implications for the current organ allocation policy. Liver Transpl 2003;9(7):684–92.

[6] Duffy JP, Vardanian A, Benjamin E, et al. Liver transplantation criteria for hepatocellular carcinoma should be expanded: a 22-year experience with 467 patients at UCLA. Ann Surg 2007;246(3):502–9.

[7] Toso C, Trotter J, Wei A.et al. Total tumor volume predicts risk of recurrence following liver transplantation in patients with hepatocellular carcinoma. Liver Transpl. 2008 Aug;14(8):1107-15.

[8] Hepatobiliary Cancers .National comprehensive cancer network 2.2012.www.nccn.org

[9] George Tsoulfas, Steven A Curley, Eddie K Abdalla, et al.Liver transplantation for hepatocellular carcinoma.uptodate 21 may 2012.www.uptodate.com

[10]   Decaens T, Roudot-Thoraval F, Bresson-Hadni S et al. Impact of pretransplantation transarterial chemoembolization on survival and recurrence after liver transplantation for hepatocellular carci- noma. Liver Transpl 2005; 11: 767–775.

[11]   Yao FY, Kinkhabwala M, LaBerge JM et al. The impact of pre- operative loco-regional therapy on outcome after liver transplan- tation for hepatocellular carcinoma. Am J Transplant 2005; 5: 795– 804.

[12]   Roayaie S, Frischer JS, Emre SH et al. Long-term results with multimodal adjuvant therapy and liver transplantation for the treat- ment of hepatocellular carcinomas larger than 5 centimeters. Ann Surg 2002; 235: 533–539.

[13]   Graziadei IW, Sandmueller H, Waldenberger P et al. Chemoem- bolization followed by liver transplantation for hepatocellular car- cinoma impedes tumor progression while on the waiting list and leads to excellent outcome. Liver Transpl 2003; 9: 557– 563.

[14]   M.Lesurtel, B.Mu llhaupt, B.C.Pestalozzi. et al. Transarterial Chemoembolization as a Bridge to Liver Transplantation for Hepatocellular Carcinoma: An Evidence-Based Analysis. *American Journal of Transplantation 2006; 6: 2644–2650*

[15]   J. Belghiti, B. I. Carr, P. D. Greig. Treatment before Liver Transplantation for HCC. Annals of Surgical Oncology 15(4):993–1000

[16]   A. James Hanje and Francis Y. Yao. Current approach to downstaging of hepatocellu- lar carcinoma prior to liver transplantation. Curr Opin Organ Transplant 13:234–240

[17]   Cheow PC, Al-Alwan A, Kachura J, et al. Ablation of hepa- toma as a bridge to liver transplantation reduces drop-out from prolonged waiting time. Hepatology 2005; 42:333A.

[18]   Shin Hwang ,Sung Gyu Lee and Jacques Belghiti.Liver transplantation for HCC: its role.Eastern and Western perspectives. J Hepatobiliary Pancreat Sci (2010) 17:443–448

[19]   Vivarelli M, Cucchetti A, Piscaglia F, La Barba G, Bolondi L, Cavallari A, et al. Analy- sis of risk factors for tumor recurrence after liver transplantation for hepatocellular carcinoma: key role of immunosuppression. Liver Transpl 2005;11:497-503.

[20]   Wang Z, Zhou J, Fan J, Tan CJ, Qiu SJ, Yu Y, et al. Sirolimus inhibits the growth and metastatic progression of hepato- cellular carcinoma. J Cancer Res Clin Oncol 2009;135:715- 722.

[21]   Schlitt HJ, Neipp M, Weimann A, et al. Recurrence patterns of hepatocellular and fi- brolamellar carcinoma after liver transplantation. J Clin Oncol 1999;17:324–331.

[22]   Ko HK, Ko GY, Yoon HK, Sung KB: Tumor response to transcatheter arterial chemo- embolization in recurrent hepatocellu- lar carcinoma after living donor liver trans- plantation. Korean J Radiol 2007;8:320–327.

[23] Michael A. Zimmerman, *et al.* Recurrence of Hepatocellular Carcinoma Following Liver Transplantation. A Review of Preoperative and Postoperative Prognostic Indicators. Arch Surg. 2008;143(2):182-188

[24] Ali Zarrinpar, Fady Kaldas and Ronald W Busuttil. Liver transplantation for hepatocellular carcinoma:an update. Hepatobiliary Pancreat Dis Int ,Vol 10,No 3 .June 15 , 2011

[25] G. C. Sotiropoulos, *et al.* META-ANALYSIS OF TUMOR RECURRENCE AFTER LIVER TRANSPLANTATION FOR HEPATOCELLULAR CARCINOMA BASED ON 1,198 CASES. Eur J Med Res (2007) 12: 527-534

[26] Sasan Roayaie, *et al.* Recurrence of Hepatocellular Carcinoma After Liver Transplant: Patterns and Prognosis. Liver Transplantation, Vol 10, No 4 (April), 2004: pp 534–540

[27] Myron Schwartz, Sasan Roayaie, Josep Llovet.How should patients with hepatocellular carcinoma recurrence after liver transplantation be treated?. J Hepatol. 2005 Oct; 43(4):584-9

[28] Peter J. Kneuertz, *et al.*Multidisciplinary Management of Recurrent Hepatocellular Carcinoma Following Liver Transplantation. J Gastrointest Surg (2012) 16:874–881

[29] Enrico Regalia ,*et al.* Pattern and management of recurrent hepatocellular carcinoma after liver transplantation. J Hep Bil Pancr Surg (1998) 5:29–34

[30] Yamashita H, Nakagawa K, Shiraishi K, et al Radiotherapy for lymph node metastases in patients with hepatocellular carcinoma: retrospective study. J Gastroenterol Hepatol 2007;22:523–527.

[31] Seong J, Koom WS, Park HC: Radiotherapy for painful bone metastases from hepatocellular carcinoma. Liver Int 2005;25:261– 265

Chapter 3

The Assessment and Management of Chemotherapy Associated Liver Injury

S. M. Robinson, J. Scott, D. M. Manas and S. A. White

Additional information is available at the end of the chapter

1. Introduction

Historically chemotherapy for the treatment of colorectal cancer consisted of the thymidy-late synthase inhibitor 5-FU (Adrucil®, Fluouracil®, Efudex®, Fluoroplex®), or more recently it's oral pro-drug Capecitabine (Xeloda®), in combination with Folinic acid. Alone these agents were associated with overall tumour response rates in the order of 20%.[10] In the last decade newer agents such as Oxaliplatin and Irinotecan have emerged on the market. These agents are not administered alone but normally in combination with a thymidylate synthase inhibitor. These combinations have seen the reported objective response to chemotherapy rise to typical rates of 50%.[11-13]

In parallel with the development of these conventional chemotherapeutics a new class of biological agents, i.e. antibody based therapies, have emerged. These agents are used to tackle specific pathways in tumour growth and development such as angiogenesis (e.g. anti-VEG-FA antibody Bevacizumab) or cellular proliferation (e.g. the anti-epidermal growth factor antibodies Cetuximab and Panitumumab). When these agents are added to Oxaliplatin or Irinotecan based chemotherapy a further 10-15% increase in overall tumour response rate can be obtained.[14-17]

This improvement in response rates has led to a resurgence of interest in utilising chemotherapy as a means of down-sizing metastatic disease to enable subsequent surgical resection – so called conversion chemotherapy.[18] This approach was initially described in 1996 in a series of 330 patients with inoperable colorectal liver metastases of whom 53 (16%) were able to undergo a subsequent liver resection with curative intent after receiving systemic chemotherapy. The five year survival for these patients was 40% which compared favourably to patients with operable disease treated with surgery alone during the same period.[19] In 2004 the same group reported the outcome of 1104 patients with initially unresectable colorectal liver metastases who were treated primarily with systemic chemotherapy over an 11 year period from 1988 – 1999. Of this cohort 138 patients had a sufficient response to chemotherapy to permit subsequent curative intent surgery with an overall 5 year survival of 33% being achieved.[20]

In a small phase II trial of 42 patients with inoperable colorectal liver metastases Alberts et al reported that systemic treatment with 5-FU/Oxaliplatin was associated with a tumour response rate of around 60% with 14 patients (33%) having a sufficient response to permit a liver resection with curative intent.[21] Similar results have been reported with a 5-FU/Irinotecan regimen by Nuzzo et al with 15 out of 42 patients (36%) with inoperable disease being able to undergo subsequent surgical treatment.[22] In an attempt to determine the most appropriate regimen for use as conversion chemotherapy the GERCOR trial randomised patients with inoperable metastatic colorectal cancer to receive either 5-FU/Irinotecan until disease progression or unacceptable toxicity and then 5-FU/Oxaliplatin or the reverse sequence (n=113 per arm). Those patients receiving first line Oxaliplatin demonstrated a higher resection rate (n=24; 22%) than those receiving first line Irinotecan (n=10; 9%) and as such this is the approach most commonly applied in UK practice.[23]

More recently studies have been designed to determine the role of the biological agents in conversion therapy. In the phase II uncontrolled BOXER trial 46 patients with inoperable colorectal liver metastases were treated with Capecitabine/Oxaliplatin in combination with Bevacizumab. 35 of these patients experienced an objective tumour response with 18 (40%) able to undergo a liver resection with curative intent. In addition 5 patients (11%) experienced a complete radiological response to systemic therapy.[24] The CRYSTAL trial randomised patients with inoperable metastatic disease to Irinotecan/5-FU either alone or in combination with Cetuximab and found that the addition of Cetuxmiab was more likely to result in patients undergoing subsequent R0 liver resection with curative intent (Odds Ratio 3.02; p=0.002).[17] It is important to note that the response to Cetuximab is primarily determined by KRAS mutation status. In the Crystal trial there was no evidence of benefit in patients with mutant KRAS who received Cetuximab as compared to those who received 5-FU/Irinotecan alone.[25]

For those patients who receive successful conversion chemotherapy and are subsequently considered for liver resection with curative intent it is important to be aware of what the likely long term outcome will be. Adam et al. reported a series of 184 patients with initially inoperable disease who underwent hepatectomy after systemic therapy. In these patients a 5 year overall survival rate of 33% was obtained although it is important to note that a significant proportion of patients in this study underwent 2 or more surgical procedures, often interspersed with further chemotherapy, before long lasting disease control was obtained.[26]

Whilst the role of conversion chemotherapy is widely accepted in the HPB community more recently the question has been asked about what role systemic therapy may play in the management of patients presenting with operable disease from the outset i.e. true neoadjuvant chemotherapy. The EPOC trial was a multicentre randomised controlled trial which allocated such patients to receive either surgery alone or 6 cycles of 5-FU/Oxaliplatin prior to surgery followed by a further 6 cycles of therapy after surgery (n=182 per arm). Of those patients randomised just over 80% of patients in both arms underwent a curative intent liver resection. When the results of this study were analysed on an intention to treat basis there was a non-significant trend to improved 3 year overall survival in the chemotherapy arm (35.4% vs. 28.1%; p=0.058) although statistical significance was only achieved when the analysis was limited to only those who underwent resection (42.4% vs. 33.2%; p=0.025).[27] The difficulty in interpretation of the EPOC trial is that it is impossible to know whether the benefits of peri-operative chemotherapy were primarily a result of the neoadjuvant or adjuvant treatment or if both are required. This important question remains, at present, unanswered.

At present most authors would agree that there is insufficient evidence to consider all patients with operable disease candidates for systemic therapy prior to surgery although it may play a role in those with poor prognostic features such as multiple tumour deposits, a large tumour size or extra-hepatic disease.[28, 29] What is clear however is that an ever increasing number of patients are presenting for surgical resection on the background of multiple cycles of chemotherapy.[30] As experience of managing this patient cohort has increased there has been a growing recognition that the use of chemotherapy can be associated with a toxic injury to the liver parenchyma.[31] The nature of this liver injury and its implication for the surgical approach to these patients will form the subject of the remainder of this chapter.

2. Chemotherapy associated liver injury

2.1. Steatosis/steatohepatitis

The presence of fatty change within the liver is increasingly prevalent in the general adult population where it is commonly associated with the presence of obesity and insulin resistance (i.e. the metabolic syndrome). Fatty liver disease represents a spectrum of changes within the liver ranging from simple steatosis through to steatohepatitis and in extreme cases cirrhosis.[32] Steatohepatitis differs from simple steatosis in that significant inflammatory infiltrates are present in the liver commonly in association with ballooning degeneration of hepatocytes.[33]

The link between chemotherapy use and fatty liver disease was first reported in the literature in 1998. In a series of 21 patients with colorectal liver metastases treated with systemic 5-FU Peppercorn et al. reported that 48% (n=10) of patients had developed radiological evidence of steatosis on follow-up imaging.[34] In a later series Pawlik et al. reported the histological findings in the liver parenchyma of 334 patients who had undergone resection of colorectal liver metastases, 153 of whom had received pre-operative chemotherapy. In this study steatosis ≥ 30% (i.e. steatosis affecting more than 30% of hepatocytes) was present in 18.4% of patients who received pre-operative chemotherapy as compared to only 3.4% of patients who were chemotherapy naive (p=0.004). In particular the authors observed that steatosis was most strongly associated with Irinotecan based chemotherapy (27.3% of patients; p<0.001) than 5-FU monotherapy (14.9%; p=0.03) and lastly Oxaliplatin based chemotherapy

(9.6%; p=0.04) suggesting that the nature of the chemotherapy regimen may be important in determining liver toxicity.[35]

In contrast however a separate series of 406 patients who underwent resection of colorectal liver metastases failed to demonstrate any association between the administration of pre-operative chemotherapy and the subsequent development of steatosis ≥ 30%. In those receiving Irinotecan based chemotherapy (n=94) there was however a dramatic increase in the incidence of steatohepatitis as compared to those patients who were chemotherapy naive (20.2% vs. 4.4%; p=0.001), a finding which was in contrast to the smaller study described above.[35, 36]

To more accurately determine the nature of the association between chemotherapy use and the development of fatty change within the liver our group undertook a systematic review and meta-analysis of the published literature. In this analysis it was not possible to demonstrate any association with chemotherapy use overall (Relative Risk 1.25; 95% confidence interval 0.99 – 1.57; p=0.15) or Oxaliplatin based chemotherapy (Relative Risk 0.98; 95% confidence interval 0.59 – 1.63; p=0.95) and the development of steatosis ≥ 30%. In the case of Irinotecan based chemotherapy there was a strong trend to an increased risk of steatosis > 30% (Relative Risk 2.51; 95% Confidence Interval 0.79 – 7.90; p=0.12) which was not statistically significant as a consequence of the heterogeneity within the included studies. In contrast there was a strong association between Irinotecan based chemotherapy and steatohepatitis (Relative Risk 3.45; 95% Confidence Interval 1.12 – 10.62; p=0.03) which was not demonstrated with other regimens.[37]

2.2. Sinusoidal obstruction syndrome

Sinusoidal obstruction syndrome (SOS; previously known as hepatic veno-occlusive disease) represents a microvascular injury to the liver characterised by the histological findings of dilatation of the hepatic sinusoids and associated atrophy of the surrounding hepatocytes. In more advanced SOS these changes are accompanied by the development of regenerative nodules within the liver and ultimately peri-sinusoidal liver fibrosis.[38] Historically SOS was described as a condition occurring after ingestion of pyrrolizidine alkaloids, a group of compounds found in plants used in traditional African herbal remedies.[39, 40] Furthermore SOS has been reported to occur in up to 50% of patients receiving myeloablative chemotherapy prior to bone marrow transplantation.[41, 42]

In a seminal paper in 2004 Rubbia-Brandt published a report of histological changes in the liver parenchyma of 153 patients who had undergone resection of colorectal liver metastases. In this study it was reported that 44 out of 87 patients treated with pre-operative chemotherapy had histological features of SOS, the majority of whom had received treatment with Oxaliplatin based regimens.[38] Similar results were reported by Vauthey et al who demonstrated a significantly increased incidence of SOS in patients receiving Oxaliplatin based chemotherapy as compared to those who were chemotherapy naive (18.9% vs. 1.9%; p<0.001) where as no such association was demonstrated with other chemotherapy regimens.[36] In our systematic review of the published literature we demonstrated a strong association between Oxaliplatin based chemotherapy and SOS (Relative Risk 2.78; 95%

Confidence Interval 1.35 – 5.69; p=0.0007) which again was not replicated in patients receiving alternative chemotherapy regimens.[37] The typical appearances of an Oxaliplatin injured liver, as encountered at laparotomy, are shown in Figure 1.

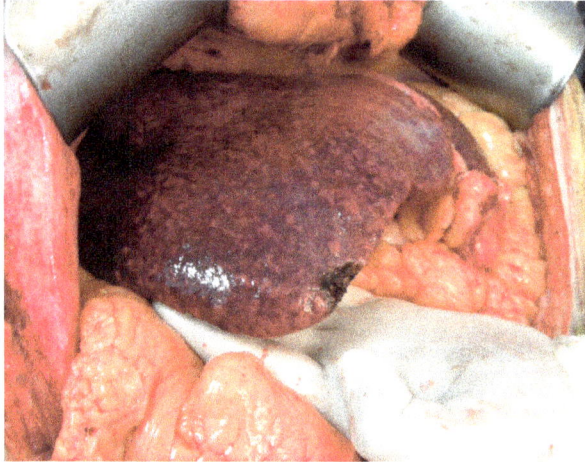

Figure 1. The classical appearance of the Oxaliplatin injured liver with SOS – commonly described as a "blue liver"

It is therefore clear from this discussion that the nature of liver injury following administration of chemotherapy to patients with colorectal liver metastases is dependent on the nature of the regimen administered. Irinotecan based regimens are primarily associated with the development of hepatic steatosis/steatohepatitis whereas Oxaliplatin based regimens are associated with the development of SOS. The assessment of the severity of this liver injury and its implications for the surgical management of these patients forms the discussion in the remainder of this chapter.

3. Assessment of the post-chemotherapy liver

Post hepatectomy liver failure (PHLF) is a feared complication of major liver resection and was recently defined as "a postoperatively acquired deterioration in the ability of the liver to maintain its synthetic, excretory and detoxifying functions"[43] whose presence is associated with a dramatic increase in the risk of post-operative mortality.[44, 45]

A key risk factor for the development of PHLF is the presence of background liver disease or injury. Belghiti et al reported, in a series of 747 patients undergoing liver resection, that the presence of either cirrhosis or steatosis affecting more than 30% of hepatocytes (n=253) was associated with a post-operative mortality of 9.5% as compared to only 1% in those with a normal liver parenchyma.[46] In a series of 406 patients undergoing resection of colorectal liver metastases Vauthey et al reported that those patients with steatohepatitis (n=34) experienced an increase in both 90 day mortality (14.7% vs. 1.6% p = 0.001) and post hepatectomy liver failure (5.8% vs. 0.8%; p=0.01).[36] The findings from these case series have been supported by a meta-analysis of the published literature which demonstrated that the presence of hepatic steatosis > 30% was associated with an increased risk of peri-operative complications (risk ratio 2.01; p<0.0001) and mortality (risk ratio 2.79; p=0.02).[47] Similarly the presence of SOS has been associated with an increased incidence of PHLF in a series of 51 patients undergoing resection of CRLM, 38 of whom had histologically proven SOS (68% vs. 23%; p=0.004)[48]

The other factor that is pivotal in determining the risk of PHLF is the volume of liver which will remain following surgery, commonly referred to as the future liver remnant or FLR, which can often be estimated pre-operatively by CT volumetry.[49] In 2003 Shoup et al reported a series of 126 patients who had undergone a liver resection to treat colorectal liver metastases. In those patients with a FLR of ≤ 25% (n=20) 90% developed PHLF as compared to 19% of those with an FLR > 25%. Logistic regression analysis demonstrated that the presence of an FLR<25% tripled the risk of PHLF (Odds Ratio 3.09; p<0.0001). Similarly in a study of 119 patients with a normal liver parenchyma undergoing major liver resection (i.e. resection of 3 or more Couinaud segments) the median FLR in the 7 patients who developed PHLF was 29.6% as compared to 42.5% in those who did not (p=0.009).[50] As a consequence of this evidence the minimum safe FLR in patients with an otherwise normal liver undergoing resection of CRLM is 25%.[51]

In those patients presenting for surgery on the background of multiple cycles of pre-operative chemotherapy it is pivotal, particularly when an extensive liver resection is planned, to minimise the risk of PHLF. When significant parenchymal injury is present it may be necessary for the FLR to be as high as 40% and this may have a significant impact on the surgical strategy employed.[52] Careful pre-operative assessment of the liver is therefore essential in these patients and the techniques which can be employed for doing this are discussed in more detail below.

3.1. Clinical/biochemical markers of chemotherapy induced liver injury

Identifying those patients at risk of steatohepatitis following Irinotecan based chemotherapy is particularly difficult not least because a significant proportion of patients in the background community will have a fatty liver as a consequence of either the metabolic syndrome, other underlying liver disease or lifestyle. This is reflected in the study of Ryan et al. which analysed histological changes in the liver of 334 patients undergoing resection of colorectal metastases. Only 8 patients in this study had histologically defined steatohepatitis the presence of which, on multivariate analysis, was found to be independently associated with a BMI > 30kg/m^2 but not the use of chemotherapy.[53] The study of Vauthey et al. reported that, in 94 patients treated with Irinotecan, the incidence of steatohepatitis was 12.1% in those with a BMI of < 25kg/m^2 but 24.6% in those with a BMI of ≥ 25kg/m^2. This study did not however undertake a multivariate analysis to identify independent risk factors associated with the presence of steatohepatitis.[36] It has been proposed that elevated serum transaminases may be of use in determining simple steatosis from steatohepatitis in patients with non-alcoholic fatty liver disease but it is not know whether this observation also holds true in those with chemotherapy associated steatohepatitis.[54-56]

Whilst one might intuitively expect that there would be a direct correlation between the number of cycles of chemotherapy received and the presence of liver injury this relationship is in fact less than clear cut. In the study of Vauthey et al. which reported the presence of liver injury in 406 patients undergoing resection of colorectal metastases there was no association between the number of cycles of chemotherapy administered and the incidence of steatohepatitis or SOS.[36] On the other hand Kishi et al., in a series of 219 patients who were treated pre-operatively with Oxaliplatin based chemotherapy, reported that SOS was present more frequently in those who received 9 or more cycles of chemotherapy than those who did not (42% vs. 26%; p=0.017).[57] Similarly the study of Aloia et al. reported that the incidence of SOS in those receiving greater than 12 cycles of chemotherapy was 50% as compared to 25% in those receiving 6-12 cycles and 10% in those who received less than 6 cycles (p=0.01).[58] Several studies have undertaken multivariate analysis to identify independent risk factors associated with the development of chemotherapy induced liver injury. Nakano et al demonstrated that the presence of SOS was independently associated with receiving 6 or more cycles of Oxaliplatin based chemotherapy (Relative Risk 3.2; p=0.048).[59] In contrast however 3 other studies have failed to demonstrate any such independent association between the number of cycles of Oxaliplatin administered and the development of SOS.[48, 60, 61] This raises the question of whether other variables, such as the presence of underlying liver disease, also make a significant contribution to the development of chemotherapy induced liver injury.

Some authors have suggested that tumour related factors may play a role in determining the development of SOS. On a univariate analysis of 78 patients treated with pre-operative Oxaliplatin based chemotherapy Soubrane et al. reported that those with SOS tended to have a larger tumour size (7.8cm vs. 5.2cm; p = 0.004) although this was not identified as an independent risk factor on multivariate analysis.[48] Tamandl et al. were able to confirm this observation in a separate study and on this occasion they were able to demonstrate that a tumour size > 5cm was independently associated with the development of SOS on multivariate analysis (Hazard Ratio 4.42; p = 0.012).[61] This clinical data is supported by experimental data from our group which suggests that the presence of tumour within the liver of mice treated with Oxaliplatin based chemotherapy accelerates changes in gene expression associated with the development of SOS.[62]

The role of various haematological and biochemical parameters to predict the presence of SOS has also been explored in several studies. Soubrane et al. reported on univariate analysis that an elevated AST (p=0.0009), ALT (p=0.02) and a low platelet count (p<0.0001) were all suggestive of the presence of SOS. On multivariate analysis they demonstrated that a high AST to platelet count ratio (APRI score) was an independent predictor for the presence of SOS (Odds Ratio 5; p<0.005).[48] Similarly a multivariate analysis from Nakano et al. demonstrated an independent association between an elevated AST and the presence of SOS (Relative Risk 3.86; p=0.044). [59] Tamandl et al. reported that on multivariate analysis on multivariate analysis an elevated alkaline phosphatase or γGT was an independent predictor of SOS (Hazard Ratio 4; p=0.038) although this was not true for AST or ALT.[61]

Whilst none of these studies have demonstrated a single factor that is reliably able to predict the presence of chemotherapy induced liver injury it is possible to begin to develop a picture of the patient characteristics which may lead to a raised index of suspicion and prompt a more thorough assessment of the liver parenchyma prior to surgery.

3.2. Radiological assessment of chemotherapy induced liver injury

The volume of data on the radiological assessment of fatty liver disease is vast and this is a reflection of the high incidence of non-alcoholic fatty liver disease in the general population. The consequence of this is that the appearances of fatty liver disease on each of the 3 main imaging modalities of the liver have been well described and is summarised in Table 1. It should be pointed out that on CT scanning hepatic steatosis is best detected on unenhanced images which are often not performed routinely in most imaging protocols in order to minimise patient radiation exposure.[63] A recent systematic review and meta-analysis of the published literature concluded that MRI represented the most accurate method for determining the extent of hepatic steatosis with a reported sensitivity of 97.4% and specificity of 76.1% for the detection of steatosis >30%.[64]

Imaging Modality	Characteristic features hepatic steatosis
Ultrasound	Intracellular fat accumulation leads to an increase in liver echogenicity [63]
Computed Tomography	Steatosis leads to a decrease in attenuation of the liver parenchyma [63, 65]
Magnetic Resonance Imaging	A loss of liver signal intensity occurs on T1 weighted gradient echo (GRE) opposed images[63, 65]

Table 1. Appearances of hepatic steatosis on the main liver imaging modalities

Several studies have attempted to identify the utility of pre-operative cross sectional imaging to identify hepatic steatosis specifically in patients undergoing liver resection. The first of these was published in 2008 by Cho et al. who conducted a retrospective analysis of 131 patients undergoing partial hepatectomy over a 4 year period who had one of either a non-contrast CT scan (n=26), contrast enhanced CT scan (n=74) or a gradient opposed MRI (n=32) with a median interval between imaging and surgery of 17 Days. The ability of these imaging modalities to predict histologically defined steatosis > 30% was determined. The authors demonstrated that of the two CT methods studied only non-contrast CT was of any utility in determining the presence of hepatic steatosis with a high degree of specificity (100%) but had low sensitivity (33%) with a corresponding positive predictive value (PPV) of 100% and negative predictive value (NPV) of 83%. In contrast MRI fared much better in excluding the presence of hepatic steatosis with an NPV of 94% but a PPV of only 44% with a sensitivity of 88% and specificity of 63%. The conclusion of this study was that cross-sectional imaging alone was not consistently able to determine the presence of hepatic steatosis and was therefore of limited utility for this purpose.[66]

In 2009 O'Rourke et al. reported a prospective study of n=37 patients undergoing resection of colorectal liver metastases who received pre-operative liver specific MRI. Again this study demonstrated a much better performance for MRI in determining the presence of hepatic steatosis > 30% with a PPV of 100%, NPV of 87% a sensitivity of 63% and a specificity of 100%.[67] A subsequent retrospective study by Marsman et al compared the ability of non-contrast enhanced CT (n=32) and MRI (n=36) to detect the presence of histologically defined steatosis > 33% in patients undergoing resection of colorectal liver metastases after receiving pre-operative chemotherapy. In this study MRI by far out performed CT in terms of sensitivity (78% vs. 70%), specificity (100% vs. 86.4%); PPV (100% vs. 70%) and NPV (93.1% vs. 86.4%) suggesting that this is the imaging modality of choice.[68]

On the basis of the currently available evidence it appears that MRI is the imaging modality of choice to assess the extent of hepatic steatosis in patients with colorectal liver metastases prior to surgery. It must be highlighted that cross-sectional imaging is not able to differentiate between simple steatosis and steatohepatitis which can only be achieved with histological assessment of the liver. Furthermore a 'normal' imaging study does not exclude the presence of hepatic steatosis and in those cases where there is a high level of clinical suspicion a further evaluation of the liver must be undertaken.

The role of cross-sectional imaging in detecting the presence of SOS is much less clear cut as compared to hepatic steatosis. It has been proposed that the development of splenomegaly on post-chemotherapy imaging may serve as a surrogate marker for the presence of SOS. Overman et al conducted a study in patients who received either 5-FU/Oxaliplatin (n=96) or 5-FU alone (n=40) as adjuvant therapy following resection of a colonic primary and compared spleen size on pre-operative imaging to that 6 weeks after the final cycle of chemotherapy. They demonstrated that the median increase in spleen size was 22% for those patients receiving 5-FU/Oxaliplatin whereas there was no increase in size in those receiving 5-FU alone (p<0.001). The authors went on to look at a subgroup of patients (n=63) who underwent a liver resection after 5-FU/Oxaliplatin and demonstrated, on multivariate analysis, that a greater than 50% increase in spleen size following chemotherapy was independently able to predict the presence of SOS (Odds Ratio 2.34; p=0.02) with a sensitivity of 43%, and specificity of 90%.[60]

Several authors have explored the utility of various MRI protocols to predict the presence of SOS. Ward et al. reported a study of 60 patients with colorectal liver metastases who underwent superparamagnetic iron oxide (SPIO) enhanced MRI prior to liver resection. Following SPIO administration SOS is characterised by reticular hyperintensity on T2*-gradient response echo weighted MRI images the presence of which the authors graded on a scale of 0 – 3 (summarised in Table 2) with a score of 2 or greater indicating the presence of SOS. Using this technique 24 of the 60 patients were thought to have SOS on the basis of MRI the presence of which was subsequently confirmed histologically in 20 patients. Of the 36 patients thought not to have SOS on the basis of MRI 3 were subsequently found to have histological features of SOS. This means that SPIO enhanced MRI, in this study, had a sensitivity of 87%, specificity of 89%, PPV of 83% and NPV of 92% for the presence of SOS.[69] In contrast to these findings however O'Rourke et al. in their study of 37 patients found that SPIO enhanced MRI had a high specificity (100%) and PPV (100%) for the presence of severe SOS but a low sensitivity (11%) with a NPV of 78% suggesting that this technique may fail to identify a significant proportion of patients with SOS.[67]

Grade	Description
0	Absent
1	Fine reticulations on a minority of sections
2	Diffuse reticulations or localised coalescent areas of high signal
3	Diffuse reticulations present on all sections or densely coalescent areas of high signal on multiple sections

Table 2. Grading of reticular hyperintensity on SPIO enhanced MRI to determine the presence of SOS[69]

Shin et al. explored the ability of Gadoxetic acid disodium (EOB-MRI; Primavist®) enhanced MRI to detect the presence of SOS prior to resection of colorectal metastases. On EOB-MRI the presence of SOS appears as reticular hypointensity which the authors graded on a scale of 1-5 with a score of 4 (probably present) or 5 (definitely present) being considered diagnostic of SOS. Of the 42 patients included in this study all 12 MRI identified cases of SOS had the diagnosis confirmed histologically and of the 30 MRI negative cases 4 had histological evidence of SOS. This resulted in a sensitivity of 75%, specificity of 100%, PPV of 100% and a NPV of 87%. The images in this study were independently reviewed by a radiological resident with a good level of agreement (weighted kappa 0.765) suggesting that this technique is subject to minimal interobserver variability.[70]

The small number of patients in these studies make it difficult to recommend the routine use of any of these MRI protocols for the sole purpose of detecting pre-operative SOS. The presence of splenomegaly on pre-operative imaging, particularly in patients who have received multiple cycles of Oxaliplatin based chemotherapy, should raise suspicion about the presence of SOS and prompt a thorough assessment of the liver parenchyma if extended resection is to be performed.

3.3. Functional assessment of the future liver remnant

A variety of techniques have been described which aim to quantitatively assess the functional reserve of the liver and thereby provide a means to determine the minimum safe FLR that is required to avoid the risk of PHLF. Perhaps the most widely described of these techniques is the Indocyanine Green (ICG) retention test. Following injection ICG is transported in the systemic circulation bound to albumin and does not leave the serum until it reaches the liver where it is taken up by hepatocytes. These hepatocytes then clear ICG by excreting the compound into the biliary system in an ATP dependent manner. ICG does not enter the portal circulation nor is it metabolised by hepatocytes prior to its excretion and therefore the clearance of ICG provides a direct measure of hepatocyte function.[71]

Typically the retention of ICG at 15 minutes is measured in a serum sample (ICGR-15) and this value is used as a measure of hepatic functional reserve with a value of <10% being considered normal. Based on their experience of using this test in a series of 1429 patients Imamura et al. described the maximum extent of liver resection they thought could be safely performed according to the ICGR-15 value (see Table 3).[72] Others however view this ICGR-15 value as too conservative and state that a cut off of <14% should be used to identify those patients in whom it is safe to perform major liver resection.[73] The use of ICG retention as a pre-operative assessment of liver function is however predominantly limited to Asia where the majority of liver resections are performed for hepatocellular carcinoma and therefore the data regarding the validity of this test in patients with colorectal liver metastases is limited.

ICGR-15 Value	Typical Safe Liver Resection
<10%	Right/Left Trisectionectomy
10 – 19%	Left hepatectomy / Right sectorectomy
20 – 29%	Segmentectomy
≥ 30%	Limited non-anatomical resection

Table 3. Typical safe liver resection volumes as recommended by Imamura et al based on ICGR-15 values[72]

Nakano et al reported the outcome of 36 patients who underwent major hepatectomy (>3 Couinaud segments) 20 of whom had histologically proven SOS and 16 who had a normal liver parenchyma. The presence of SOS in these patients was independently associated with an ICGR-15 of >10%. It is of note that these patients experienced an increased risk of perioperative complications (40% vs. 6.3%; p=0.026) and a longer mean hospital stay (17 days vs. 11 days; p = 0.006).[59] Experimental studies have also suggested that ICGR-15 may be a useful measure of hepatocyte function in the context of hepatic steatosis.[74] In a series of 101 patients undergoing liver resection for colorectal metastases Klinger et al reported that the use of preoperative chemotherapy (n=83; all regimens) was associated with a longer ICGR-15 (7.3% vs. 3.5%; p = 0.005). Similarly those who had received pre-operative chemotherapy were more likely to have an ICGR-15 ≥ 10% (27.7% vs. 0%; p=0.011) and this was associated with an increased rate of post-operative complications (39.1% vs. 12.8%; p=0.005). No attempt was made in this study to correlate ICGR-15 values with histological changes within the liver parenchyma.[75]

The LiMAx test has recently been described as an alternative means of assessing the hepatic functional reserve. This test measures the cytochrome P450 mediated metabolism of ^{13}C labelled methacetin into acetaminophen and $^{13}CO_2$ which is exhaled. The test measures changes in the ratio of exhaled $^{13}CO_2 : ^{12}CO_2$ over a 60 minute period – the greater the $^{13}CO_2$ excretion the greater the functional reserve of the liver.[76] The authors have demonstrated that low post-operative LiMAx values (<80μg/kg/h) are correlated with an unacceptable risk of post-operative morbidity. On the basis of this they have proposed an algorithm to determine the safety of liver surgery based upon pre-operative measurement of the LiMAx to calculate the likely post-operative LiMAx using CT volumetric calculations of the FLR. This strategy has not however been proven in an independent prospective cohort and therefore cannot currently be recommended for routine clinical use.[77]

A final technique for assessing the functional reserve of the liver is hepatobiliary scintigraphy using ^{99m}Tc-mebrofenin. Following injection ^{99m}Tc-mebrofenin is taken up by hepatocytes and excreted directly into the biliary system without prior intracellular metabolism in a similar manner to ICG. The hepatic uptake and excretion of ^{99m}Tc-mebrofenin is determined using images obtained with a gamma camera and from this it is possible to determine the total liver uptake, corrected for body surface area, as a %/min/m^2 of the total injected dose (referred to as the total liver function or TL-F). In addition the FLR uptake function (FLR-F) can be calculated as a function of the TL-F based on uptake in the calculated.[78]

De Graaf et al. reported a series 55 patients judged to be at high risk of post-operative complications following liver resection assessed with ^{99m}Tc-mebrofenin scintigraphy prior to liver resection. They demonstrated that TL-F was significantly reduced in those patients with background parenchymal disease (7.4 vs. 8.5 %/min/m^2; p=0.007). In addition the FLR-F was significantly lower in those patients who developed PHLF as compared to those who did not (2.2 vs. 4.3%/min/m^2; p=0.001).[79] Whilst this technology needs further evaluation in prospective studies it is likely that the emerging ability to perform single photon emission computed tomography (SPECT) thereby enabling quantification of tracer compound activity in combination with standard CT will lead to renewed interest in the technique.

At present none of these technologies have been adequately characterised in patients with colorectal metastases undergoing liver resection. Whilst they undoubtedly have potential merit in identifying those patients with an impaired hepatocyte mass it is not known whether the information they add is superior to that obtained standard clinical and radiological assessment. This must be established before the routine integration of these technologies into the assessment of this cohort of patients can be recommended.

4. Surgical management of the chemotherapy injured liver

When either clinical suspicion or pre-operative imaging suggest the presence of a chemotherapy induced injury to the liver it may no longer be possible to resect all metastatic disease whilst maintaining an adequate FLR to avoid the risk of liver failure. In this situation two key surgical strategies have been described to reduce the risk of surgery i.e. pre-operative portal vein embolisation and two-stage hepatectomy and these are discussed in more detail below.

4.1. Pre-operative portal vein embolisation

Portal vein embolisation (PVE) is a particularly useful technique in patients who have disease which is technically resectable in a single operation but where so doing would lead to a compromised FLR. As early as 1920 Rous and Larimore observed that if they ligated a single branch of the portal vein in a rabbit there was atrophy of the ipsilateral lobe and hypertrophy of the contralateral lobe.[80] As a clinical technique PVE was initially described by Kinoshita et al. in 1986 as a means of limiting the extension of tumour thrombus in patients with hepatocellular carcinoma.[81] Subsequently in 1990 Makuuchi et al. demonstrated the safety and efficacy of this technique as a means of increasing the FLR in a series of 14 patients undergoing resection of hilar cholangiocarcinoma.[82] In a prospective study Farges et al. performed CT volumetry on patients undergoing pre-operative PVE and demonstrated that in those patients with no underlying parenchymal disease the typical increase in FLR was 16% whereas in those with chronic liver disease the typical increase in FLR was 9%.[83]

In 2010 Wicherts et al. reported a retrospective series of 67 patients who underwent liver resection for colorectal metastases after pre-operative PVE with a cohort of 297 patients who did not receive PVE. The authors observed that those patients treated with pre-operative PVE demonstrated a significantly higher complication rate (55.5% vs. 41.1%; p = 0.035) although there was no difference in surgical mortality between groups. Whilst this difference in morbidity is striking it is difficult to interpret since whilst all patients in the study underwent a major hepatectomy (≥3 Couinaud segments) 54% of those in the PVE group underwent a right trisectionectomy as compared to only 28% in the control group. What was striking in this study however was that 32 of the patients treated with PVE did not proceed to surgery and amongst these patients there were no 3 year survivors as compared to a 3 year survival rate of 44% in those who did undergo surgery.[84]

A similarly designed study by Pamecha et al. compared the outcome of 36 patients treated with pre-operative PVE with 65 patients who did not receive PVE all of whom had a diagnosis of colorectal metastases. Of the 36 patients treated with PVE 12 did not progress to surgery and had a median survival of 14 months as compared to 42 months in those who did progress to surgery (p<0.0001). Again there was a tendency to higher morbidity in the PVE group (36% vs. 20%) but in a similar manner to the study of Wicherts et al. more of these patients had undergone a right trisectionectomy (22% vs. 11%).[85]

The most important finding in both of these series is that nearly a third of all patients selected to undergo pre-operative portal vein embolisation do not undergo subsequent surgery and this is primarily a consequence of disease progression.[84, 85] It is likely that the most important factor driving this disease progression is the compensatory increase in arterial blood flow which occurs in the embolised lobe.[86] The blood supply of colorectal metastases is predominantly derived from the hepatic artery[87] and it is probable that the increase in arterial flow results in increased oxygen and nutrient supply to the tumour. In addition following PVE there is an increase in the hepatic production of a wide variety of cytokines, growth factors and other humoral factors that mediate liver regeneration and it may be that these also contribute to the progression of metastatic disease.[88, 89]

In summary PVE is a potentially useful technique for increasing the FLR in patients in whom this is likely to be compromised there is a significant risk that the procedure will result in disease progression rendering the patient inoperable and therefore must not be embarked upon lightly.

4.2. Two-stage hepatectomy

For a proportion of patients presenting with bilobar disease it is not possible to clear the entire tumour burden by an extended resection alone (e.g. right trisectionectomy) but rather it is necessary to combine an anatomical resection (e.g. or the right lobe) with multiple metastectomies from the contralateral lobe potentially resulting in an insufficient FLR, particularly in patients with a background liver injury (Figure 2). In such circumstances a PVE alone would not be appropriate because of the significant risk of tumour progression in the FLR and therefore a two stage resection should be considered. In the scenario described above this would typically consist of an initial operation to clear the left liver of tumour using multiple metastectomies followed several weeks later by a right hepatectomy. If it was felt at the time of the primary operation that the hypertrophy induced by surgery alone would not leave an adequate FLR for the second operation then it may be desirable to perform either intra-operative ligation of the right portal vein or post-operative percutaneous portal vein embolisation.[90] In this situation it is the authors preference to perform the latter procedure thereby avoiding unnecessary dissection of the hilum prior to right hepatectomy.

Wicherts et al. reported the outcomes of 59 patients considered to be inoperable using a single stage procedure who were selected for a two stage approach. All of these patients underwent a primary surgical procedure which in the majority of cases consisted of a minor hepatectomy (<3 Couinaud segments resected) the aim of which was to clear the left liver of tumour. Subsequently 42 patients underwent a second procedure which was typically a major hepatic resection (≥3 Couinaud segments) and typically this took place 3 months after the initial surgical procedure. It is of note that 17 patients selected for this approach did not undergo a second procedure primarily as a consequence of disease progression. The overall 5 year survival in this series was 31% when analysed on an intention to treat basis and this did not differ, in a statistically significantly manner, from patients undergoing a single stage hepatectomy over the same period in the authors unit.[91]

More recently Narita et al. reported the outcome of 79 patients treated using a two stage approach. After the initial surgical procedure 75 of these patients were considered appropriate to proceed to the second operation although the majority (92%) were thought to require portal vein embolisation to facilitate this. Of that cohort of patients 61 (78% of the original cohort) eventually underwent a successful second operation. The main reasons for patients not proceeding to a second procedure were tumour progression in 10 cases and insufficient regeneration of the FLR in a further 5 cases. It is of note that almost 1:6 of the patients who underwent a second surgical procedure were found to have new disease in the previously cleared FLR although this was dealt with at the time of surgery in all cases. In those patients who underwent a successful two stage resection the overall 5 year survival was 32%. Of the 61 patients who were treated successfully by a two stage approach 11 went on to have a subsequent resection of lung metastases although this had no effect on overall survival when compared to the 50 patients who did not.[92]

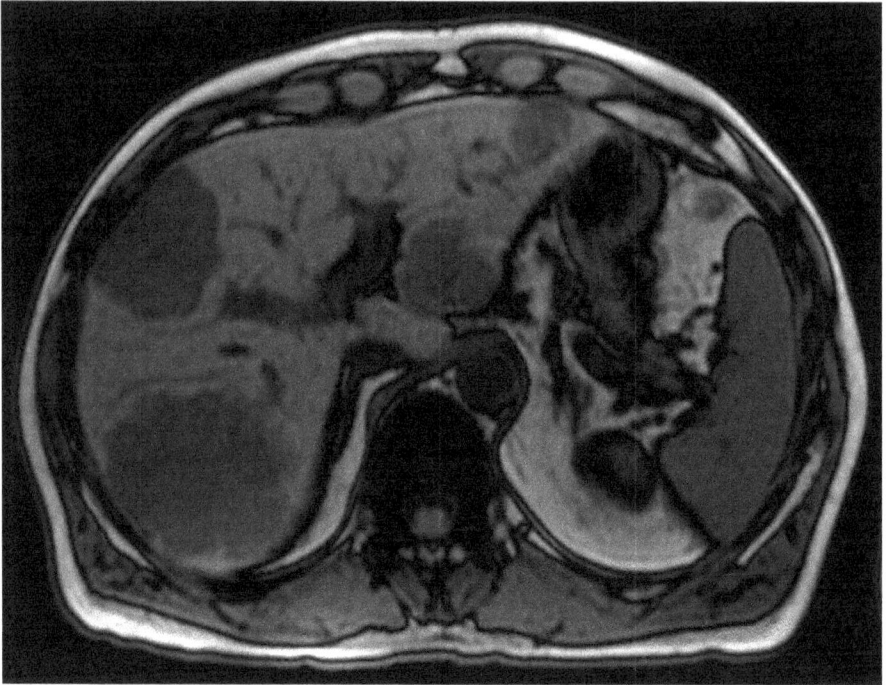

Figure 2. Typical MRI scan of patient with bilobar disease who would be considered suitable for a two staged approach to liver resection. With this distribution of disease a one stage approach would not leave an adequate FLR.

In a similar manner to PVE alone a two stage hepatectomy is a major undertaking and before embarking on this both surgeon and patient should be aware that there is a significant risk of not being able to complete the planned course of treatment. Despite this it does provide an opportunity to achieve a meaningful long term survival in selected patients with advanced disease.

5. The long term consequences of chemotherapy associated liver injury

Whilst the primary focus of this chapter is on the effects of chemotherapy associated liver injury on the surgical management of patients with colorectal liver metastases it would not be complete without some mention of the emerging evidence that this injury may have an effect on long term disease specific outcomes. Tamandl et al. have suggested that the presence of the histological features of SOS within the resected liver of patients with colorectal liver metastases may have a negative impact on long term disease specific survival. In particular patients with SOS demonstrated a significantly poorer 3 year progression free survival (6.7% vs. 22.7%; p=0.006) a finding which was upheld on multivariate analysis (Hazard Ratio 2.20; p=0.006). Specifically patients with SOS demonstrated a higher rate of intra-hepatic recurrence following surgery (66.7% vs. 30.5%; p=0.003) and not surprisingly this was associated with an increased risk of early all cause mortality on multivariate analysis (Hazard Ratio 2.90; p<0.001).[61]

A major criticism of the study of Tamandl et al. is that it includes only small numbers of patients (n=20 with SOS) and therefore it is difficult to draw definitive conclusions.[61] None the less a recent paper by Vreuls et al. has reported that the development of SOS may be associated with a poorer tumour response to Oxaliplatin based chemotherapy which the authors propose may be a consequence of tissue hypoperfusion leading to diminished leading to impaired delivery of chemotherapy to the tumour.[93] An alternative explanation may be that SOS is associated with increased expression of the chemokine CCL20 within the liver which is known to act as a chemo-attractant for colorectal cancer cells.[94] At the same time as this is occurring within the liver Oxaliplatin chemotherapy also results in increased expression of the CCL20 receptor CCR6 within colorectal liver metastases thereby increasing the migration and proliferation of tumour cells in response to CCL20.[95, 96] It may therefore be that the presence of SOS leads to the establishment of an autocrine signalling loop which favours the further growth and development of colorectal liver metastases.[97]

This emerging evidence is clearly a cause for concern and, if proven to be true, would add further impetus to the drive to develop strategies for the prevention of liver injury in patients being treated with systemic chemotherapy.

6. Conclusion

Advances in chemotherapy over the last decade or so have revolutionised the care for patients with colorectal liver metastases with the end result that patients who historically would have been considered inoperable are now able to undergo potentially curative surgical resection. The pay off for this advance has been the development of a chemotherapy associated injury to the liver the nature of which is determined the specific regimens used.

There is no specific test that is able to reliably detect the presence of an injured liver parenchyma and ultimately surgeons must maintain a high index of suspicion for its presence particularly in patients who have received multiple cycles of chemotherapy over a prolonged period of time. When a liver injury is present it is important that the surgical approach is considered carefully and makes allowances for the possibility of an impaired FLR with a subsequent risk of post operative liver failure. In those situations where there is a high risk of an insufficient FLR it may be appropriate to utilise techniques such as PVE or two stage hepatectomy although there is a risk with both these techniques of treatment failure as a consequence of disease progression.

Author details

S. M. Robinson[1], J. Scott[2], D. M. Manas[3] and S. A. White[3]

*Address all correspondence to: s.m.robinson@newcastle.ac.uk

1 Institute of Cellular Medicine, Newcastle University, Framlington Place, Newcastle upon Tyne, UK

2 Department of Radiology, Freeman Hospital, Newcastle upon Tyne, UK

3 Department of HPB Surgery, Freeman Hospital, Newcastle upon Tyne, UK

References

[1] Cancer Research UK. CancerStats - Bowel Cancer. Cancer Research UK; 2011 (updated 2011; cited 13/11/2011); Available from: http://info.cancerresearchuk.org/cancerstats/types/bowel/.

[2] Leporrier J, Maurel J, Chiche L, Bara S, Segol P, Launoy G. A population-based study of the incidence, management and prognosis of hepatic metastases from colorectal cancer. Br J Surg. 2006 Apr;93(4):465-74.

[3] Kopetz S, Chang GJ, Overman MJ, Eng C, Sargent DJ, Larson DW, et al. Improved survival in metastatic colorectal cancer is associated with adoption of hepatic resection and improved chemotherapy. J Clin Oncol. 2009 Aug 1;27(22):3677-83.

[4] Pawlik TM, Abdalla EK, Ellis LM, Vauthey JN, Curley SA. Debunking dogma: surgery for four or more colorectal liver metastases is justified. J Gastrointest Surg. 2006 Feb;10(2):240-8.

[5] Scheele J, Stangl R, Altendorf-Hofmann A. Hepatic metastases from colorectal carcinoma: impact of surgical resection on the natural history. Br J Surg. 1990 Nov;77(11):1241-6.

[6] Poston G, Adam R, Vauthey JN. Downstaging or downsizing: time for a new staging system in advanced colorectal cancer? J Clin Oncol. 2006 Jun 20;24(18):2702-6.

[7] Brouquet A, Vauthey JN, Contreras CM, Walsh GL, Vaporciyan AA, Swisher SG, et al. Improved survival after resection of liver and lung colorectal metastases compared with liver-only metastases: a study of 112 patients with limited lung metastatic disease. J Am Coll Surg. 2011 Jul;213(1):62-9; discussion 9-71.

[8] Neeff H, Horth W, Makowiec F, Fischer E, Imdahl A, Hopt UT, et al. Outcome after resection of hepatic and pulmonary metastases of colorectal cancer. J Gastrointest Surg. 2009 Oct;13(10):1813-20.

[9] Pawlik TM, Schulick RD, Choti MA. Expanding criteria for resectability of colorectal liver metastases. Oncologist. 2008 Jan;13(1):51-64.

[10] Van Cutsem E, Twelves C, Cassidy J, Allman D, Bajetta E, Boyer M, et al. Oral capecitabine compared with intravenous fluorouracil plus leucovorin in patients with metastatic colorectal cancer: results of a large phase III study. J Clin Oncol. 2001 Nov 1;19(21):4097-106.

[11] Giacchetti S, Perpoint B, Zidani R, Le Bail N, Faggiuolo R, Focan C, et al. Phase III multicenter randomized trial of oxaliplatin added to chronomodulated fluorouracil-leucovorin as first-line treatment of metastatic colorectal cancer. J Clin Oncol. 2000 Jan;18(1):136-47.

[12] de Gramont A, Figer A, Seymour M, Homerin M, Hmissi A, Cassidy J, et al. Leucovorin and fluorouracil with or without oxaliplatin as first-line treatment in advanced colorectal cancer. J Clin Oncol. 2000 Aug;18(16):2938-47.

[13] Saltz LB, Cox JV, Blanke C, Rosen LS, Fehrenbacher L, Moore MJ, et al. Irinotecan plus fluorouracil and leucovorin for metastatic colorectal cancer. Irinotecan Study Group. N Engl J Med. 2000 Sep 28;343(13):905-14.

[14] Hochster HS, Hart LL, Ramanathan RK, Childs BH, Hainsworth JD, Cohn AL, et al. Safety and efficacy of oxaliplatin and fluoropyrimidine regimens with or without bevacizumab as first-line treatment of metastatic colorectal cancer: results of the TREE Study. J Clin Oncol. 2008 Jul 20;26(21):3523-9.

[15] Hurwitz H, Fehrenbacher L, Novotny W, Cartwright T, Hainsworth J, Heim W, et al. Bevacizumab plus irinotecan, fluorouracil, and leucovorin for metastatic colorectal cancer. New England Journal of Medicine 2004 Jun 3;350(23):2335-42.

[16] Bokemeyer C, Bondarenko I, Makhson A, Hartmann JT, Aparicio J, de Braud F, et al. Fluorouracil, leucovorin, and oxaliplatin with and without cetuximab in the first-line treatment of metastatic colorectal cancer. J Clin Oncol. 2009 Feb 10;27(5):663-71.

[17] Van Cutsem E, Kohne CH, Hitre E, Zaluski J, Chang Chien CR, Makhson A, et al. Cetuximab and chemotherapy as initial treatment for metastatic colorectal cancer. N Engl J Med. 2009 Apr 2;360(14):1408-17.

[18] Khatri VP, Chee KG, Pertrelli NJ. Modern multimodality approach to hepatic colorectal metastases: Solutions and controversies. Surgical Oncology. 2007;16:71-83.

[19] Bismuth H, Adam R, Levi F, Farabos C, Waechter F, Castaing D, et al. Resection of nonresectable liver metastases from colorectal cancer after neoadjuvant chemotherapy. Ann Surg. 1996 Oct;224(4):509-20; discussion 20-2.

[20] Adam R, Delvart V, Pascal G, Valeanu A, Castaing D, Azoulay D, et al. Rescue surgery for unresectable colorectal liver metastases downstaged by chemotherapy: a model to predict long-term survival. Ann Surg. 2004 Oct;240(4):644-57; discussion 57-8.

[21] Alberts SR, Horvath WL, Sternfeld WC, Goldberg RM, Mahoney MR, Dakhil SR, et al. Oxaliplatin, fluorouracil, and leucovorin for patients with unresectable liver-only metastases from colorectal cancer: a North Central Cancer Treatment Group phase II study. Journal of Clinical Oncology. 2005;23(36):9243-9.

[22] Nuzzo G, Giuliante F, Ardito F, Vellone M, Pozzo C, Cassano A, et al. Liver resection for primarily unresectable colorectal metastases downsized by chemotherapy. J Gastrointest Surg. 2007 Mar;11(3):318-24.

[23] Tournigand C, Andre T, Achille E, Lledo G, Flesh M, Mery-Mignard D, et al. FOL-FIRI followed by FOLFOX6 or the reverse sequence in advanced colorectal cancer: a randomized GERCOR study. J Clin Oncol. 2004 Jan 15;22(2):229-37.

[24] Wong R, Cunningham D, Barbachano Y, Saffery C, Valle J, Hickish T, et al. A multi-centre study of capecitabine, oxaliplatin plus bevacizumab as perioperative treatment of patients with poor-risk colorectal liver-only metastases not selected for upfront resection. Ann Oncol. 2011 Sep;22(9):2042-8.

[25] Van Cutsem E, Kohne CH, Lang I, Folprecht G, Nowacki MP, Cascinu S, et al. Cetuximab plus irinotecan, fluorouracil, and leucovorin as first-line treatment for metastatic colorectal cancer: updated analysis of overall survival according to tumor KRAS and BRAF mutation status. J Clin Oncol. May 20;29(15):2011-9.

[26] Adam R, Wicherts DA, de Haas RJ, Oriana C, Levi F, Paule B, et al. Patients with Initially Unresectable Colorectal Liver Metastases: Is There a Possibility of Cure. Journal of Clinical Oncology. 2009;27(11):1829-935.

[27] Nordlinger B, Sorbye H, Glimelius B, Poston GJ, Schlag PM, Rougier P, et al. Perioperative chemotherapy with FOLFOX4 and surgery versus surgery alone for resectable liver metastases from colorectal cancer (EORTC Intergroup trial 40983): a randomised controlled trial. Lancet. 2008 Mar 22;371(9617):1007-16.

[28] Fong Y, Fortner J, Sun RL, Brennan MF, Blumgart LH. Clinical score for predicting recurrence after hepatic resection for metastatic colorectal cancer: analysis of 1001 consecutive cases. Ann Surg. 1999 Sep;230(3):309-18; discussion 18-21.

[29] Adam R, Bhangui P, Poston G, Mirza D, Nuzzo G, Barroso E, et al. Is Perioperative Chemotherapy Useful for Solitary, Metachronous, Colorectal Liver Metastases. Annals of Surgery. 2010;252(5):774-87.

[30] Adam R, Frilling A, Elias D, Laurent C, Ramos E, Capussotti L, et al. Liver resection of colorectal metastases in elderly patients. Br J Surg. 2010 Mar;97(3):366-76.

[31] Nordlinger B, Benoist S. Benefits and risks of neoadjuvant therapy for liver metastases. Journal of Clinical Oncology. 2006;24(31):4954-5.

[32] Anstee QM, McPherson S, Day CP. How big a problem is non-alcoholic fatty liver disease? BMJ. 2011;343:d3897.

[33] Kleiner DE, Brunt EM, Van Natta M, Behling C, Contos MJ, Cummings OW, et al. Design and validation of a histological scoring system for nonalcoholic fatty liver disease. Hepatology. 2005 Jun;41(6):1313-21.

[34] Peppercorn PD, Reznek RH, Wilson P, Slevin ML, Gupta RK. Demonstration of hepatic steatosis by computerized tomography in patients receiving 5-fluorouracil-based therapy for advanced colorectal cancer. Br J Cancer. 1998 Jun;77(11):2008-11.

[35] Pawlik TM, Olino K, Gleisner AL, Torbenson M, Schulick R, Choti MA. Preoperative chemotherapy for colorectal liver metastases: impact on hepatic histology and postoperative outcome. J Gastrointest Surg. 2007 Jul;11(7):860-8.

[36] Vauthey JN, Pawlik TM, Ribero D, Wu TT, Zorzi D, Hoff PM, et al. Chemotherapy regimen predicts steatohepatitis and an increase in 90-day mortality after surgery for hepatic colorectal metastases. Journal of Clinical Oncology. 2006;24(13):2065-72.

[37] Robinson SM, Wilson CH, Burt AD, Manas DM, White SA. Chemotherapy Associated Liver Injury in Patients with Colorectal Liver Metastases : A Systematic Review and Meta-Analysis. Annals of Surgical Oncology. 2012.

[38] Rubbia-Brandt L, Audard V, Sartoretti P, Roth AD, Brezault C, Le Charpentier M, et al. Severe hepatic sinusoidal obstruction associated with oxaliplatin-based chemotherapy in patients with metastatic colorectal cancer. Ann Oncol. 2004 Mar;15(3): 460-6.

[39] Willmot FC, Robertson GW. Senecio disease, or cirrhosis of the liver due to senecio poisoning. Lancet. 1920;2:848-9.

[40] DeLeve LD, Shulman HM, McDonald GB. Toxic injury to hepatic sinusoids: sinusoidal obstruction syndrome (veno-occlusive disease). Semin Liver Dis. 2002 Feb;22(1): 27-42.

[41] McDonald GB, Hinds MS, Fisher LD, Schoch HG, Wolford JL, Banaji M, et al. Veno-occlusive disease of the liver and multiorgan failure after bone marrow transplantation: a cohort study of 355 patients. Ann Intern Med. 1993 Feb 15;118(4):255-67.

[42] Hasegawa S, Horibe K, Kawabe T, Kato K, Kojima S, Matsuyama T, et al. Veno-occlusive disease of the liver after allogeneic bone marrow transplantation in children with hematologic malignancies: incidence, onset time and risk factors. Bone Marrow Transplant. 1998 Dec;22(12):1191-7.

[43] Rahbari NN, Garden OJ, Padbury R, Brooke-Smith M, Crawford M, Adam R, et al. Posthepatectomy liver failure: A definition and grading by the International Study Group of Liver Surgery (ISGLS). Surgery. 2011 Jan 13.

[44] Mullen JT, Ribero D, Reddy SK, Donadon M, Zorzi D, Gautam S, et al. Hepatic insufficiency and mortality in 1,059 noncirrhotic patients undergoing major hepatectomy. J Am Coll Surg. 2007 May;204(5):854-62; discussion 62-4.

[45] Reissfelder C, Rahbari NN, Koch M, Kofler B, Sutedja N, Elbers H, et al. Postoperative course and clinical significance of biochemical blood tests following hepatic resection. Br J Surg. 2011 Jun;98(6):836-44.

[46] Belghiti J, Hiramatsu K, Benoist S, Massault P, Sauvanet A, Farges O. Seven hundred forty-seven hepatectomies in the 1990s: an update to evaluate the actual risk of liver resection. J Am Coll Surg. 2000 Jul;191(1):38-46.

[47] de Meijer VE, Kalish BT, Puder M, Ijzermans JN. Systematic review and meta-analysis of steatosis as a risk factor in major hepatic resection. Br J Surg. 2010 Sep;97(9): 1331-9.

[48] Soubrane O, Brouquet A, Zalinski S, Terris B, Brezault C, Mallet V, et al. Predicting high grade lesions of sinusoidal obstruction syndrome related to oxaliplatin-based chemotherapy for colorectal liver metastases: Correlation with post-hepatectomy outcome. Annals of Surgery. 2010;251(3):454-60.

[49] Karlo C, Reiner CS, Stolzmann P, Breitenstein S, Marincek B, Weishaupt D, et al. CT-and MRI-based volumetry of resected liver specimen: comparison to intraoperative volume and weight measurements and calculation of conversion factors. Eur J Radiol. 2010 Jul;75(1):e107-11.

[50] Ferrero A, Vigano L, Polastri R, Muratore A, Eminefendic H, Regge D, et al. Postoperative liver dysfunction and future remnant liver: where is the limit? Results of a prospective study. World J Surg. 2007 Aug;31(8):1643-51.

[51] Garden OJ, Rees M, Poston GJ, Mirza D, Saunders M, Ledermann J, et al. Guidelines for resection of colorectal cancer liver metastases. Gut. 2006 Aug;55 Suppl 3:iii1-8.

[52] Kubota K, Makuuchi M, Kusaka K, Kobayashi T, Miki K, Hasegawa K, et al. Measurement of liver volume and hepatic functional reserve as a guide to decision-making in resectional surgery for hepatic tumors. Hepatology. 1997 Nov;26(5):1176-81.

[53] Ryan P, Nanji S, Pollett A, Moore M, Moulton CA, Gallinger S, et al. Chemotherapy-induced liver injury in metastatic colorectal cancer: semiquantitative histologic analysis of 334 resected liver specimens shows that vascular injury but not steatohepatitis is associated with preoperative chemotherapy. American Journal of Surgical Pathology. 2010;34(6):784-91.

[54] Anty R, Iannelli A, Patouraux S, Bonnafous S, Lavallard VJ, Senni-Buratti M, et al. A new composite model including metabolic syndrome, alanine aminotransferase and cytokeratin-18 for the diagnosis of non-alcoholic steatohepatitis in morbidly obese patients. Aliment Pharmacol Ther. Dec;32(11-12):1315-22.

[55] Boza C, Riquelme A, Ibanez L, Duarte I, Norero E, Viviani P, et al. Predictors of non-alcoholic steatohepatitis (NASH) in obese patients undergoing gastric bypass. Obes Surg. 2005 Sep;15(8):1148-53.

[56] Neuschwander-Tetri BA, Clark JM, Bass NM, Van Natta ML, Unalp-Arida A, Tonascia J, et al. Clinical, laboratory and histological associations in adults with nonalcoholic fatty liver disease. Hepatology. Sep;52(3):913-24.

[57] Kishi Y, Zorzi D, Contreras CM, Maru DM, Kopetz S, Ribero D, et al. Extended preoperative chemotherapy does not improve pathologic response and increases postoperative liver insufficiency after hepatic resection for colorectal liver metastases. Annals of Surgical Oncology. 2010;17(11):2870-6.

[58] Aloia T, Sebagh M, Plasse M, Karam V, Levi F, Giacchetti S, et al. Liver histology and surgical outcomes after preoperative chemotherapy with fluorouracil plus oxaliplatin in colorectal cancer liver metastases.[see comment]. Journal of Clinical Oncology. 2006 Nov 1;24(31):4983-90.

[59] Nakano H, Oussoultzoglou E, Rosso E, Casnedi S, Chenard-Neu MP, Dufour P, et al. Sinusoidal injury increases morbidity after major hepatectomy in patients with colorectal liver metastases receiving preoperative chemotherapy. Annals of Surgery. 2008;247(1):118-24.

[60] Overman MJ, Maru DM, Charnsangavej C, Loyer EM, Wang H, Pathak P, et al. Oxaliplatin-mediated increase in spleen size as a biomarker for the development of hepatic sinusoidal injury. Journal of Clinical Oncology. 2010;28(15):2549-55.

[61] Tamandl D, Klinger M, Eipeldauer S, Herberger B, Kaczirek K, Gruenberger B, et al. Sinusoidal obstruction syndrome impairs long-term outcome of colorectal liver metastases treated with resection after neoadjuvant chemotherapy. Ann Surg Oncol. 2011 Feb;18(2):421-30.

[62] Robinson SM, Mann J, Burt AD, Manas DM, Mann DA, White SA. Does a pro-thrombotic environment contribute to the development of chemotherapy associated liver injury in patients with colorectal liver metastases? British Journal of Surgery. 2012;99(S4).

[63] Schwenzer NF, Springer F, Schraml C, Stefan N, Machann J, Schick F. Non-invasive assessment and quantification of liver steatosis by ultrasound, computed tomography and magnetic resonance. J Hepatol. 2009 Sep;51(3):433-45.

[64] Bohte AE, van Werven JR, Bipat S, Stoker J. The diagnostic accuracy of US, CT, MRI and 1H-MRS for the evaluation of hepatic steatosis compared with liver biopsy: a meta-analysis. Eur Radiol. Jan;21(1):87-97.

[65] Robinson PJ. The effects of cancer chemotherapy on liver imaging. Eur Radiol. 2009 Jul;19(7):1752-62.

[66] Cho CS, Curran S, Schwartz LH, Kooby DA, Klimstra DS, Shia J, et al. Preoperative radiographic assessment of hepatic steatosis with histologic correlation. J Am Coll Surg. 2008 Mar;206(3):480-8.

[67] O'Rourke TR, Welsh KFS, Tekkis PP, Mustajab A, John TG, Peppercorn D, et al. Accuracy of liver-specific magnetic resonance imaging as a predictor of chemotherapy-

associated hepatic cellular injury prior to liver resection. European Journal of Surgical Oncology. 2009;35(10):1085-91.

[68] Marsman HA, Van Der Pool AE, Verheij J, Padmos J, Ten Kate FJW, Dwarkasing RS, et al. Hepatic steatosis assessment with CT or MRI in patients with colorectal liver metastases after neoadjuvant chemotherapy. Journal of Surgical Oncology.104(1): 10-6.

[69] Ward J, Guthrie JA, Sheridan MB, Boyes S, Smith JT, Wilson D, et al. Sinusoidal ob-structive syndrome diagnosed with superparamagnetic iron oxide-enhanced mag-netic resonance imaging in patients with chemotherapy-treated colorectal liver metastases. Journal of Clinical Oncology. 2008;26(26):4304-10.

[70] Shin NY, Kim MJ, Lim JS, Park MS, Chung YE, Choi JY, et al. Accuracy of gadoxetic acid-enhanced magnetic resonance imaging for the diagnosis of sinusoidal obstruc-tion syndrome in patients with chemotherapy-treated colorectal liver metastases. Eur Radiol. Apr;22(4):864-71.

[71] Garcea G, Ong SL, Maddern GJ. Predicting liver failure following major hepatecto-my. Dig Liver Dis. 2009 Nov;41(11):798-806.

[72] Imamura H, Sano K, Sugawara Y, Kokudo N, Makuuchi M. Assessment of hepatic reserve for indication of hepatic resection: decision tree incorporating indocyanine green test. J Hepatobiliary Pancreat Surg. 2005;12(1):16-22.

[73] Fan ST, Lai EC, Lo CM, Ng IO, Wong J. Hospital mortality of major hepatectomy for hepatocellular carcinoma associated with cirrhosis. Arch Surg. 1995 Feb;130(2): 198-203.

[74] Seifalian AM, El-Desoky A, Davidson BR. Hepatic indocyanine green uptake and ex-cretion in a rabbit model of steatosis. Eur Surg Res. 2001 May-Jun;33(3):193-201.

[75] Krieger PM, Tamandl D, Herberger B, Faybik P, Fleischmann E, Maresch J, et al. Evaluation of chemotherapy-associated liver injury in patients with colorectal cancer liver metastases using indocyanine green clearance testing. Ann Surg Oncol. Jun; 18(6):1644-50.

[76] Stockmann M, Lock JF, Riecke B, Heyne K, Martus P, Fricke M, et al. Prediction of postoperative outcome after hepatectomy with a new bedside test for maximal liver function capacity. Ann Surg. 2009 Jul;250(1):119-25.

[77] Stockmann M, Lock JF, Malinowski M, Niehues SM, Seehofer D, Neuhaus P. The Li-MAx test: a new liver function test for predicting postoperative outcome in liver sur-gery. HPB (Oxford). Mar;12(2):139-46.

[78] de Graaf W, van Lienden KP, van Gulik TM, Bennink RJ. (99m)Tc-mebrofenin hepa-tobiliary scintigraphy with SPECT for the assessment of hepatic function and liver functional volume before partial hepatectomy. J Nucl Med. Feb;51(2):229-36.

[79] de Graaf W, van Lienden KP, Dinant S, Roelofs JJ, Busch OR, Gouma DJ, et al. Assessment of future remnant liver function using hepatobiliary scintigraphy in patients undergoing major liver resection. J Gastrointest Surg. Feb;14(2):369-78.

[80] Rous P, Larimore LD. Relation of the Portal Blood to Liver Maintenance : A Demonstration of Liver Atrophy Conditional on Compensation. J Exp Med. 1920 Apr 30;31(5):609-32.

[81] Kinoshita H, Sakai K, Hirohashi K, Igawa S, Yamasaki O, Kubo S. Preoperative portal vein embolization for hepatocellular carcinoma. World J Surg. 1986 Oct;10(5): 803-8.

[82] Makuuchi M, Thai BL, Takayasu K, Takayama T, Kosuge T, Gunven P, et al. Preoperative portal embolization to increase safety of major hepatectomy for hilar bile duct carcinoma: a preliminary report. Surgery. 1990 May;107(5):521-7.

[83] Farges O, Jagot P, Kirstetter P, Marty J, Belghiti J. Prospective assessment of the safety and benefit of laparoscopic liver resections. J Hepatobiliary Pancreat Surg. 2002;9(2):242-8.

[84] Wicherts DA, de Haas RJ, Andreani P, Sotirov D, Salloum C, Castaing D, et al. Impact of portal vein embolization on long-term survival of patients with primarily unresectable colorectal liver metastases. Br J Surg. 2010 Feb;97(2):240-50.

[85] Pamecha V, Glantzounis G, Davies N, Fusai G, Sharma D, Davidson B. Long-term survival and disease recurrence following portal vein embolisation prior to major hepatectomy for colorectal metastases. Ann Surg Oncol. 2009 May;16(5):1202-7.

[86] Denys AL, Abehsera M, Leloutre B, Sauvanet A, Vilgrain V, O'Toole D, et al. Intrahepatic hemodynamic changes following portal vein embolization: a prospective Doppler study. Eur Radiol. 2000;10(11):1703-7.

[87] Archer SG, Gray BN. Vascularization of small liver metastases. Br J Surg. 1989 Jun; 76(6):545-8.

[88] Uemura T, Miyazaki M, Hirai R, Matsumoto H, Ota T, Ohashi R, et al. Different expression of positive and negative regulators of hepatocyte growth in growing and shrinking hepatic lobes after portal vein branch ligation in rats. Int J Mol Med. 2000 Feb;5(2):173-9.

[89] Yokoyama Y, Nagino M, Nimura Y. Mechanisms of hepatic regeneration following portal vein embolization and partial hepatectomy: a review. World J Surg. 2007 Feb; 31(2):367-74.

[90] Jaeck D, Oussoultzoglou E, Rosso E, Greget M, Weber JC, Bachellier P. A two-stage hepatectomy procedure combined with portal vein embolization to achieve curative resection for initially unresectable multiple and bilobar colorectal liver metastases. Ann Surg. 2004 Dec;240(6):1037-49; discussion 49-51.

[91] Wicherts DA, Miller R, de Haas RJ, Bitsakou G, Vibert E, Veilhan LA, et al. Long-term results of two-stage hepatectomy for irresectable colorectal cancer liver metastases. Ann Surg. 2008 Dec;248(6):994-1005.

[92] Narita M, Oussoultzoglou E, Bachellier P, Rosso E, Pessaux P, Jaeck D. Two-stage hepatectomy procedure to treat initially unresectable multiple bilobar colorectal liver metastases: technical aspects. Dig Surg. 2011;28(2):121-6.

[93] Vreuls CP, Van Den Broek MA, Winstanley A, Koek GH, Wisse E, Dejong CH, et al. Hepatic sinusoidal obstruction syndrome (SOS) reduces the effect of oxaliplatin in colorectal liver metastases. Histopathology. May 9.

[94] Rubbia-Brandt L, Tauzin S, Brezault C, Delucinge-Vivier C, Descombes P, Dousset B, et al. Gene expression Profiling Provides Insights into Pathways of Oxaliplatin Related Sinusoidal Obstruction Syndrome in Humans. Mol Cancer Ther. 2011 Feb 17;10(4):687-96.

[95] Rubie C, Frick VO, Ghadjar P, Wagner M, Justinger C, Graeber S, et al. Effect of pre-operative FOLFOX chemotherapy on CCL20/CCR6 expression in colorectal liver metastases. World J Gastroenterol. Jul 14;17(26):3109-16.

[96] Brand S, Olszak T, Beigel F, Diebold J, Otte JM, Eichhorst ST, et al. Cell differentiation dependent expressed CCR6 mediates ERK-1/2, SAPK/JNK, and Akt signaling resulting in proliferation and migration of colorectal cancer cells. J Cell Biochem. 2006 Mar 1;97(4):709-23.

[97] Robinson SM, White SA. Hepatic Sinusoidal Obstruction Syndrome (SOS) reduces the effect of Oxaliplatin in colorectal liver metastases. Histopathology. 2012;In Press.

Chapter 4

Liver Tumors in Infancy

Julio C. Wiederkehr, Izabel M. Coelho,
Sylvio G. Avilla, Barbara A. Wiederkehr and
Henrique A. Wiederkehr

Additional information is available at the end of the chapter

1. Introduction

Hepatic tumors in children are relatively rare, accounting for 1 to 4% of all pediatric solid tumors. [1] Primary liver masses constitute the third most common group of solid abdominal tumors of childhood [2] with an incidence of 0.4 to 1.9 per million children each year. [3,4]

Liver masses in children can be malignant, benign, or indeterminate and they are a diverse group of epithelial and mesenchymal tumors whose incidence can vary considerably with patient age. [5] Two thirds of liver tumors in children are malignant. [6] Unlike liver tumors in adults, in which the predominant histology is hepatocellular carcinoma, hepatoblastoma accounts for two thirds of liver tumors in children. [7] Other liver malignancies in children include sarcomas, germ cell tumors, and rhabdoid tumors, as well as the more familiar hepatocellular carcinoma. Benign tumors of the liver in children include vascular tumors, hamartomas, adenomas, and focal nodular hyperplasia. The histology and anatomy of a pediatric liver tumor guides the treatment and prognosis. [8]

In this chapter we outline the epidemiology, etiology, pathology, clinical presentation, diagnosis and management of each of the most important types of liver tumor. Also aspects of the surgical anatomy and resection techniques and other ways to improve ressecability in liver tumors in childhood will be described such as portal vein thrombosis, chemotherapy and transarterial chemoembolization (TACE).

2. Epidemiology

The incidence of hepatic tumors in childhood is consistently quoted from many series as being in the region of 0.5-2.5 per million population [9] and approximately 100–150 new cases of liver tumors are diagnosed in the U.S. annually. [7] Two thirds of liver tumors in children are malignant. [6] acounting for slightly more than 1% of all pediatric malignancies and among those there is a male preponderance of 1.8 : 1. [7,10]

Hepatoblastoma presents in a younger age group, being a uncommon diagnosis over the age of 4 years. Hepatocellular carcinoma has its peak onset in early adolescence, although the range is wide. The older age at onset for hepatocarcinoma may well reflect its close association with other underlying disease processes. [10]

There are several suggestions that the incidence of malignant liver tumors is increasing in the U.S. Surveillance, Epidemiology, and End Results data from 1972–1992 showed a 5% annual increase. [7] Liver cancer represented 2% of all malignancies in infants in the early 1980s with the incidence doubling to 4% 10 years later. [11]

At a population level, there has been a dramatic increase in survival in countries in which a modern health system has been implemented, although the increased survival is lower for hepatocarcinoma in comparison with hepatoblastomas. [10] According to Litten & Tomlinson [8], it has been suggested that the improvements in technology, care, and outcomes for premature infants have been driving forces in the increase of the incidence in hepatic tumors. Hepatoblastoma is more commonly diagnosed in children with a history of prematurity than in full-term infants. Interestingly, those tumors that arise in ex-premature infants do not present at a younger age than those of term infants. [8]

3. Hepatoblastoma

Hepatoblastoma is the most common malignant tumor of the liver in children and is an embryonal tumor in the classic sense of incomplete differentiation; [12] accounts for 1% of all pediatric malignancies and for 79% of all liver cancers in children under age. [13] Its overall incidence is 0.5–1.5 per million, however the incidence in children under the age of 18 months is 11.2 cases per million. [14]

Hepatoblastoma is diagnosed in very young children with a peak in the newborn period reflecting those tumors that developed prenatally, and an overall median age at diagnosis of 18 months; 90 percent of cases are manifest by the fourth birthday, several have been present at birth, and there is an hypothesized association with prematurity. [15] Only 5% of new hepatoblastoma cases are diagnosed in children >4 years of age. [8]

The increased incidence of HB in children born before 28 weeks gestation (with birth weight <1500 g) compared with term gestations, may be explained by the exposure of rapidly dividing hepatoblasts to endogenous metabolites and hormones as well as exogenous chemicals that would normally be eliminated via the placenta. Inefficiency and compromise of the immature detoxification mechanisms could produce multiple somatic mutations and epigenetic (ie, methylation) modifications of the genome. [16, 17]

For poorly understood reasons, hepatoblastoma occurs in males significantly more frequently than it does in females with a male:female ratio that ranges from 1.2 to 3.6:1. [14] Most commonly, these tumors present in the right lobe of the liver. [18] There is an increased incidence of hepatoblastoma in Beckwith-Wiedemann Syndrome, which has a relative risk of 2280 suggesting a role for genetic aberrations of chromosome 11 in the pathogenesis of hepatoblastoma,[19, 20] hemihypertrophy, and familial adenomatous polyposis (FAP) witch has a relative risk of 1220 suggesting a role for aberrations of chromosome 5 in the pathogenesis. [21] Screening for cases in FAP kindred families is recommended by testing for germline mutations in the APC tumor suppressor gene. [22, 23] Inactivation of the APC tumor-suppressor gene (found on chromosome 5) is found in 67–89% of sporadic hepatoblastoma [24, 25] This gene is known to regulate B-catenin and modulate the wnt signaling pathway, suggesting a role for this signaling pathway in the development of hepatoblastoma. [26] Additional biologic markers may include Trisomy 2, 8, and 20 and translocation of the NOTCH2 gene on chromosome 1. [27]

Many etiological factors have been linked with the development of malignant hepatic tumors in childhood (Table 1). Broadly speaking, genetic influences are particularly important in the development of hepatoblastoma, whereas environmental factors and coexisting liver disease are strongly associated with hepatocellular carcinoma. [10]

Hepatoblastoma	Hepatocellular carcinoma
Beckwith-Wiedemann Syndrome	Hepatitis B
Hemihypertrophy	Hepatitis C
Familial adenomatous polyposis (FAP)	Hereditary tyrosinemia
	α_1-Antitrypsin deficiency
Gardner syndrome	Cirrhosis secondary to biliary atresia
Glycogen storage disease type I	Glycogen storage disease type I
Trisomy 18	Neurofibromatosis
Fetal alcohol syndrome	
Prematurity and low birth weight	Familial adenomatous polyposis
Maternal exposure to:	Drug/toxin exposure:
Oral contraceptives	Androgens
Gonadotropins	Oral contraceptives
Metals	Methotrexate
Petroleum products	Aflatoxins
Paints and pigments	
Paternal exposure to:	Fanconi anemia
Metals	
Meckel diverticulum	

Table 1. Conditions associated with hepatoblastoma and hepatocellular carcinoma.

Hepatoblastomas are composed of cells resembling the developing fetal and embryonic liver, hence the classification as an embryonal tumor. Indeed, the cells comprising hepatoblastoma mark similarly to hepatic stem cells, defined as pluripotent hepatoblasts capable of differentiating into hepatocytes or cholangiocytes. [28, 29]

According to the Childhood Epithelial Liver Tumors – International Criteria (CELTIC) group, the pathology of hepatoblastoma is classified into four groups based on the work of Weinberg and Finegold: fetal, embryonal, macrotrabecular and small-cell undifferentiated. [10]

Histologically, these tumors can be divided into epithelial (56%) or mixed epithelial/ mesenchymal tissue. The epithelial group is further subdivided into fetal (31%), embryonal (19%), macrotrabecular (3%) and small-cell undifferentiated subtypes (3%). Thema- jority of hepatoblastomas is epithelial and consist of a mixture of embryonal and fetal cell types (Fig. 1). [8, 30]

Hepatoblastoma Histology

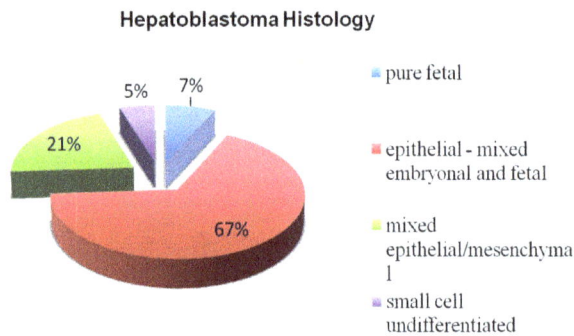

Figure 1. Distribution of histologic subtypes of hepatoblastoma. The majority are epithelial and consist of embryonal and fetal cell types. Pure fetal histology accounts for approximately 7% of hepatoblastomas and is associated with a favorable prognosis. Small cell undifferentiated hepatoblastoma accounts for 5% of hepatoblastoma cases and is associated with a poor prognosis. [8]

Of the five histologic subtypes—pure fetal, embryonal, mixed epithelial, mesenchymal/ macrotrabecular, and small cell undifferentiated—fetal carries the most favorable prognosis. [31] Approximately 5% of hepatoblastomas are of the small cell undifferentiated subtype. This subtype is associated with a worse prognosis. [32] In the mixed epithelial/ mesenchy- mal type, the presence of mesenchymal elements is associated with improved prognosis and the most common mesenchymal elements are cartilage and osteoid. [33]

Hepatoblastomas usually presents as a palpable asymptomatic mass with abdominal disten- sion. [10] Less common presentations include weight loss, anorexia, emesis and abdominal pain and usually indicate advanced disease. [34] One of the more unusual presenting features of hepatoblastoma is its association with sexual precocity due to the release of human chorion- ic gonadotropic hormone (β-HCG) by the tumor. Osteoporosis is said to occur in up to 20% of the cases and when severe can lead to bone fractures and vertebral compression. [35] The tu- mor may rupture spontaneously, producing an acute abdomen and hemoperitoneum. [10]

Approximately 90% of patients demonstrate elevated serum AFP levels and there is a correlation between AFP levels and extent of disease. [36]

The right lobe of the liver is most commonly involved with disease but in 35% of patients there is bilateral disease. [37] Distant metastasis are present in 20% of patients at the time of diagnosis with the lung being the most common site of metastasis; other common sites are the brain and bone and metastasis occur more commonly with disease relapse. [38]

	Hepatoblastoma (%)	Hepatocellular carcinoma (%)
Abdominal mass	71	58
Weight loss	24	21
Anorexia	22	22
Pain	18	16
Vomiting	13	10
Jaundice	7	10

Table 2. Signs and symptoms of liver tumors in children. [10]

Overall, the diagnosis is based on laboratory tests (such as full blood count, liver function tests, α-Fetoprotein – AFP and other markers), imaging (abdominal radiography, ultrasonography, computer tomography, magnetic resonance imaging, hepatic angiography, chest radiography and positron-emission tomography – PET) and biopsy.

The full blood count can reveal anemia (usually normocytic, normochromic) in at least 50% of children with hepatoblastoma. [13, 39] The platelet count is also often abnormal with up to one-third of patients demonstrating thrombocytosis and fewer patients having thrombocytopenia. Thrombocytosis is thought to be related to increased levels of circulating thrombopoietin. [40]

Liver function tests are commonly normal in hepatoblastoma. [10] The serum alpha-fetoprotein (AFP) level is elevated in 90% of children with hepatoblastoma and tumors that fail to express AFP at diagnosis are felt to be biologically more aggressive. [41, 42] AFP levels must be interpreted with caution because AFP is commonly elevated in normal neonates up to 6 months of age and may be slightly elevated in other tumors, as well as after hepatic damage or during regeneration of liver parenchyma.

The imaging study is important in evaluation liver neoplasms. CT, MRI and ultrasound are the most commonly used modalities for pediatric doctors in their medical researches as well as their clinical practice. Ultrasound is accepted as a first-line imaging method because of its less irradiation, greater convenience and better real-time. [43] Ultrasound is extremely valuable in detecting much smaller lesions, especially in detecting fluid and blood-flow in a lesion, and it also can evaluate the hepatic vascular anatomy.[44] As a rule, the initial diagnosis of live tumor is usually made by the abdominal ultrasound examination, which will identify the liver as the organ of origin. Hepatoblastoma are seen as a hyperechoic, solid, intrahepatic mass on US. [45]

Both CT and MRI define the extent of tumor involvement showing its segmental extension and its proximity to the portal vein, to help determine the resectability. Evaluation with CT demonstrates a delineated hypoattentuated mass compared with the surrounding normal tissue and allows identification of calcifications. [46] The use of contrast allows assessment of vascular involvement by the tumor. Combined MRI and contrast enhanced MR-angiography gives the best evaluation of the vascular structures and the tumor blood supply, and this best enables the planning of a resection. A diagnostic biopsy is recommended in all children with a suspected hepatoblastoma. Given the potential side effects of chemotherapy, it is not a good clinical practice to start therapy in a patient in the absence of a tissue diagnosis. Additionally, it is necessary to rule out HCC. Although it is rare, HCC have been reported in children under the age of three and they carry a worse prognosis. [47]

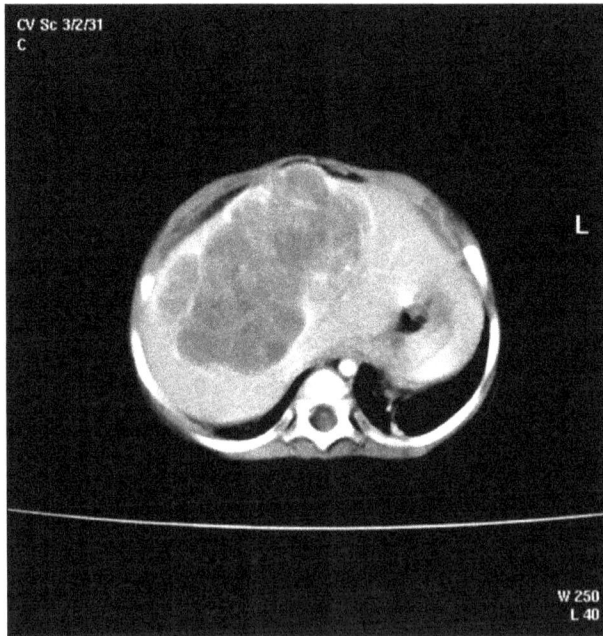

Figure 2. CT scan of an infant with a large central hepatoblastoma.

Large multinodular expansile masses, hepatoblastomas radiographically appear well demarcated from the normal liver but are not encapsulated. They may invade hepatic veins, disseminate to the lungs, or penetrate the liver capsule to reach contiguous tissues. [12]

Historically, North Americans have staged liver tumors similar to other solid tumors, staging system continues to be used by the children's oncology group (COG) and depends upon extent of surgery at the time of initial diagnosis.

Relative number of patients presenting in each stage in the COG trial 9645 (1999–2003) is as follows: Stage I (22%) indicates complete resection at diagnosis, Stage II (0.5%) microscopic residual after attempted complete resection at diagnosis, Stage III (53%) biopsy at diagnosis with gross residual tumor, and Stage IV (23%) metastatic disease at diagnosis.[48, 49] The traditional COG staging system has been criticized for being rather subjective, depending to a large extent on the surgeon rather than the tumor.[12, 50] To address this concern specific surgical guidelines have been proposed by the COG liver tumor committee which define the anatomic and biologic characteristics of a tumor for which resection at diagnosis is recommended. In addition the upcoming COG hepatoblastoma (AHEP 0731) protocol will add a risk-based stratification of treatment as follows: low risk (Stage I/II lacking any unfavorable biologic feature); intermediate risk (Stage III or Stage I/II with small cell undifferentiated histology); and high risk (Stage IV or Stage I/II/III with AFP <100 at diagnosis). [12]

3.1. Stage Information

There are two standard surgical staging systems for pediatric liver tumors. The Childhood Liver Tumour Strategy Group (SIOPEL) uses a presurgical-based staging system, while the Children's Oncology Group (COG) uses a postsurgical-based staging system. The staging systems support different treatment strategies. The presurgical staging system is used with neoadjuvant chemotherapy followed by definitive surgery (with the exception of Pretreatment Extent of Disease [PRETEXT] stage 1), while the postsurgical staging system has surgery as the initial strategy.

Both systems are used in the United States. In a retrospective comparison of the two staging systems at diagnosis using data from patients entered on a North American randomized trial, both staging systems predicted outcome. The presurgical PRETEXT staging system may add prognostic information for patients staged postsurgically at stage 3. [51] The COG is investigating the use of PRETEXT stage before and after chemotherapy to determine the optimal surgical approach. [52]

3.2. Presurgical Staging for Hepatoblastoma and Hepatocellular Carcinoma

The PRETEXT staging system for hepatoblastoma categorizes the primary tumor based on extent of liver involvement at diagnosis. The staging system was devised for use in an international hepatoblastoma treatment program in which only children with PRETEXT stage 1 hepatoblastoma undergo initial resection of tumor. All others are treated with chemotherapy prior to attempted resection of the primary tumor. The liver tumors are staged by interpretation of computerized tomography or ultrasound with or without additional imaging by magnetic resonance. The presence or absence of metastases is noted in addition to the PRETEXT stage, but does not alter the PRETEXT stage. Tumor involvement of the vena cava, hepatic veins, and portal vein, and extrahepatic extension are also noted.

The imaged liver is divided into four quadrants and involvement of each quadrant with tumor is determined. Stage increases and prognosis decreases as the number of quadrants radiologically involved with tumor increases from one to four. [53, 50] Experienced radiologist review is important because it may be difficult to discriminate between real invasion beyond the anatomic border of a given sector and displacement of the anatomic border. [50, 43]

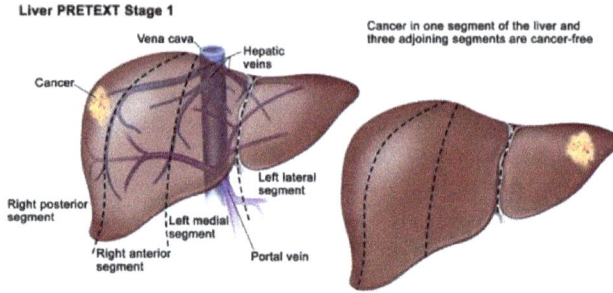

Figure 3. Pretext stage 1 - Tumor involves only one quadrant; three adjoining liver quadrants are free of tumor. [http://www.cancer.gov/PublishedContent/MediaLinks/308970.html]

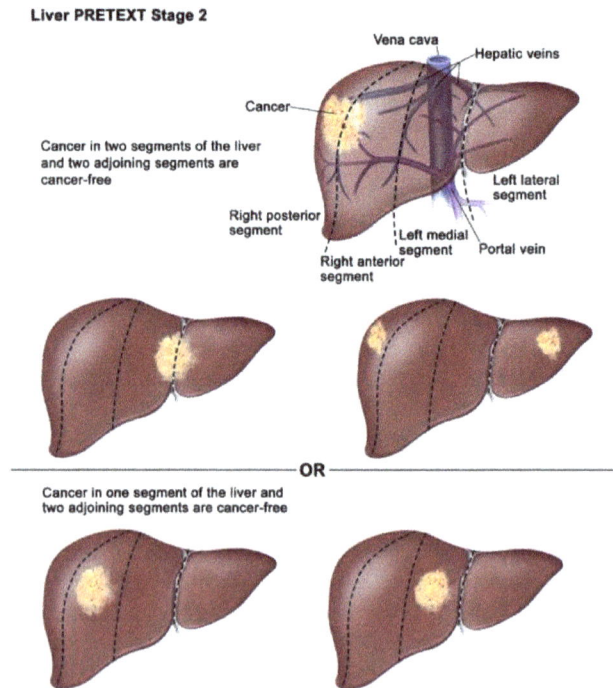

Figure 4. Pretext stage 2 - Tumor involves one or two quadrants; two adjoining quadrants are free of tumor. [http://www.cancer.gov/PublishedContent/MediaLinks/308970.html]

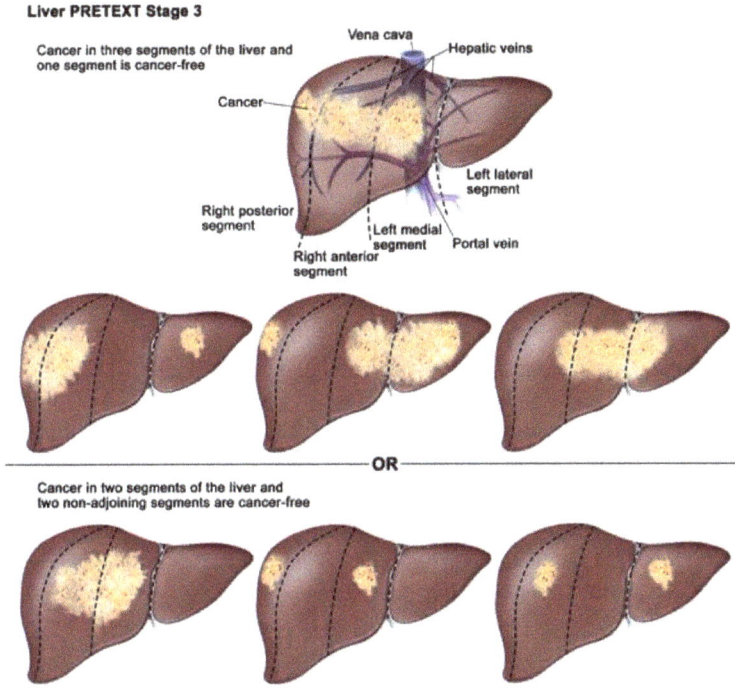

Figure 5. Pretext stage 3 - Tumor involves three quadrants and one quadrant is free of tumor or tumor involves two quadrants and two nonadjoining quadrants are free of tumor. [http://www.cancer.gov/PublishedContent/MediaLinks/308970.html]

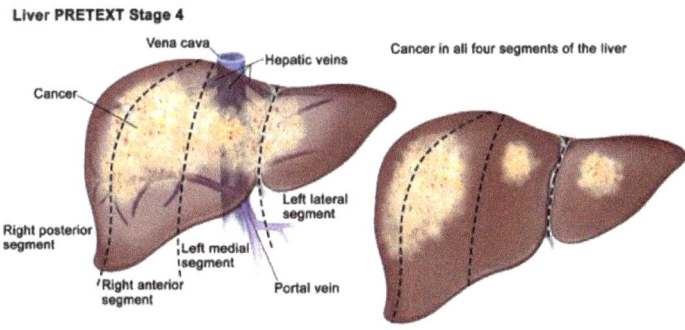

Figure 6. Pretext stage 4 - Tumor involves all four quadrants; there is no quadrant free of tumor. [http://www.cancer.gov/PublishedContent/MediaLinks/308970.html]

3.3. Treatment - Chemotherapy

During the past 30 years, there has been an improved survival for patients with HB based on refinements in surgical techniques, a better understanding of the hepatic segmental anatomy, advances in chemotherapy, and the advent of liver transplantation as a therapeutic modality for patients with unresectable disease. HB is a surgical neoplasm and only complete tumor resection results in a realistic hope for cure. Long-term disappearance of tumor with complete remission with chemotherapy alone has been anecdotally observed. However, chemotherapy is a cornerstone in the management of HB. [55]

Although chemosensitivity varies between patients, it is an essential component of the management and complementary to radical surgical resection to affect a cure. In general, surgeons agree that preoperative chemotherapy helps to reduce the size of most tumors and obtains better demarcation between the tumor and surrounding liver tissue. [56, 57, 58] Consequently, tumors are more likely to be completely resected without increasing perioperative morbidity or mortality. It is also speculated that residual microscopic disease may behave more aggressively under the influence of hepatotrophic factors stimulating liver regeneration if preoperative chemotherapy has not been used. [58] On the other hand, von Schweinitz et al. [59] have shown that there is little to be gained from prolonging chemotherapy beyond the planned treatment regimen, which incurs the risk of developing chemoresistance. [55]

Even if unresectable at diagnosis, most hepatoblastomas are unifocal and chemosensitive, especially to "platinum" derivative chemotherapeutic agents. With the routine addition of cisplatin to the chemotherapy in the late 1980s, overall survival in hepatoblastoma increased from 30% to 70%. [60, 61] Twenty years later, cisplatin remains the backbone of the chemotherapy regimen. In current trials by COG (America), SIOPEL (Europe, South America), GPOH (German), and JPLT (Japan) chemotherapeutic agents used in combination with cisplatin have differed slightly. Although most use some form of doxorubicin, COG currently recommends Cisplatin/5FU/Vincristin (C5V) for low-risk tumors, C5V+Doxorubicin for intermediate risk, and hopes to investigate new agents with up-front window therapy in high-risk tumors. [48, 49] Irinotectan, with or without doxorubicin, has been used in both America and Europe for patients with relapse. [62] Because tumor cells may become resistant to chemotherapy over prolonged exposure [63] and because cumulative chemotherapy toxicity may be unwarranted, prolonged (44 cycles) courses of neoadjuvant chemotherapy are discouraged by all study groups. Early referral for complex surgical planning may be indicated for large invasive tumors potentially requiring transplantation. [12]

Two principle strategies exist. In the United States, tumor resection at diagnosis, whenever prudently possible, has been advocated with the argument that toxicity of chemotherapy can be reduced by avoidance of unnecessary neoadjuvant chemotherapy, that some tumors may become resistant to prolonged courses of chemotherapy [64] and the highest survival rates have historically been observed in patients with initially resected tumors—although these tumors also tend to be the smaller more favorable tumors. Proposed COG Surgical guidelines advocate definitive surgical resection at diagnosis for localized, unifocal PRE-TEXT I and II tumors followed by chemotherapy. When the tumor is large (PRETEXT III or IV), multicentric, shows radiographic evidence of portal or hepatic venous invasion, or pulmonary metastatic lesions the chance of curative resection may be improved neoadjuvant chemotherapy and delayed primary resection. Alternatively, the SIOPEL study group discourages resection of hepatoblastoma at diagnosis favoring neoadjuvant chemotherapy in all patients with the argument that the chemotherapy renders most tumors smaller, better demarcated, and more likely to be completely resected, and that the toxicity of neoadjuvant chemotherapy is offset by the increased rates of surgical resectability. Both COG and SIO-PEL have invested considerable effort in attempts to decrease the significant ototoxiciy attendant to the use of cisplatin based chemotherapy in young infants and toddlers. [12]

In the Intergroup Hepatoblastoma/ Hepatocellular Carcinoma Study, 28% of HB tumors were completely resected at diagnosis (Stage I) and 4% (Stage II) were incompletely excised. These patients had a 91% and 100% 5-year survival, respectively. However, the surgical guidelines of the protocol lacked clear recommendations regarding which tumor should or should not be resected at diagnosis. The study compared the use of cisplatin and doxorubicin in one treatment arm to cisplatin, vincristine, and 5-fluorouracil (5-FU) in the other arm. The overall 3- year survival rates were 63% and 71%, respectively. [65] Although the difference between the groups was not significant, the cisplatin/ doxorubicin group had a higher toxicity rate. A significant response to preoperative chemotherapy was observed in Stage III patients allowing complete tumor resection in 70–80% of these cases. Pre-operative chemotherapy had no effect on operative mortality; however, increased transfusion requirement and a higher operative morbidity was observed in patients that received chemotherapy preoperatively. [55]

The studies coordinated by the SIOPEL group have concentrated on using preoperative chemotherapy. [56, 66] In SIOPEL-1, all patients were treated preoperatively with four courses of cisplatin and doxorubicin (PLADO); surgical resection was followed by two more courses of chemotherapy. If the tumor was judged unresectable by imaging after four courses of chemotherapy, attempting surgical resection was delayed until after the sixth course. If the tumor remained localized to the liver but was still unresectable, liver transplantation was recommended as the primary operative procedure if some response to chemotherapy had been obtained in the absence of extrahepatic tumor extent or metastatic disease. The SIO-PEL-2 pilot study [67]was designed to test the efficacy and toxicity of two chemotherapy regimens, one for patients with HB confined to the liver and involving no more then three hepatic sections "standard-risk (SR) HB", and one for instances of HB extending into all four sections and/or with lung metastases or intra-abdominal extrahepatic spread or tumor rupture at presentation or with serum AFP < 100 units at presentation "high-risk (HR) HB". Those with SR-HB were treated with four courses of cisplatin monotherapy, delayed surgery, and then two more courses of cisplatin. Patients with HR-HB were given cisplatin alternating with carboplatin and doxorubicin, pre- and postoperatively. For SR-HB patients (n = 77), and HR-HB patients (n = 58), the 3-year progression-free survival rates were 89% and 48%, respectively. For SR-HB patients, the efficacy of cisplatin monotherapy and the cisplatin/doxorubicin combination are now being compared in a prospective randomized trial (SIOPEL-3 study). For HR-HB patients, intensified chemotherapy with cisplatin, doxorubicin, and carboplatin is being investigated in a SIOPEL-4 study. [55]

In unifocal HB, PRETEXT grouping based on imaging studies at diagnosis in some cases may lead to overstaging the tumor from PRETEXT III to PRETEXT IV when the anatomic border separating a lateral section from the sections of the liver harboring the bulging mass is simply displaced (due to compression) but not invaded. [56, 68] Indeed, repeat imaging studies after chemotherapy, when the tumor has shrunken, can demonstrate that the ana- tomic border is free from invasion and allow for correct staging and performance of a partial hepatectomy (right or left trisegmentectomy). In multifocal HB with lesions scattered in the different sections of the liver, clearance of one section, (e.g. the left lateral section) [69] can apparently be achieved by chemotherapy in some cases, tempting the surgeon to perform a partial rather than a total hepatectomy. However, this strategy is not recommended because of the high-risk of leaving viable malignant tumor cells in the remaining section. Therefore, in multifocal hepatoblastoma, liver transplantation is the best treatment option, whatever the apparent result of chemotherapy. Further intensification of chemotherapy when the re- sponse to completion of full courses of chemotherapy according to protocol is considered unsatisfactory, and hazardous attempts at partial liver resection in order to avoid liver trans- plantation "at any cost" are no longer justified since the efficacy of primary liver transplan- tation for unresectable HB has been validated during the last decade. [55]

Even patients presenting with metastatic disease are potentially curable with a combination of chemotherapy, complete tumor resection by partial hepatectomy or transplantation, and pul- monary metastasectomy. The role of pulmonary metastasectomy has yet to be clearly defined, although it appears that surgical resection of lung deposits may be more likely to cure patients with disease present at diagnosis but persistent after neoadjuvant therapy rather than patients with pulmonary relapse. [12] Data from the most recent COG study, 9645, show 3-year event- free survival of 90% for Stage I–II, 50% for Stage III, and only 20% for Stage IV (Malogolowkin et al., 2007). In the European SIOPEL II 3-year survival for standard risk tumors was 90% and for high-risk tumors was 50%. Cure from hepatoblastoma mandates a complete gross resection of the primary tumor at some point during the treatment regimen. [12]

3.4. Surgical resection

The objective of the surgical procedure is to obtain a complete resection of the tumor, both macro- and microscopically, which is paramount for cure of HB (and other liver cancers). The surgical strategy should be based on a sound knowledge of segmental liver anatomy as described by Couinaud, [70] vascular occlusion techniques and expertise in performing the different types of liver resections, including the most extensive procedures (left or right tri- segmentectomies). Intraoperative ultrasound is useful in confirming the location of major vessels and other structures. Nonanatomical, atypical resections are best avoided, except in rare cases (i.e., pedunculated tumor), because of an increased risk of incomplete tumor re- moval and a higher incidence of postoperative complications. [58] Very extensive liver re- sections (up to 80% of the liver mass) can be tolerated by young children with HB and hepatic regeneration can be complete within 3 months, despite the administration of toxic agents since they usually have no underlying liver disease and excellent hepatic reserve. [71] Liver function rapidly returns to normal without long-term sequelae. Complete tumor resection can be easily achieved with a partial hepatectomy when the intrahepatic extent is limited to one or two sections (PRETEXT I and II). When the tumor involves three sections (PRETEXT III), preoperative neoadjuvant chemotherapy can make lesions initially considered "unresectable" become resectable with a trisegmentectomy. [55]

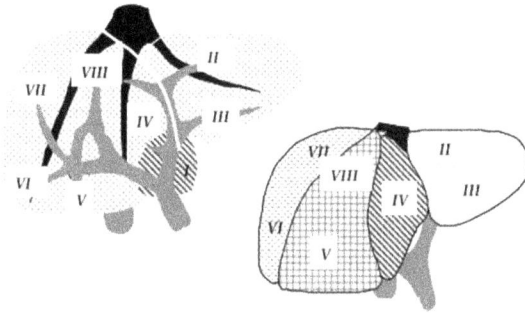

Figure 7. Couinaud's liver segmentation.

In centrally located HB, resection of Couinaud's segments 4, 5 and 8 ("central hepatectomy") can occasionally be performed by expert hands. When an accessory right hepatic vein of appropriate size is present to drain remaining segments 5–7, subtotal hepatectomy removing segments 1–4 and 8 can be successfully performed. [55]

3.5. Liver transplantation

A growing experience with liver transplantation has shown that liver transplant is a good treatment option in children with unresectable primary tumors and without demonstrable metastatic disease after neoadjuvant chemotherapy and pulmonary metastasectomy if necessary. In large solitary, and especially multifocal, hepatoblastomas invading all four sectors of the liver, transplantation has resulted in long-term disease free survival in up to 80% of children. [73] While most agree that "extreme" resection of tumors without liver transplant will avoid the need for long-term immunosuppressive therapy, hazardous attempts at partial hepatectomy in children with major venous involvement or with extensive multifocal tumors should be discouraged. [56, 69, 74, 75, 76] Extensive hepatic surgery in children should be carried out in centers that have a facility for liver transplant, where surgical expertise, as well as willingness to embark on more radical surgery with a transplant "safety net" is likely to be greater. [76]

Previous studies have validated the concept of total hepatectomy and primary orthotopic liver transplantation (OLT) for unresectable HB. In SIOPEL-1, [77] 12 patients (8% of all patients enrolled from 1990 to 1994) underwent liver transplantation as the primary surgical option (after appropriate preoperative chemotherapy) in seven children, and as a rescue procedure in five children because of incomplete partial resection or tumor relapse after partial hepatectomy. The long-term, disease-free patient survival was 66% for the entire series and 85% and 40% for primary transplants and rescue transplants, respectively. Current follow up is >10 years for all patients. All eight patients with PRETEXT IV tumors and all six patients with multifocal HB were cured of their disease. Of the seven patients with macroscopic extension into the portal vein and/or the hepatic veins/vena cava, 71% became long-term, disease-free survivors, as well as four of five (80%) children who had lung metastases at presentation with complete clearance of lung lesions after chemotherapy. [55]

An extensive review of the world experience collected 147 cases of liver transplantation for HB. [77] Data were contributed by 24 centers (12 in North America, 10 in Europe, 1 in Japan and Australia each). Twenty-eight (19% of the total) patients presented with macroscopic venous extension and 12 (8%) with lung metastases. A total of 106 patients (72%) underwent a primary transplant and 41 (28%) received a rescue transplant, either for incomplete resection with partial hepatectomy or for tumor relapse after previous partial hepatectomy. Twenty-eight (19%) received a live, donor-related liver transplant, and 119 (81%) received a deceased donor liver graft. Median follow up since diagnosis for surviving patients was 38 months (range 1– 121 months). Overall disease-free survival at 6 years post-transplant was 82% and 30% for primary transplants and for rescue transplants, respectively. Multivariate statistical analysis showed no difference in regard to gender, age, and lung metastases at presentation or type of transplant. For primary transplants, the only parameter significantly related to overall survival was macroscopic venous invasion (P = 0.045). Remarkably, the 6-year, disease-free survival (82%) for the 106 patients who received a primary transplant was similar to the 3-year, progression-free survival (89%) for the 77 HB patients with standard-risk hepatoblastoma confined to the liver and involving no more than 3 hepatic sections that were enrolled in the SIOPEL-2 study. [67] In a recent review of the UNOS database in the USA concerning liver transplantation in 135 children transplanted for unresectable or recurrent HB (1987–2004), the one, five, and 10-year survival was 79%, 69%, and 66% respectively. [78] The median age at transplantation was 2.9 ± 2.5 years. Sixteen percent received a graft from a live donor. Fifty-five percent of the deaths were due to metastases or recurrent disease. The latest ELTR report, including 129 patients transplanted for HB has shown a 1- and 5-year survival of 100% and 74%, respectively. [55, 79]

3.6. Timing of transplantation

Timing of liver transplantation should not be delayed in excess of a few weeks after the last course of chemotherapy (as per protocol). An expeditious access to organ donors is required to meet this requirement. If this is not possible with deceased donors (including split liver grafts), a live-related donor is a valuable option. [55]

According to the results of published studies, the following guidelines have been developed for early consultation with a transplant surgeon: [55]

1. Multifocal PRETEXT IV HB is a clear and undisputed indication for primary liver transplantation, whatever the result of chemotherapy. Apparent clearance of one liver lobe should not distract from this guideline because of the high probability of persistent microscopic viable neoplastic cells. Pediatric oncologists should resist the temptation to in-

tensify chemotherapy in a vain effort to avoid transplantation. These patients should be treated within the same protocol as patients with localized tumors amenable to partial hepatectomy, with as many cycles of chemotherapy before and after transplantation as patients submitted to partial hepatectomy for a localized HB.

2. Primary liver transplantation may be the best option for large, solitary PRETEXT IV HB, involving all four sections of the liver, unless tumor downstaging is clearly demonstrated after initial chemotherapy. If this is the case, a clear retraction of the tumor from the anatomic border of one lateral sector would allow performance of a radical trisegmentectomy.

3. Unifocal, centrally located PRETEXT II and III tumors involving main hilar structures or all three main hepatic veins should be considered for primary liver transplantation because these venous structures would presumably not become free of tumor after chemotherapy. Heroic attempts at partial hepatectomy would be best avoided because of the risk of incomplete resection of malignant tissue.

3.7. Contraindications

Persistence of viable extrahepatic tumor deposit after chemotherapy, not amenable to surgical resection, is the only absolute contraindication for liver transplantation. Macroscopic venous invasion (portal vein, hepatic veins, vena cava) is not a contraindication if complete resection of the invaded venous structures can be accomplished. When there is evidence or suspicion of invasion of the retrohepatic vena cava, it should be resected "en-bloc" and reconstructed. Review of the world experience showed that venous extent was associated with a significantly shorter survival ($P = 0.045$). [77] Of the nine TNM IV A/IVB patients (eight with major intrahepatic venous invasion) reported by Reyes and associates, seven were alive and disease-free 21–146 months after transplantation. [80]

Patients with lung metastases at presentation should not be excluded from liver transplantation if the metastases clear completely after chemotherapy and/or surgical resection. Long-term, disease-free survival was obtained in 80% of such patients in the SIOPEL-l study and 58% in the world experience. Complete eradication of metastatic lesions by chemotherapy and surgical resection of any suspicious remnant after chemotherapy is a paramount pre-requisite for transplantation. [81] When tumor resection by partial hepatectomy is incomplete or when intrahepatic relapse is observed after a previous partial hepatectomy, performing a rescue liver transplantation may be a relative contraindication because of the disappointing results observed in the SIOPEL-l study and in the reported world experience. [55]

3.8. Outcomes

In experienced surgical units, major intraoperative complications of liver resection for HB such as severe bleeding, air embolism, and unrecognized bile duct injury are infrequent and operative mortality is very low, even after extended hepatectomies, since children with HB have no underlying liver disease. As an example, summarizes the 25 years (1978–2003) of experience gained at Cliniques Saint-Luc, Brussels [82] with 53 children treated for HB.

There were 39 partial hepatectomies, including 23 right or left trisegmentectomies, and 13 primary liver transplants (two from deceased donors and 11 from living related donors). Only one child died from surgical complications (extensive portal vein thrombosis present at diagnosis). Postoperative bleeding requiring reoperation was encountered in 2 patients (3.5%). The incidence of biliary complications was 7.6% after partial hepatectomy and 23% following liver transplantation. Actuarial disease-free survival was 89% and 79% in transplant patients and in children treated with partial hepatectomy, respectively. [55]

Although individual centers treat relatively small numbers of patients with liver cancer, the best overall survival rates are obtained in experienced units that include liver transplantation in their surgical armamentarium. [55, 83, 84, 85]

The most recent report from King's college, London [86] confirms that the modern strategy of combining chemotherapy and radical tumor resection enables the majority of children with HB to be cured. From October 1993 to February 2007, 25 liver transplantations were performed for HB: 18 from deceased donors and 7 from living donors. Fifteen and ten patients were PRETEXT IV and III, respectively. All patients received preoperative chemotherapy following the successive SIOPEL protocols. Patient and graft survival after cadaveric transplantation was 91%, 77.6% and 77.6% after 1, 5 and 10 years, respectively, without retransplantation. Patient and graft survival after living related liver transplantation was 100%, 83.3% and 83.3%, respectively. All surviving children but one remain disease-free, with a median follow up of 6.8 years (range: 0.9–14.9). There were five deaths at a median of 13 months post-OLT, secondary to tumor recurrence in 4 and respiratoryfailure in one. [55]

A remote data entry system is accessible online, worldwide, and free of charge. Registration is open for patients transplanted since January 1st, 2006 (http://www.pluto.cineca.org). PLUTO stands for Pediatric Liver Unresectable Tumor Observatory and was developed by the SIOPEL strategy group. This will allow online registration of children undergoing liver transplantation for a malignant liver tumor. The aim is to establish an international multi-center database with prospective registration of children (<18 years) presenting with unresectable tumor (HB, HCC, epithelioid hemangioendothelioma and other rare malignant tumors) undergoing primary orrescue liver transplantation.

4. Hepatocellular carcinoma

Hepatocellular carcinoma (HCC) in childhood is rare and accounts for less than 0.5% of all pediatric malignancies, [87, 88] is the second most common malignant hepatic neoplasm in children. HCC presents at an older age than does hepatoblastoma, with most HCC cases diagnosed in children older than 5 years. [89] Its relative frequency is 0.5 to 1.0 cases per million children. It is more frequently encountered in older children and teenagers than in infants. [88,90] HCC is more often encountered in males and older children between age 10 and 14 yr and the median age of onset is 12 year. [88]

Previous reports from Southeast Asia cite an annual incidence of pediatric hepatic tumors that is roughly four times higher than western reports in children with less than 15 years of age. [91] This finding is largely based on the high hepatitis carrier rate, with a Taiwanese report stating that 80% of primary liver tumors in children were hepatocellular carcinoma. With the introduction of hepatitis B vaccine in Southeast Asia, however, there has been a marked reduction in the incidence of hepatocellular carcinoma, although the impact of the hepatitis B vaccine has mainly reduced the incidence of liver tumors in males. [92] Occasionally, malignant tumors in children are seen with features of both hepatocellular carcinoma and hepatoblastoma. These tumors are more common in children with a diagnosis at later ages than that typical of hepatoblastoma.

There is an association with pediatric HCC and pre-existing liver cirrhosis, most often because of biliary atresia, Fanconi's syndrome, and hepatitis B. However, most pediatric HCC are de novo tumors and are not necessarily related to cirrhosis. [75] In certain metabolic diseases such as hereditary tyrosinemia and glycogen storage disease type IA, there is an increased incidence of HCC. Hereditary tyrosinemia, caused by a deficiency in fumarylacetoacetate hydrolase, results in a greatly increased susceptibility to HCC. This is because of the accumulation of toxic metabolites in the liver, and the incidence of HCC is 50% by age two. Current medical therapies for tyrosinemia markedly reduce but do not eliminate the risk of development of HCC. Glycogen storage disease type IA is caused by a deficiency in glucose- 6-phosphatase. This results in the development of hepatic adenomas in 50% of patients, and about 11% of patients with adenomas because of glycogen storage disease type IA will undergo malignant transformation into HCC. [93] Other risk factors for HCC include previous treatment with androgenic steroids, oral contraceptives and methotrexate. [94] Unlike adult HCC, pediatric HCC often demonstrate reduced levels of cyclin D1 expression. [95] Whether this is involved in the pathogenesis of pediatric HCC is still unclear. [96]

HCC is a malignancy of hepatocyte origin. The tumor is noted to have a fibrous capsule and is also predisposed to vascular invasion. [97] There are two distinct groups of HCC patients in childhood: those developing HCC in the context of advanced chronic liver disease (CLD), and children who develop sporadic HCC without preceding liver disease. The latter group typically affects older children. Their clinical behavior and biologic behavior are similar to HCC in adults. Approximately 26% of cases are histologically of a fibrolamellar type, [98] which does not appear to make a prognostic difference. Sporadic HCC in children has a relatively poor outcome, [75] while the several small series that report on HCC developing in CLD do so in the context of liver transplantation (LT) [82, 99, 100, 101, 102] The fibrolamellar subtype of HCC (FLHCC) accounts for 3% of HCCs and is not associated with underlying liver disease. FLHCC lesions are solitary, encapsulated, and well defined. Up to 75% of patients will have elevated serum AFP levels. [89, 97].

As for the pathology, HCC macroscopically are usually multifocal and invasive, commonly involving both lobes and frequently associated with vascular invasion, extrahepatic extension, or both at the time of diagnosis. Areas of hemorrhage and necrosis are common, and the lesions themselves vary in consistency from soft to firm. This significantly reduces the resectability rate. Czauderna et al report only a 36% complete tumor resection rate in a series of 39 children recorded by the International Society of Pediatric Oncology over a 4-year time period. [75] The microscopic features distinguishing hepatocellular carcinoma from hepato-

blastoma are the presence of tumor cells larger than normal hepatocytes, broad cellular trabeculae, considerable nuclear pleomorphism, nucleolar predominance, frequent tumor giant
cells, and absence of hemopoiesis. [33,94] The fibrolamellar variant of HCC is probably a
separate clinical entity. Histologically, the tumor cells are plump, with deeply eosinophilic
cytoplasm and a marked fibrous stroma separating epithelial cells into trabeculae. [103]

HCC often present as abdominal swelling associated with dull aching pain and discomfort.
Other frequent complaints are of rapid weight loss and weakness. [75] The most common
clinical sign is hepatomegaly. HCC frequently presents at the time of diagnosis with metastatic spread, most commonly to the regional lymph nodes, lungs and bones. [96]

4.1. Laboratory findings

Although most children with HB have an elevated serum AFP level, this marker is elevated
in 50–70% of patients with HCC and less markedly than in HB. Approximately 60–80% of
HCC present with significantly elevated AFP levels. [96] All children with HCC should be
screened for exposure to viral hepatitis B and C. Similar to HB, some children with HCC
may be anemic and others may demonstrate thrombocytosis. Children with cirrhosis-associ-
ated HCC may present with elevated serum liver enzyme levels (AST) and those with splenomegaly may show pancytopenia. Careful assessment of hepatic functional reserve in
children with cirrhosis is important prior to embarking on major hepatic resection. However, no specific data are available for children regarding tests used in adults (Iodocyanine-
green (ICG) dye clearance, galactose elimination capacity). Therefore, the evaluation of the
hepatic functional reserve in children is based on standard liver tests including total bilirubin, prothrombine time and INR. [55]

4.2. Imaging

The diagnostic imaging in children with HCC is not different from HB. HCC is often multifocal and may present with a variable number and distribution of tumor nodules. While
identifying larger nodules is not difficult, recognizing lesions less than 1.0 cm is still a challenge. Positron emission tomography (PET) using 18- fluorodeoxyglucose may be useful in
identifying unsuspected extrahepatic disease. [104]

Three-dimensional CT image analysis techniques are now available to estimate tumor volume and provide detailed intrahepatic anatomy that resembles the actual intraoperative
findings. CT volumetry may permit calculation of resected tumor volume and anticipated
size of the remnant liver in planning resection. [105] Diagnostic laparoscopy is useful to determine if extra- hepatic disease is present and may avoid unnecessary attempts at resection.
Plain radiograph and CT of the chest should be obtained to rule out lung metastases. Hepatic arteriography is currently limited to instances of HCC managed by hepatic artery infusion
or transcatheter chemoembolization which can be performed in older children. [55]

On US imaging, HCC may appear as a solitary or multicentric mass most commonly involving the right lobe of the liver, or as a diffusely infiltrating lesion. At diagnosis, these masses
appear solid, rarely contain calcification, and have variable echogenicity. Small lesions ap-

pear homogeneous and are most often hypoechoic. The capsule can be seen as a hypoechoic halo. Larger lesions become necrotic, and therefore demonstrate a more heterogeneous appearance. Doppler US may detect the high-velocity flow that is related to neovascularity, but Doppler US is most useful for identifying venous invasion. Portal venous invasion is identified in up to 60% of cases, [106] with hepatic venous invasion identified less commonly. Doppler US may differentiate neoplastic thrombus from bland (benign) thrombus by detecting internal neovascularity in the former. [97]

Potentially curative therapies can treat the very early and early stages of the disease. However, less than 30% of HCC patients are detected with the disease in those stages. [107] Another 20% of patients with terminal stage HCC receive recommendations for the best supportive treatment. Since HCC is unresectable in the majority of patients at the time of the first diagnosis, patients are often directed to nonsurgical treatments. Physicians have long overlooked radiotherapy (RT) for HCC as radiation might induce fatal hepatic toxicity at doses lower than the therapeutic doses. [108] However, such limitation has been overcome by recent developments in RT technology involving precise delivery of focused high-dose on partial volume of the liver. [109, 110, 111, 112, 113, 114] According to the Korean Liver Cancer Study Group (KLCSG) practice guidelines, RT is considered appropriate for unresectable, locally advanced HCC without extrahepatic metastasis, Child-Pugh class A or B, and tumors occupying less than two-thirds of the liver. [115]

4.3. Results of resection

Based on recent experience, the optimal treatment should have been total hepatectomy and liver transplantation. Katzenstein et al. reported on 46 children enrolled in the POG and CCG studies - 8 with stage I, 25 with stage III, 13 with stage IV. [49] The overall event-free survival at 5 years was 17%. The outcome was not more favorable in 10 children with FL-HCC. No difference in survival was observed whatever the chemotherapy regimen was given. 369 The German Cooperative Liver Study Group [116] reported the results of two prospective trials. The survival rate of HCC was 33% and 25% in HB-89 (12 patients – 1989–1993) and 25% in HB-94 (25 patients – 1994–1998), respectively. The SIOPEL-1 study (1990–1994) enrolled 39 patients with HCC who were treated with neoadjuvant chemotherapy (PLADO). Thirty-one percent had metastases, 39% had extrahepatic extension/vascular invasion, 56% had multifocal HCC while 31% had pre-existing liver disease. A partial response to PLADO was observed in 49%, a complete tumor resection was possible in 36% (2 with liver transplantation). The 5-year event-free survival was 17%. Adverse prognostic factors included multifocality, metastases and vascular invasion. In SIOPEL-2 pilot study (1994–1998), 21 patients were treated with "super-PLADO" (carboplatin, cisplatin and doxorubicine). Eighteen percent had metastases, 35% had extrahepatic extension/vascular invasion and 53% had multifocal HCC. Partial response to SUPER-PLADO was observed in 46%; complete tumor resection was performed in 47% (one with liver transplantation). The 3-year overall survival was 22%. In SIOPEL-3 (1999–2004), 65 patients were treated with SUPER-PLADO with a partial response in 40%. Thirteen underwent primary surgery. Forty-four percent were never resectable. The 3-year event-free survival was 10%. Currently, the new

SIOPEL-5 study is evaluating non-cirrhotic HCC patients staged according to the PRETEXT system and receiving neoadjuvant PLADO chemotherapy and thalidomide (an anti-angiogenic agent) followed by surgery and postoperative metronomic chemotherapy.

4.4. Liver transplantation for hepatocellular carcinoma

Experience with liver transplantation in children with unresectable HCC is somewhat limited but results have significantly improved over the recent years. Beaunoyer et al. reported on 10 children with underlying liver disease in 5 and cirrhosis in 5. Six had one nodule >5 cm and 7 had >3 nodules. The 5-year actuarial survival was 83%; two died, one of recurrence, while 2 with macrovascular invasion survived. Number and size of lesions or gross vascular invasion did not significantly impact survival. [82] Reyes et al. reported on 19 children with HCC who underwent total hepatectomy and liver transplantation in 1989–1998; two thirds had underlying liver disease. [80] The 5-year disease-free survival was 63% (3/6 died of recurrent HCC). In their experience, risk factors for recurrence were tumor size, vascular invasion and lymphnode involvement. [80] Austin et al. analyzed the aggregated outcome for OLT in HCC in 41 children <18 years (UNOS data). Patient survival was 63% at 5 year and 58% at 10 year. Recurrence was the primary cause of death in 86%. [78]

The most conventional criteria for transplantation are the so-called Milan criteria: [117] no more than three tumors, each not more than 3 cm in size, or a single tumor, not more than 5 cm in diameter, and no evidence of extrahepatic disease or vascular invasion. Recent studies suggest that, in an otherwise normal liver, the present cut-off for tumor size might be expanded to 6.5 cm or 7 cm. [118, 119] The evidence supports the moderate expansion of the Milan criteria although findings from different studies lack consistency and prospective validation by pretransplant imaging. [79] There are no hard data implying that Milan criteria can appropriately select children with a low risk of recurrence of HCC after transplantation. Indeed, Milan criteria are derived from experience in adults with cirrhosis, whereas the majority of children with HCC have no underlying cirrhosis. There is no prospective trial in children while the role of OLT in non-cirrhotic liver is unknown. Moreover, there are differences in biology [120] between adult and pediatric HCC with different molecular findings: mutation of c- met gene in children with HCC, not in adults, level of glycin D1 (regulatory protein of G1 phase cycle) expression is lower in children, loss of heterozygosity on chromosomal arm, 13q, higher in children. There is evidence that childhood HCC might be less chemoresistant than adult HCC; a partial response was observed in 49% enrolled in SIOPEL-1 study. [75] The SIOPEL group has launched in 2005 a new SIOPEL-5 trial directed to non-cirrhotic hepatocellular carcinoma in children and adolescents. It is based on the hypothesis that the addition of an antiangiogenic drug (Thalidomide) to PLADO will result in an improvement of survival with acceptable toxicity. Most likely, Sorafenib will be substituted for Thalidomide on the basis of data obtained in adults with advanced HCC. [121]

Patients with unresectable disease restricted to the liver will be submitted to liver transplantation. Since the majority of children with HCC in western countries have no underlying liver disease, recent data suggest that liver transplantation may be quite useful treatment in carefully selected unresectable cases. [78, 80, 82] Unlike the adult population, the frequency of HCC in the pediatric population is low; therefore, the experience in the application of liver transplantation in the pediatric population for HCC is limited. [122, 123, 124, 125] In patients whose disease is confined to the liver, the use of liver transplantation is indicated. Because chemotherapy is not beneficial at present in this group, results in patients with more extensive disease are poor. [126]

5. Benign tumors

In general, benign tumors of the liver may arise from hepatocytes, bile duct epithelium, the supporting mesenchymal tissue, or a combination of two or more of these. In addition to true neoplastic conditions of the liver, a variety of nodular diseases may occur that resemble, and must therefore be differentiated from, tumours. Although most patients with benign hepatic tumors are asymptomatic, a minority may present with symptoms that may be local or systemic. In these patients, the relationship between the symptoms and the hepatic lesions may be difficult to correlate, and additional evaluation is necessary to rule out other causes for the patients complaints. In most cases patients with benign hepatic lesions have no preexisting liver disease, and the finding of a coexisting chronic liver disease such as cirrhosis, chronic hepatitis B or C, or hemochromatosis should raise a suspicion for a malignant tumor. A conclusive diagnosis of a focal hepatic lesion is essential because it may represent a primary or secondary malignancy, which may require immediate treatment. In addition, some benign lesions carry specific risks such as rupture, bleeding, malignant transformation, consumptive coagulopathy, and disseminated intravascular coagulation. [127]

Primary liver masses constitute the third most common group of solid abdominal tumors of childhood, [2, 128, 129] with an incidence of 0.4 to 1.9 per million children each year. [129, 130] Benign primary liver masses described in children include hemangioma/infantile hepatic hemangioendothelioma, focal nodular hyperplasia, simple hepatic cysts, mesenchymal hamartomas, adenomas, nodular regenerative hyperplasia, hematomas, arterial venous malformations, granulomas, and lymphangiomas. [2, 12, 128, 129, 130, 131, 132, 133]

Infantile hepatic hemangioendothelioma is a tumor derived from vascular endothelial cells, which is the most diagnosed benign hepatic tumor in children. Hence it accounts for approximately 12% of all childhood hepatic tumors,the most common benign vascular tumor of the liver in infancy, and the most common symptomatic liver tumor during the first 6 months of life. [134, 135, 136, 137]

While the majority of benign masses may be of little consequence, morbidity and mortality can occur from benign masses, mass effect from a tumor can cause pain, biliary obstruction and inferior vena cava obstruction, limit lung capacity, or cause feeding difficulty. [2, 12, 129, 138] Most of the recent radiology literature concerning the liver has focused on lesions detection or identification of specific features (enhancement patterns) that may help distinguish benign from malignant hepatic tumours. Except for hemangioma and focal nodular hyperplasia (FNH), little is know about imaging characteristics that can help identify and distinguish among the many less common bening liver masses. [139]

5.1. Infantile hepatic hemangioendothelioma

More than 90% are diagnosed before the age of 6 years. The typical presentation is of hepatomegaly, hemangiomas of the skin, and heart failure resulting from massive arteriovenous shunting. [127, 140] In addition to heart failure, this tumor may cause consumption coagulopathy (Kasabach–Merritt syndrome) and obstructive jaundice. [127, 141] Although well circumscribed, this tumor is not encapsulated and often has scattered calcifications. Microscopically, this tumor consists of multiple small vessels lined by plump endothelial cells and surrounded by fibrous stroma.

Ultrasonography usually shows hepatomegaly and solitary or multiple hepatic lesions, which may vary from anechoic to hyperechoic. The unenhanced CT scan demonstrates the lesion as a well-defined hypo-attenuating mass, occasionally with calcifications. After contrast injection, the lesion may show enhancement resembling hemangioma and may become isodense on delayed images. Angiography shows dilated, irregular vascular lakes that commonly persist beyond the venous phase. 99mTc-sulfur colloid scintigraphy shows the lesion as a cold spot because of a lack of Kupffer cells within the tumor. [127]

The prognosis of this lesion is dependent on its size and its effect on the heart function. Spontaneous regression is frequent but death may occur within the first 6 months of life because of cardiac failure or replacement of the normal hepatic parenchyma. [127, 142] The prognosis is usually good if heart failure is managed successfully.

Treatment is dictated by tumor-related symptoms produced by tumor size. Management of congestive heart failure may be sufficient in some cases. If symptoms are not relieved, treatment should be aimed at decreasing the tumor size. [127]

Other treatments include hepatic artery ligation, transcatheter endovascular embolization, and radiation therapy. [127, 143, 144] Liver transplant is increasingly recognized as a viable treatment modality for infantile hemangioendothelioma when other treatments fail. [127, 145]

5.2. Focal Nodular Hyperplasia (FNH)

FNH is very rare in pediatric population with an age prevalence in children 7-8 years old, although some cases are diagnosed in early childhood or even in the prenatal period. [146, 147] The female sex is predominant with a M/F ratio of less than 1/10 in one of the largest series. [147, 148]

The majority (70-90%) of FNH at presentation is asymptomatic and the most common way that the disease is discovered is when, during an occasional physical examination, hepatomegaly or a palpatory abdominal mass are detected. The lesion is more often unique, but about 8% of cases may show multiple nodules, up to 30. The diameter of lesions is extremely variable, from less than 1 cm to more than 15 cm but usually is less than 5 cm. [147]

The diagnosis in the majority of cases could be by Ultrasound, CT Scan and MRI. Needle biopsy or open air biopsy are necessary when the radiological investigations are doubtful, above all in case of absence of the central scar, and not rarely the differential diagnosis from other nodular lesions of liver may be difficult. The differential diagnosis includes different nodular lesions of the liver. [147]

The natural evolution of FNH is unpredictable. In about 2/3 of cases, remain stable and in about 1/3-1/4 of cases show a gradual spontaneous improvement as far as a complete remission. In rare instances an increase in number as well as in size may occur [9]. The recent studies in molecular biology have confirmed that FNH is not a pre-neoplastic lesion: the tissue parenchymal organization is pretty the same of usual liver tissue and, moreover, even though in some cases a clonal origin of FNH nodules have been demonstrated, until now no somatic mutation in the β-catenin gene or in the other genes implicated in the hepatocellular adenoma (where a malignant transformation is possible) have been discovered. [147, 149, 150]

About the management the first step is, of course, the stop of oral contraceptive. Considering the body of evidence that FNH doesn't undergo malignant transformation and that there are only sporadic cases followed by spontaneous rupture and consequent abdominal bleeding, we agree with the opinion that in asymptomatic cases it is opportune a careful follow-up with an ultrasound scan every 6-12 months, and that elective surgery has probably to be limited to the patients suffering of abdominal pain or with a voluminous or growing mass. [147, 149]

5.3. Nodular regenerative Hyperplasia (NRH)

Nodular regenerative hyperplasia (NRH) is a disease characterized by multiple nodules composed by hepatocytes, without a fibrous tissue or central scar. The rare pediatric cases are mostly in association with the congenital absence of portal vein (sometimes complicated by heart disease or multi-cystic kidney dysplasia). Indeed, only about 200 cases have been reported. Symptoms, when present, are mainly associated with the complication of portal hypertension. [151, 152, 153, 154]

CT presentation is really different from FNH, as there are multiple hypodense lesions with poor or absent enhancement after contrast administration. [147, 155] The typical imaging showing anechoic and regular profile of the mass at ultrasound, easily recognize cystic lesions: however CT and MRI may be necessary in selected cases. [147]

5.4. Hamartomas

Mesenchymal hamartoma is a rare, benign, developmental tumor of the liver, with occasional risk of malignancy. Histologically, it appears as a disordered arrangement of the mesenchyme, bile ducts, and hepatic parenchyma. Cords of normal appearing hepatocytes are separated by zones of loose, poorly cellular mesenchyme. The porous nature of the mesenchyme permits accumulation of fluid. [156, 157] Grossly, it has stromal and cystic components with no capsules, and can grow to large sizes. [157, 158] The typical presentation is one of asymptomatic, rapid abdominal distention with a palpable mass on physical examination. The rapid expansion of the tumor is believed to be due to degeneration of the mesenchyme and fluid accumulation. Other uncommon associated symptoms are vomiting, fever, constipation, diarrhea, and weight loss. [156, 157] Laboratory investigations usually reveal normal liver function with elevated alpha-fetoprotein, which is believed to be secreted by the proliferating hepatocytes within the tumor. [157, 159] The radiological appearance is one of a large, uni or multi-cystic, avascular mass occupying part of the liver. [157, 158] Surgical resection has been the standard treatment for this tumor.

6. Sarcoma

The third most common hepatic malignancy, after hepatoblastoma and hepatocellular carcinoma, is undifferentiated embryonal sarcoma. [8, 160, 161] It is believed to be a primitive mesenchymal neoplasm, which usually behaves in a highly malignant fashion. [162] It was first recognized as a clinicopathologic entity by Stocker and Ishak in 1978. [156] Before their report, this tumor had been described under different names such as embryonal sarcoma [163] mesenchymoma, [164] primary sarcoma [165] or fibromyxosarcoma. [166]

These tumors occur in children 5–10 years of age and are mesenchymal in appearance. [8, 167] Diagnosis of primary hepatic sarcoma is challenging due to the lack of specific presenting symptoms, lack of serological markers, non-specific findings on radiological imaging and the rarity of the disease. [86] However, leukocytosis and elevated aspartate aminotransferase and alkaline phosphatase are not uncommon laboratory findings. [156, 161, 162, 168, 169] The serum α-fetoprotein level is always normal. [156, 161, 162, 169] There is no correlation with hepatitis B or C virus infection. Most tumors have prominent areas of cystic degeneration. [161, 162] Multinucleated giant tumor cells with eosinophilic cytoplasm and frequent mitosis are usually present. (Stocker and Ishak,1978 and [162] et al.,2001) PAS-positive, diastase-resistant hyaline globules, which are believed to be lysosomes or apoptotic bodies, are frequently seen within tumor cells as well as in extracellular stromata. [156, 162, 168, 170, 171]

Regarding the radiological imaging, undifferentiated embryonal sarcoma often show a misleading cystic appearance on CT and magnetic resonance imaging (MRI) in contrast to a predominantly solid appearance on ultrasound. [86, 172]

Undifferentiated embryonal sarcoma of the liver behaves in a highly malignant fashion, [162, 173] and the median survival has been less than a year. [156, 162] Complete surgical resection is the key to a favorable outcome. However, despite apparent complete resectability in somecases, local recurrence and distant metastases have been major impediments to achieving long-term disease-free survival. [162, 173] Multidisciplinary treatment (chemotherapy and radiotherapy) has been used to achieve superior and local control and disease-free survival in patients with Undifferentiated embryonal sarcoma of the liver. [160, 167, 173]

Author details

Julio C. Wiederkehr[1,2*], Izabel M. Coelho[1,2], Sylvio G. Avilla[1,2], Barbara A. Wiederkehr[2] and Henrique A. Wiederkehr[2]

*Address all correspondence to: julio.wieder@uol.com.b

1 Federal University of Paraná, Curitiba, Brazil

2 Hospital Pequeno Príncipe, Curitiba, Brazil

References

[1] Kim, E. H., Koh, K. N, Park, M, Kim, B. E, Im, H. J, & Seo, J. J. (2011). Clinical features of infantile hepatic hemangioendothelioma. *Korean Journal of Pediatrics*, 54(6), 260, doi:10.3345/kjp.2011.54.6.260.

[2] Luks, F. I., Yazbeck, S., Brandt, M. L., et al. (1991). Benign liver tumors in children: a 25- year experience. *J Pediatr Surg*, 26, 1326-30.

[3] Reymond, D., Plaschkes, J., Luthy, A. R., et al. (1995). Focal nodular hyperplasia of the liver in children: review of follow-up and outcome. *J Pediatr Surg*, 30, 1590-3.

[4] Ehren, H., Mahour, G. H., & Isaacs, H., Jr. (1983). Benign liver tumors in infancy and childhood. Report of 48 cases. *Am J Surg*, 145, 325-9.

[5] Emre, S., & Mc Kenna, G. J. (2004). Liver tumors in children. *Pediatric transplantation*, 8(6), 632-8.

[6] Weinberg, AG, & Finegold, MJ. (1983). Primary hepatic tumors of childhood. *Hum Pathology*, 14, 512-537.

[7] Multerys, M., Goodman, M. T., Smith, MA, et al. (1999). Hepatic Tumors. In Ries LAG, SmithMA,GurneyJGet al. (eds). Cancer Incidence, SurvivalamongChildren, Adolescents: United States SEER Program 1975-1995. *SEER Program, NIH Pub.* [99-4649], Bethesda, MD, National Cancer Institute, 91-97.

[8] Litten, J. B., & Tomlinson, G. E. (2008). Liver tumors in children. *The oncologist*, 13(7), 812-20.

[9] Dimmick, J. E., Rogers, P. C. J., & Blair, G. (1994). Hepatic Tumors. *In: Pochedly C, ed. Neoplastic Siseases of Childhood*, Chur, Switzerland, Harwood Academic, 973-1010.

[10] Kelly, D. (2008). *Diseases of the Liver and Biliary System in Children ed.*, Wiley-Black-well, Oxford.

[11] Kenney, LB, Miller, B. A., Ries, L. A., et al. (1998). Incidence of cancer in infants in the U.S.: 1980-1990. *Cancer*, 82, 1396-1400.

[12] Meyers, R. L. (2007). Tumors of the liver in children. *Surgical oncology*, 16(3), 195-203.

[13] Mann, J. R., Kasthuri, N., Raafat, F., et al. (1990). Malignant hepatic tumours in children: incidence, clinical features and aetiology. *Paediatr Perinat Epidemiol*, 4, 276-289.

[14] Bulterys, M., Goodman, M. T., Smith, M. A., et al. (1999). Cancer Inci- dence and Survival Among Children and Adolescents: United States SEER Program1975-1995. *National Cancer Institute SEER Program. NIHPublication* [99-4649], 91-97.

[15] Owe, T., Kubota, A., Okuyama, H., et al. (2003). Hepatoblastoma in children of extremely low birth weight: a report from a single prenatal center. *Journal of Pediatric Surgery*, 38, 134-7.

[16] Honda, S., Haruta, M., Sugawara, W., et al. (2008). The methylation status of RASSF1A promoter predicts responsiveness to chemotherapy and eventual cure in hepatoblastoma patients. *Int J Cancer*, 5, 1117-25.

[17] Sakamoto, L. H., De Camargo, B., Cajaiba, M., et al. (2010). MT1G hypermethylation: a potential prognostic marker for hepatoblastoma. *Pediatr Res*, 67, 387-93.

[18] Exelby, P. R., Filler, R. M., & Grosfeld, J. L. (1975). Liver tumors in children in the particular reference to hepatoblastoma and hepatocellular carcinoma: American Academy of pediatrics surgical section survey- 1974. *Journal of pediatric surgery*, Saunders, Retrieved from, http://linkinghub.elsevier.com/retrieve/pii/0022346875900950? showall=true.

[19] DeBaun, M. R., & Tucker, M. A. (1998). Risk of cancer during the first four years of life in children from the Beckwith-Wiedemann Syndrome Registry. *J Pediatr*, 132, 398-400.

[20] Steenman, M., Westerfeld, A., & Mannens, M. (2000). Genetics of Beckwith-Weidemann Syndrome associated tumours: common genetic pathways. *Genes Chromosomes Cancer*, 28, 1-13.

[21] Giardello, F. M., Offerhaus, G. J., Krush, A. J., et al. (1991). Risk of hepatoblastoma in familial adenomatous polyposis. *J Pediatr*, 119, 766-768.

[22] Aretz, S., Koch, A., Uhlhaas, S., et al. (2006). *Pediatric Blood Cancer*, 47, 811-8.

[23] Hirschman, B. A., Pollock, B. H., & Tomlinson, G. E. (2005). The spectrum of APC mutations in children with hepatoblastoma from familial adenomatous polyposis kindreds. *Journal of Pediatrics*, 147, 263-6.

[24] Wei, Y., Fabre, H., Branchereau, S., et al. (2000). Activation of B-catenin in epithelial and mesenchymal hepatoblastomas. *Oncogene*, 19, 498-506.

[25] Jeng, Y. M., Wu, M. Z., Chang, M. H., et al. (2000). Somatic mutations of B-catenin play a crucial role in the tumorigenesis of sporadic hepatoblastoma. *Cancer*, 152, 45-5.

[26] Udatsu, Y., Kusafuka, T., Kuroda, S., et al. (2001). High frequency of beta catenin mutations in hepatoblastoma. *Pediatr Surg Int*, 17, 508-512.

[27] Tomlinson, G. E., Douglass, E. C., Pollock, B. H., et al. (2006). Cytogenetic analysis of a large series of hepatoblastoma: numerical aberrations with recurring translocations involving 1q12-21. *Genes Chromosomes Cancer*, 44, 177-8

[28] Ruck, P., Xiao, J. C., Pietsch, T., et al. (1997). Hepatic stem-like cells in hepatoblasto-ma: Expression of cytokeratin 7, albumin and oval cell associated antigens detected by OV-1 and OV-. *Histopathology*, 31, 324-329.

[29] Ruck, P., & Xiao, J. C. (2002). Stem-like cells in hepatoblastoma. *Med Pediatr Oncol*, 39, 504-507.

[30] Stocken, J. T. (1994). Hepatoblastoma. *Semin Diagn Pathol*, 11, 136-143.

[31] Malogolowkin, M. H., Katzenstein, H. M., Krailo, M., et al. (2006). Intensified plati-num therapy is an ineffective strategy for improving outcome in pediatric patients with advanced hepatoblastoma. *Journal of Clinical Oncology*, 24, 2879-84.

[32] Haas, J. E., Feusner, J. H., & Finegold, M. J. (2001). Small cell undifferentiated histolo-gy in hepatoblastoma may be unfavorable. *Cancer*, 92, 3130-4.

[33] Hass, J. E., Mczynski, K. A., Krailo, M., et al. (1989). Histopathology and prognosis in childhood hepatoblastoma and hepatocellular carcinoma. *Cancer*, 64, 1082-1095.

[34] Perilongo, G., & Shafford, E. A. (1999). Liver tumours. *Eur J Cancer*, 19, 953-958.

[35] Teng, C. T., Daeschner, C. W., Jr., Singleton, E. B., Rosenberg, H. S., Cole, V. W., Hill, L. L., & Brennan, J. C. (1961). Liver disease and osteoporosis in children. I. Clinical observations. *Journal of Pediatrics*, 59, 684-702.

[36] Van Tornout, J. M., Buckley, J. D., Quinn, J. J., et al. (1997). Timing and magnitude of decline in alpha-fetoprotein levels in tested children with unresectable or metastatic hepatoblastoma are predictors of outcome: a report from the Children's Cancer Group. *J Clin Oncol*, 15, 1190-1197.

[37] Hartley, A. L., Birch, J. M., Kelsey, A. M., et al. (1990). Epidemiological and familial aspects of hepatoblastoma. *Med Pediatr Oncol*, 18, 103-119.

[38] Feusner, J. R., Krailo, M. A., Hass, J. E., et al. (1993). Treatment of pulmonary meta-stasis of initial stage I hepatoblastoma in child- hood: report from the children's can-cer group. *Cancer*, 71, 859-864.

[39] Lack, E. E., Neave, C., & Vawter, G. F. (1982). Hepatoblastoma- A clinical and patho-logic study of 54 cases. *Am J Suj Pathol*, 6, 693-705.

[40] Nickerson, H. J., Silberman, T. L., & McDonald, T. P. (1980). Hepatoblastoma, throm-bocytosis and increased thrombopoetin. *Cancer*, 315-7.

[41] Meyers, R. L., Katzenstein, H. M., Rowland, J. H., et al. (2008). PRETEXT and other prognostic factors in hepatoblastoma. *Pediatric Blood Cancer*.

[42] Perilongo, G. (2006). State of the art: Treatment of childhood liver tumors. Geneva, Switzerland. *In: 38th annual meeting of SIOP*.

[43] Roebuck, D. J., Olsen, O., & Pariente, D. (2006). Radiological staging in children with hepatoblastoma. *Pediatr Radiol*, 36, 176-82.

[44] Roebuck, D. (2008). Focal liver lesion in children. *Pediatr Radiol*, 38(3), 518-22.

[45] De Campo, M., & De Campo, J. F. (1988). Ultrasound of primary hepatic tumors in childhood. *Pediatric Radiol*, 19, 19-24.

[46] Helmberger, J. R., Ros, P. R., Medgo, P. J., et al. (1999). Pediatric liver neoplasms: a radiology-pathological correlation. *Eur Radiol*, 9, 1339-1347.

[47] Von Schweiniz, D., Burger, D., Weiner, P., et al. (1992). Therapy of malignant liver tumors in childhood. An intermittent report of the HB-89 multicenter. *Clin Pediatr*, 204, 214-220.

[48] Katzenstein, H. M., Krailo, M., Malogolowkin, M. H., et al. (2007, February). Biology and treatment of children with all stages of hepatoblastoma: COG proposal AHEP-0731. *submitted to CTEP and NCI*.

[49] Katzenstein, H. M., Krailo, M., Malogolowkin, M. H., et al. (2002). Hepatocellular carcinoma in children and adolescents: results from the Pediatric Oncology Group and the Children's Cancer Group intergroup study. *J Clin Oncol*, 20(12), 2789-97.

[50] Aronson, D. C., Schnater, J. M., Staalman, C. R., et al. (2005). Predictive value of pre-treat- ment extent of disease system in hepatoblastoma: Results from the International Society of Pediatric Oncology Liver Tumor Study Group SIOPEL-1 study. *J Clin Oncol*, 23, 1245-1262.

[51] Meyers, R. L., Rowland, J. R., Krailo, M., et al. (2009). Predictive power of pretreatment prognostic factors in children with hepatoblastoma: a report from the Children's Oncology Group. *Pediatr Blood Cancer*, 53(6), 1016-22.

[52] Douglass, E. C., Reynolds, M., Finegold, M., et al. (1993). Cisplatin, vincristine, and fluorouracil therapy for hepatoblastoma: a Pediatric Oncology Group study. *J Clin Oncol*, 11(1), 96-9.

[53] Brown, J., Perilongo, G., Shafford, E., et al. (2000). Pretreatment prognostic factors for children with hepatoblastoma-- results from the International Society of Paediatric Oncology (SIOP) study SIOPEL 1. *Eur J Cancer*, 36(11), 1418-25.

[54] http://www.cancer.gov/PublishedContent/MediaLinks/308970.html.

[55] Otte, J. B. (2010). Progress in the surgical treatment of malignant liver tumors in children. *Cancer treatment reviews*, 36(4), 360-71, Elsevier Ltd.

[56] Czauderna, P., Otte, J. B., Aronson, D. C., et al. (2005). Guidelines for surgical treatment of hepatoblastoma in the modern era : recommendations from the childhood liver tumour strategy group of the international society of paediatric oncology (SIOPEL). *European Journal of Cancer*, 41, 1031-6.

[57] Stringer, M. (2006). Liver tumors. *Semin Pediatr Surg*, 9, 196-208.

[58] Fuchs, J., Rydzynski, J., Hecker, H., et al. (2002). The influence of preoperative chemotherapy and surgical technique in the treatment of hepatoblastoma-a report from

the German cooperative liver tumours studies HB-89 and HB-94. *Eur J Pediatr Surg*, 12, 255-61.

[59] Von Schweinitz, D., Faundez, A., Teichmann, B., et al. (2000). Hepatocyte growth-factor- scatter-factor can stimulate postoperative tumor-cell proliferation in childhood hepatoblastoma. *Int J Cancer*, 85, 151-9.

[60] Ortega, J. A., Douglass, E. C., Feusner, J. H., et al. (2000). Randomized comparison of cisplatin/vincristin/5-fluorouracil and cisplatin/doxorubicin for the treatment of pediatric hepatoblastoma (HB): a report from the Children's cancer group and the pediatric oncology group. *Journal of Clinical Oncology*, 18, 2665-75.

[61] Schnater, J. M., Aronson, D. C., Plaschkes, J., et al. (2002). Surgical view of the treatment of patients with hepatoblastoma. *Cancer*, 94, 1111-20.

[62] Malogolowkin, M. H., Katzenstein, H. M., Krailo, M., et al. Redefining the role of doxorubicin for the treatment of children with hepatoblastoma. *Journal of Clinical Oncology*.

[63] Von Schweinitz, D., & Haberle, B. (2007, March). German liver tumor study: HB 99. Poland, Gdansk. *In: First international symposium childhood hepatoblastoma*.

[64] Von Schweinitz, D., Hecker, H., Harms, D., et al. (1995). Complete resection before development of drug resistance is essential for survival from advanced hepatoblastoma-a report fro the German cooperative pediatric liver tumor study HB-89. *Journal of Pediatric Surgery*, 30, 845-52.

[65] Ortega, J. A., Douglass, E., Feusner, J., et al. (1994). A randomized trial of cisplatin/ vincristine/5-fluorouracil vs. CCP/doxorubicin continuous infusion for the treatment of hepatoblastoma: results from the pediatric inter-group hepatoma study (abstr). *Proc Am Soc Clin Oncol (ASCO)*, 13, 416.

[66] Pritchard, J., Brown, J., Shafford, E., et al. (2000). Cisplatin, doxorubicin and delayed surgery for childhood hepatoblastoma: a successful approach-results of the first prospective study of the International Society of Pediatric Oncology. *J Clin Oncol*, 18, 3819-28.

[67] Perilongo, G., Shafford, E., Maibach, R., et al. (2004). Risk-adapted treatment for childhood hepatoblastoma Final report of the second study of the International Society of Pediatric Oncology- SIOPEL 2. *Eur J Cancer*, 40, 411-21.

[68] Meyers, R. L., Malogolowkin, M. H., Rowland, J. M., & Krailo, M. (2006, May 27). Predictive value of the PRETEXT staging system in children with hepatoblastoma. *In: Presented at the 37th annual meeting American Pediatric Surgical Association, Hilton Head, SC*.

[69] Dall'Igna, P., Cecchetto, G., Toffolutti, T., et al. (2003). Multifocal hepatoblastoma is there a place for partial hepatectomy? *Med Pediatr Oncol*, 40, 113-6.

[70] Couinaud, C. (1992). The anatomy of the liver. *Ann Ital Chir*, 63, 693-7.

[71] Wheatley, J. M., Rosenfield, N. S., Berger, L., & La Quaglia, M. P. (1996). Liver regeneration in children after major hepatectomy for malignancy-evaluation using a computer-aided technique of volume measurement. *J Surg Res*, 61, 183-9.

[72] Von Schweinitz, D. (2006). Management of liver tumors in childhood. *Semin Pediatr Surg*, 15, 17-24.

[73] Otte, J. B., & De Ville de Goyet, J. (2005). The contribution of transplantation to the treatment of liver tumors in children. *Semin Pediatr Surg*, 14, 233-8.

[74] Chardot, C., Sant Martin, C., Gilles, A., et al. (2002). Living related liver transplantation and vena cava reconstruction after total hepatectomy including the vena cava for hepatoblastoma. *Transplantation*, 73, 90-2.

[75] Czauderna, P., Mac Kinley, G., Perilongo, G., et al. (2002). Hepatocellular carcinoma in children: results of the first prospective study of the international society of pediatric oncology group. *Journal of Clinical Oncology*, 20, 2798-804.

[76] Millar, A. J. W., Hartley, P., Khan, D., et al. (2001). Extended hepatic resection with transplantation back-up for an unresectable tumor. *Pediatric Surgery International*, 17, 378-81.

[77] Otte, J. B., Pritchard, J., Aronson, D. C., et al. (2004). Liver transplantation for hepatoblastoma: Results from the International Society of Pediatric Oncology (SIOP) study SIOPEL-1 and review of the world experience. *Pediatr Blood Cancer*, 42, 74-83.

[78] Austin, M. T., Leys, C. M., Feurer, I. D., et al. (2006). Liver transplantation for childhood hepatic malignancy: a review of the United Network for Organ Sharing (UNOS) database. *J Pediatr Surg*, 41, 182-6.

[79] Hoti, E., & Adam, R. (2008). Liver transplantation for primary and metastatic liver cancers. *Transplant Int*, 21, 1107-17.

[80] Reyes, J. D., Carr, B., Dvorchik, I., et al. (2000). Liver transplantation and chemotherapy for hepatoblastoma and hepatocellular cancer in childhood and adolescence. *J Pediatr*, 136(6), 795-804.

[81] Perilongo, G., Brown, J., Shafford, E., et al. (2000). Hepatoblastoma presenting with lung metastases: treatment results of the first cooperative, prospective study of the International Society of Pediatric Oncology on childhood liver tumors. *Cancer*, 89, 1845-53.

[82] Beaunoyer, M., Vanatta, J. M., Ogihara, M., et al. (2007). Outcomes of transplantation in children with primary hepatic malignancy. *Pediatr Transplant*, 11(6), 655-60.

[83] Pimpalwar, A. P., Sharif, K., Ramani, P., et al. (2002). Strategy for hepatoblastoma management: transplant versus nontransplant surgery. *J Pediatr Surg*, 37, 240-5.

[84] Tiao, G. M., Bobey, N., Allen, S., et al. (2005). The current management of hepatoblastoma: a combination of chemotherapy, conventional resection, and liver transplantation. *J Pediatr*, 146, 204-11.

[85]   Molmenti, E. P., Wilkinson, K., Molmenti, H., et al. (2002). Treatment of unresectable hepatoblastoma with liver transplantation in the pediatric population. *Am J Transplant*, 6, 535-8.

[86]   Faraj, W., Mukherji, D., El Majzoub, N., Shamseddine, A., Shamseddine, A., & Khalife, M. (2010). Primary undifferentiated embryonal sarcoma of the liver mistaken for hydatid disease. *World journal of surgical oncology*, 8(58).

[87]   Moore, S. W., Hesseling, P. B., Wessels, G., et al. (1997). Hepatocellular carcinoma in children. *Pediatr Surg Int*, 12, 266-70 .

[88]   Bellani, F. F., & Massimino, M. (1993). Liver tumors in childhood: Epidemiology and clinics. *J Surg Oncol*, 3, 119-121.

[89]   Dubois, J., Garel, L., Russo, P., et al. (1993). Pediatric case of the day. *Radiographics*, 13, 691-2.

[90]   Parkin, D. M., Stiller, C. A., Draper, G. J., et al. (1988). The international incidence of childhood cancer. *Int J Cancer*, 42, 511-520.

[91]   Chen, J. C., Chang, M. L., Lin, J. N., et al. (2005). Comparison of childhood hepatic malignancies in a hepatitisBhyper-endemic area. *World J Gastroenterol*, 11, 5289-5294.

[92]   Chang, M. L., Chen, J. C., Lai, M. S., et al. (1997). Universal hepatitis B vaccination in Taiwan and the incidence of hepatocellular carcinoma in children. Taiwan Childhood Hepatoma Study Group. *N Engl J Med*, 336, 1855-1859.

[93]   Howell, R. R., Stevenson, R. E., Ben-Menachem, Y., et al. (1976). Hepatic adenoma in type I glycogen storage disease. *JAMA*, 236, 1481-1489.

[94]   Weinberg, A. G., & Finegold, M. J. (1983). Primary Hepatic Tumor of Childhood. *Hum Pathol*, 14, 512-537.

[95]   Kim, H., Lee, M. J., Kim, M. R., et al. (2000). Expression of cyclin D1, cyclin E, cdk4 and loss of heterozygosity of 8p13q 17p in hepatocellular carcinoma. *Comparison study of childhood and adult hepatocellular carcinoma. Liver*, 20, 173-178.

[96]   Emre, S., & Mc Kenna, G. J. (2004). Liver tumors in children. *Pediatric transplantation*, 8(6), 632-8.

[97]   Varich, L. (2010). Ultrasound of Pediatric Liver Masses. *Ultrasound Clinics*, 5(1), 137-152, Elsevier Ltd.

[98]   Katzenstein, H. M., Krailo, M. D., Malogolowkin, M. H., et al. (2003). Fibrolamellar hepatocellular carcinoma in children and adolescents. *Cancer*.

[99]   Arikan, C., Kilic, M., Nart, D., et al. (2006). Hepatocellular carcinoma in children and effect of living-donor liver transplantation on outcome. *Pediatr Transplant*, 10, 42-7.

[100] Sevmis, S., & Karakayali, H. (2008). Ozc carcinoma in children. *Pediatr Transplant*, 12, 52-6.

[101] Hadzic, N., Quaglia, A., Portmann, B., et al. (2011). Hepatocellular carcinoma in children with biliary atresia; King's College Hospital Experience. *J Pediatr*.

[102] Hadzic, N., & Finegold, M. J. (2011). Liver neoplasia in children. *Clinics in liver disease*, 15(2), 443-62, vii-x., Elsevier Ltd.

[103] Craig, J. R., Peters, R., Edmondson, H. A., & Omata, M. (1980). Fibrolamellar carcinoma of the liver: a tumor of adolescentes and Young adults with distinctive clinicopathologic features. *Cancer*, 46, 372-9.

[104] Hain, S. F., & Fogelman, I. (2004). Recent advances in imaging hepatocellular carcinoma: diagnosis, staging and response assessment functional imaging. *Cancer J*, 10, 121-7.

[105] Shoup, M., Gonen, M., D'Angelica, M., et al. (2003). Volumetric analysis predicts hepatic dysfunction in patients undergoing major liver resection. *J Gastrointest Surg*, 7, 325-30.

[106] Rumack, C. M., Wilson, S. R., & Charboneau, J. W. (2005). *Diagnostic ultrasound* (3rd edition), St Louis (MO), Mosby.

[107] Bruix, J., & Sherman, M. (2005). Practice Guidelines Committee, American Association for the Study of Liver Diseases. Management of hepatocellular carcinoma. *Hepatology*, 42, 1208-1236.

[108] Cochrane, A. M., Murray-Lyon, I. M., Brinkley, D. M., & Williams, R. (1977). Quadruple chemotherapy versus radiotherapy in treatment of primary hepatocellular carcinoma. *Cancer*, 40, 609-6.

[109] Lawrence, T. S., Tesser, R. J., & ten Haken, R. K. (1990). An application of dose volume histograms to the treatment of intrahepatic malignancies with radiation therapy. *Int J Radiat Oncol Biol Phys*, 19, 1041-1047.

[110] Lawrence, T. S., Ten Haken, R. K., Kessler, M. L., et al. (1992). The use of 3-D dose volume analysis to predict radiation hepatitis. *Int J Radiat Oncol Biol Phys*, 23, 781-788.

[111] Robertson, J. M., Mc Ginn, C. J., Walker, S., et al. (1997). A phase I trial of hepatic arterial bromodeoxyuridine and conformal radiation therapy for patients with primary hepatobiliary cancers or colorectal liver metastases. *Int J Radiat Oncol Biol Phys*, 39, 1087-1092.

[112] Seong, J., Keum, K. C., Han, K. H., et al. (1999). Combined transcatheter arterial chemoembolization and local radiotherapy of unresectable hepatocellular carcinoma. *Int J Radiat Oncol Biol Phys*, 43, 393-397.

[113] Shim, S. J., Seong, J., Han, K. H., et al. (2005). Local radiotherapy as a complement to incomplete transcatheter arterial chemoembolization in locally advanced hepatocellular carcinoma. *Liver Int*, 25, 1189-1196.

[114] Park, W., Lim, D. H., Paik, S. W., et al. (2005). Local radiotherapy for patients with unresectable hepatocellular carcinoma. Int J Radiat Oncol Biol Phys , 61, 1143-1150.

[115] Park, JW. (2004). Korean Liver Cancer Study Group and National Cancer Center. Practice guideline for diagnosis and treatment of hepato- cellular carcinoma. *Korean J Hepatol*, 10, 88-98.

[116] Von Schweinitz, D. (2004). Treatment of liver tumors in children. *In: Clavian PA, Fong Y, Lyerly H, et al. editors. Liver tumors: current and emerging therapies*, Boston, Jones and Bartlett.

[117] Mazzaferro, V., Regalia, E., Doci, R., et al. (1996). Liver transplantation for the treatment of small hepatocellular carcinoma in patients with cirrhosis. *New Engl J Med*, 334, 693-9.

[118] Yao, F. Y., Ferrell, L., Bass, N. M., et al. (2001). Liver transplantation for hepatocellular carcinoma: expansion of the tumor size limits does not adversely impact survival. *Hepatology*, 33, 1394-403.

[119] Roayaie, S., Frischer, J. S., Emre, S. H., et al. (2002). Long-term results with multimodal adjuvant therapy and liver transplantation for the treatment of hepatocellular carcinoma larger than 5 centimetres. *Ann Surg*, 235, 533-9.

[120] Terracciano, L., & Tornillo, L. (2003). Cytogenetic alteration in liver cell tumors as detected by comparative genomic hybridization. *Pathologica*, 95, 71-82.

[121] Llovet, J. M., Ricci, S., Mazzaferro, V., et al. (2008). Sorafenib in advanced hepatocellular carcinoma. *New Engl J Med*, 359, 420-2.

[122] Srinivasan, P., Mc Call, J., Pritchard, J., et al. (2002). Orthotopic liver transplantation for unresectable hepatoblastoma. *Transplantation*, 74, 652-5.

[123] Tagge, E. P., Tagge, D. U., Reyes, J., et al. (1992). Resection, including transplan- tation, for hepatoblastoma and hepatocellular carcinoma: impact on survival. *J Pediatr Surg*, 27, 292-6, discussion 297.

[124] Freeman, R. B., Jr., & Edwards, E. B. (2000). Liver transplant waiting time does not correlate with waiting list mortality: implications for liver allocation policy. *Liver Transplant*, 6, 543-52.

[125] Organ Procurement and Transplantation Network-HRSA. (1998). Final rule with comment period. *Fed Regist*, 63, 16296-338.

[126] Tiao, G. M., Alonso, M. H., & Ryckman, F. C. (2006). Pediatric liver transplantation. *Seminars in pediatric surgery*, 15(3), 218-27.

[127] Schiff, E. R., Maddrey, W. C., & Sorrel, M. F. (2011). *Schiff's Disease of the Liver* (11th ed.), Wiley-Blackwell.

[128] Ehren, H., Mahour, G. H., & Isaacs, H., Jr. (1983). Benign liver tumors in infancy and childhood. *Report of 48 cases. Am J Surg*, 145, 325-9.

[129] Kochin, M. D., Tamir, A., Miloh, M. D., Ronen Arnon, M. D., Kishore, R., Iyer, M. D., Frederick, J., Suchy, M. D., Nanda Kerkar, M., Zenge, J. P., Fenton, L., Lovell, M. A.,

Grover, T. R., et al. (2002). Case report: infantile hemangioendothelioma. *Curr Opin Pediatr*, 14, 99-102.

[130] Reymond, D., Plaschkes, J., Luthy, A. R., et al. (1995). Focal nodular hyperplasia of the liver in children: review of follow-up and outcome. *J Pediatr Surg*, 30, 1590-3.

[131] Bakshi, P., Srinivasan, R., Rao, K. L., et al. (2006). Fine needle aspiration biopsy in pediatric space- occupying lesions of liver: a retrospective study evaluating its role and diagnostic efficacy. *J Pediatr Surg*, 41, 1903-8.

[132] Schwartz, M. E., Konstadoulakis, M. M., Roayaie, S., et al. (2008). The Mount Sinai experience with orthotopic liver transplantation for benign tumors: brief report and literature review: case reports. *Transplant Proc*, 40, 1759-62.

[133] Finegold, M. J., Egler, R. A., Goss, J. A., et al. (2008). Liver tumors: pediatric population. *Liver Transpl*, 14, 1545-56.

[134] Zenge, J. P., Fenton, L., Lovell, M. A., & Grover, T. R. (2002). Case report: infantile hemangioendothelioma. *Curr Opin Pediatr*, 14, 99-102.

[135] Mortelé, K. J., Vanzieleghem, B., Mortelé, B., Benoit, Y., & Ros, P. R. (2002). Solitary hepatic infantile hemangioendothelioma: dynamic gadolinium-enhanced MR imaging findings. *Eur Radiol*, 12, 862-865.

[136] Ingram, J. D., Yerushalmi, B., Connell, J., Karrer, F. M., Tyson, R. W., & Sokol, R. J. (2000). Hepatoblastoma in a neonate: a hypervascular presentation mimicking hemangioendothelioma. *Pediatr Radiol*, 30, 794-797.

[137] Roos, J. E., Pfiffner, R., Stallmach, T., Stuckmann, G., Marincek, B., & Willi, U. (2003). Infantile hemangioendothelioma. *Radiographics : a review publication of the Radiological Society of North America*, 23(6), 1649-55.

[138] Stringer, M. D., & Alizai, N. K. (2005). Mesenchymal hamartoma of the liver: a systematic review. *J Pediatr Surg*, 40, 1681-90.

[139] Horton, K. M., Bluemke, D. A., Ralph, H., Soyer, P., & Fishman, E. K. (1999). *CT and MR Imaging of Benign Hepatic*, 431-451.

[140] Zafrani, E. S. (1989). Update on vascular tumours of the liver. *J Hepatology*, 8(1), 125-30.

[141] Linderkamp, O., Hopner, F., Klose, H., et al. (1976). Solitary hepatic hemangioma in a newborn infant complicated by cardiac failure, consumption coagulopathy, microangiopathic hemolytic anemia, and obstructive jaundice. Case report and review of the literature. *Eur J Pediatr*, 125(1), 239.

[142] Hobbs, K. E. (1990). Hepatic hemangiomas. *World J Surg*, 14(4), 468-71.

[143] DeLorimier, A. A., Simpson, E. B., Baum, R. S., et al. (1967). Hepatic-artery ligation for hepatic hemangiomatosis. *N Engl J Med*, 277(7), 333-7.

[144] Warmann, S., Bertram, H., Kardorff, R., et al. (2003). Interventional treat- ment of infantile hepatic hemangioendothelioma. *J Pediatr Surg*, 38(8), 1177-81.

[145] Walsh, R., Harrington, J., Beneck, D., et al. (2004). Congenital infantile hepatic hemangioendothelioma type II treated with orthotopic liver transplantation. *J Pediatr Hematol Oncol*, 26(2), 121-3.

[146] Lack, E. E., & Ornvold, K. (1986). Focal nodular hyperplasia and hepatic adenoma: a review of eight cases in the pediatric age group. *J Surg Oncol*, 33, 129-35.

[147] Farruggia, P., Alaggio, R., Cardella, F., Tropia, S., Trizzino, A., Ferrara, F., & D'Angelo, P. (2010). Focal nodular hyperplasia of the liver: an unusual association with diabetes mellitus in a child and review of literature. *Italian journal of pediatrics*, 36, 41, doi: 10.1186/1824-7288-36-41.

[148] Luciani, A., Kobeiter, H., Maison, P., Cherqui, D., Zafrani, E. S., Dhumeaux, D., & Mathieu, D. (2002). Focal nodular hyperplasia of the liver in men: is presentation the same in men and women? *Gut*, 50, 877-80.

[149] Rebouissou, S., Bioulac-Sage, P., & Zucman-Rossi, J. (2008). Molecular pathogenesis of focal nodular hyperplasia and hepatocellular adenoma. *J Hepatol*, 48, 163-170.

[150] Raidl, M., Pirker, C., Schulte-Hermann, R., Aubele, M., Kandioler-Eckersberger, D., Wrba, F., Micksche, M., Berger, W., & Grasl-Kraupp, B. (2004). Multiple chromosomal abnormalities in human liver (pre)neoplasia. *J Hepatol*, 40, 660-668.

[151] Vernier-Massouille, G., Cosnes, J., Lemann, M., Marteau, P., Reinisch, W., Laharie, D., & Cadiot, G. (2007). Nodular regenerative hyperplasia in patients with inflammatory bowel disease treated with azathioprine. *Gut*, 56(10), 1404-9.

[152] Stromeyer, F. W., & Ishak, K. G. (1981). Nodular transformation (nodular "regenerative" hyperplasia) of the liver.A clinicopathologic study of 30 cases. *Hum Pathol*, 12, 60-71.

[153] Wanless, I. R., Godwin, T. A., Allen, F., et al. (1980). Nodular regenerative hyperplasia of the liver in hematologic disorders: a possible response to obliterative portal venopathy. A morphometric study of nine cases with an hypothesis on the pathogenesis. *Medicine*, 59, 367-79.

[154] Naber, A. H., Van Haelst, U., & Yap, S. H. (1991). Nodular regenerative hyperplasia of the liver: an important cause of portal hypertension in non-cirrhotic patients. *J Hepatol*, 12, 94-9.

[155] Reshamwala, P. A., Kleiner, D. E., & Heller, T. (2006). Nodular regenerative hyperplasia: not all nodules are created equal. *Hepatology*, 44, 7-14.

[156] Stocker, J. T., & Ishak, K. G. (1983). Mesenchymal hamartoma of the liver: Report of 30 cases and review of the literature. *Pediatr Pathol*, 1, 245-67.

[157] Gupta, R., Parelkar, S. V., & Sanghvi, B. (2009). Mesenchymal hamartoma of the liver. *Indian J Med Paediatr Oncol*, 30, 141-143, doi:.

[158]   Kirks, D. R., & Griscom, N. T. (1990). Practical pediatric imaging. Lippincott Williams
        and Wilkins, 3rd ed, Boston, Little, Brown, *Diagnostic radiology of infants and children*,
        808-815.

[159]   Ito, H., Kishikawa, T., Toda, T., Arai, M., & Muro, H. (1984). Hepatic mesenchymal
        hamartoma of an infant. *J Pediatr Surg*, 19, 315-7.

[160]   Bisogno, G., Pilz, T., Perilongo, G., et al. (2002). Undifferentiated sarcoma of the liver
        in childhood: A curable disease. *Cancer*, 94, 252-257.

[161]   Lack, E. E., Schloo, B. L., Azumi, Net, et al. (1991). Undifferentiated (embryonal) sar-
        coma of the liver.Clinical and pathological study of 16 cases with emphasis on immu-
        nohistochemical features. *Am J Surg Pathol*, 15, 1-16.

[162]   Chuang, W.-yu., Lin, J.-nan., Hung, I.-jih., & Hsueh, C. (2001). *Undifferentiated Sarco-
        ma of the Liver*, 399-404.

[163]   Foster, J. H., & Berman, M. M. (1977). *Solid Liver Tumors*, Philadelphia, W. B. Saun-
        ders, 198-202.

[164]   Donovan, E. J., & Santulli, T. V. (1946). Resection of the left lobe of the liver for mes-
        enchymoma- Report of case. *Ann Surg*, 124, 90-3.

[165]   Willeford, G., & Stembridge, V. A. (1950). Primary sarcoma of liver- Report of a case.
        Am J Dis Child, 80, 404-7.

[166]   Dintzman, M., Reiss, R., & Haimoff, H. (1966). Right hepatectomy. *Isr J Med Sci*, 2,
        743-9.

[167]   Noguchi, K., Yokoo, H., Nakanishi, K., Kakisaka, T., Tsuruga, Y., Kamachi, H., Mat-
        sushita, M., et al. (2012). A long-term survival case of adult undifferentiated embry-
        onal sarcoma of liver. *World journal of surgical oncology*, 10(1), 65.

[168]   Walker, N. I., Horn, M. J., Strong, R. W., Lynch, S. V., Cohen, J., Ong, T. H., & Harris,
        O. D. (1992). Undifferentiated (embryonal) sarcoma of the liver: Pathologic findings
        and long-term survival after complete surgical resection. *Cancer*, 69(1), 52-59.

[169]   Aoyama, C., Hachitanda, Y., Sato, J. K., Said, J. W., & Shimada, H. (1991). Undifferen-
        tiated (embryonal) sarcoma of the liver. A tumor of uncertain histogenesis showing
        divergent differentiation. *Am J Surg Pathol*, 15, 615-24.

[170]   Chou, P., Mangkornkanok, M., & Gonzalez-Crussi, F. (1990). Undifferentiated (em-
        bryonal) sarcoma of the liver: ultrastructure, immunohistochemistry, and DNA ploi-
        dy analysis of two cases. *Pediatr Pathol*, 10, 549-62.

[171]   Keating, S., & Taylor, G. P. (1985). Undifferentiated (embryonal) sarcoma of the liver:
        ultrastructural and immunohistochemical similarities with malignant fibrous histio-
        cytoma. *Hum Pathol*, 16, 693-9

[172] Buetow, P. C., Buck, J. L., Pantongrag-Brown, L., Marshall, W. H., Ros, P. R., Levine, M. S., & Goodman, Z. D. (1997). Undifferentiated embryonal sarcoma of the liver: pathological basis of imaging findings in 28 cases. *Radiology*, 203, 779-783.

[173] Urban, C. E., Mache, C. J., Schwinger, W., Pakisch, B., Ranner, G., Riccabona, M., Schimpl, G., Brandesky, G., Messner, H., Pobegen, W., Becker, H., & Grienberger, H. (1993). Undifferentiated (embryonal) sarcoma of the liver in childhood. Successful combined-modality therapy in four patients. *Cancer*, 72, 2511-6.

[174] Newman, K. D., Schisgall, R., Reaman, G., & Guzzetta, P. C. (1989). Malignant mesenchymoma of the liver in cildren. *J Pediatr Surg*, 24, 781-3.

[175] Kirks, D. R., & Griscom, N. T. (1990). Practical pediatric imaging. editors. Lippincott Williams and Wilkins, 3rd ed., Boston, Little, Brown, *Diagnostic radiology of infants and children*, 808-815.

Chapter 5

Liver Tumors in Infancy and Children

Chunbao Guo and Mingman Zhang

Additional information is available at the end of the chapter

1. Introduction

The liver is the third-most-common site for intra-abdominal malignancy in children, follow-ing adrenal neuroblastoma and wilms tumor. Although the overall incidence of childhood cancer has been slowly increasing since 1975, cancer in children and adolescents is still rare, the incidence of primary malignant liver tumors per year is 1-1.5 per million children in the United States [1, 2, 3, 4]. This yields a relative low rate for hepatic tumors (1.3% of all pedia-tric malignancies). Tumors of the liver may be either malignant or benign. Two thirds of liv-er tumors in children are malignant. Of these malignant tumors, hepatoblastoma (HB) and hepatocellular carcinoma (HCC) are the most common and account for 70 persent of all hep-atic neoplasms. Unlike liver tumors in adults, in which the predominant histology is hepato-cellular carcinoma, hepatoblastoma accounts for two thirds of liver tumors in children. Other liver malignancies in children include sarcomas, germ cell tumors, as well as rhab-doid tumors. Benign tumors of the liver in children include vascular tumors, hamartomas, adenomas, and focal nodular hyperplasia (FNH). The histology and anatomy of a pediatric liver tumor guides the treatment and prognosis [5, 6, 7, 8].

Recently, dramatic improvements in survival have been achieved for children and adoles-cents with liver cancer. Children and adolescents with liver cancer should be referred to multidisciplinary team incorporates the skills of the primary care physician, pediatric surgi-cal subspecialists, radiation therapists, pediatric oncologists/hematologists, rehabilitation specialists, pediatric nurse specialists, social workers, and others to ensure that children re-ceive treatment, supportive care, and rehabilitation that will achieve optimal survival and quality of life. Almost all liver masses in children are surgically treated, either primarily or following systemic chemotherapy [9, 10]. The conditions that eventuate in this choice of therapy, when and how to accomplish it, and the medical and surgical consequences for children of transplantation for tumors are described in guidelines for pediatric cancer cen-ters and their role in the treatment of pediatric patients with cancer by the American Academy of Pediatrics [11, 12, 13]. Clinical trials for children and adolescents with cancer are generally designed to compare potentially better therapy with therapy that is currently accepted as standard. Clinical trials are available in many clinical institutes for liver cancer that occur in children and adolescents, and the opportunity to participate in these trials is offered to most patients/families [14].

2. Epidemiology of pediatric hepatic tumors

Benign lesions in children represent 30% of hepatic tumors and are most commonly vascular in origin (eg, hemangiomas, hemangioendotheliomas). Two-thirds of hepatic neoplasms in children are malignant. Liver cancer is also rare malignancy in children and adolescents and account for approximately 1% of all pediatric malignancies. The malignant liver tumor is divided into two major histologic subgroups: hepatoblastoma, affecting around 80% of children, and hepatocellular carcinoma (HCC) [15, 16]. The age of onset of liver cancer in children is related to tumor histology. Hepatoblastoma usually occur before the age of 3 years, and approximately 90% of malignant liver tumors in children aged 4 years and younger are hepatoblastomas. There are 2 distinct groups of HCC patients in childhood: children who develop sporadic HCC without preceding liver disease, and those developing HCC in the context of advanced chronic liver disease (CLD). Sporadic HCC in children has a relatively poor outcome, while the several small series that report on HCC developing in CLD do so in the context of liver transplantation (LT). Some biologic differences may exist between HCCs developing in adults and children. One study reported an high radiological response (49%) in pediatric HCC, higher than adult HCC [17].

The incidence of hepatocellular carcinoma is negligible in children aged 14 years and younger. In china, the incidence of hepatic tumors in children 14 years and younger is 2.6 per 100,000, of which 81 persent are hepatoblastoma. The incidence of hepatoblastoma in the United States increased in the last 25 years, whereas the incidence of hepatocellular carcinoma in the United States has not changed appreciably over time. The cause for the increase in incidence of hepatoblastoma is unknown, but the increasing survival of very low birth weight premature infants, which is known to be associated with hepatoblastoma, may contribute. In Japan, the risk of hepatoblastoma in children who weighed less than 1,000 g at birth are 15 times the risk in normal birth weight children. Other data has confirmed the high incidence of hepatoblastoma in very low birth weight premature infants. In several asian countries, the incidence of hepatocellular carcinoma in children is 10 times more than that in North America. The high incidence appears to be related to the incidence of perinatally acquired hepatitis B, which can be prevented in most cases by vaccination and administration of hepatitis B immune globulin to the newborn [18, 19].

Additional rare malignant liver tumors in children are sarcoma, including its 3 variants rhabdomyosarcoma, embryonal or undifferentiated sarcoma, and angiosarcoma predominantly presenting in early childhood. Also included is the exceedingly uncommon cholangiocarcinoma, which can present at any age, often in the context of chronic biliary disease.The overall survival rate for children with hepatoblastoma is 70%, but is only 25% for those with hepatocellular carcinoma.

3. Clinical presentation and diagnosis

Most children with liver tumors commonly present insidiously with nonspecific abdominal discomfort, a palpable abdominal mass, feeding difficulties, and abdominal distension. Chronic fatigue secondary to anemia thrombocytopenia, and leukocytosis and lack of appetite are often reported. Jaundice and biochemical derangement are signs of advanced neoplastic change. Children with both HB and HCC may also present with weight loss, fever, and anorexia [20, 21, 22].

Fetal and neonatal presentations include hydramnios, fetal hydrops, congestive heart failure, and respiratory distress. Occasionally, the child may present acutely with vomiting, fever and clinical signs of abdominal irritation, often suggestive of tumor rupture with intraperitoneal spread. Patients with congestive heart failure have been shown to have lower survival rates. Very rarely HB can present with signs of precocious puberty/virilization due to b-HCG secretion by the tumor. Laboratory studies are performed to assess baseline CBC count, electrolyte levels, liver enzyme levels, liver synthetic function, and α -fetoprotein (AFP) levels Serum AFP remains the key clinical marker of malignant neoplastic change, response to the treatment, and relapse. AFP levels are elevated in 50%-70% of children with hepatic neoplasms, and multiple studies confirm that AFP is a valuable surveillance marker in children who have previously undergone hepatic resection for malignancy. However, there are some variants of both HB and HCC that have low or normal AFP. These variants may have distinct histologic features and poorer prognoses [23, 24]. The initial workup for hepatic masses includes radiographic assessment using ultrasonography.

All children with a palpable abdominal mass usually undergo an initial ultrasound to confirm the location and to characterize the consistency as cystic or solid. Cystic or vascular lesions may not require any further imaging. However, definitive characterization of the mass requires a computed tomography (CT) or magnetic resonance imaging (MRI) scan. Calcifications can be seen in a minority of liver tumors. Hypervascularized hepatic lesions with delayed contrast excretion are highly suspicious of a malignant tumor.
Abdominal ultrasonography usually demonstrates a large mass, possibly with some satellite lesions and areas of hemorrhage within the tumor. CT scanning of the abdomen and chest are used for indeterminate or solid lesions to further delineate the location and to assess resectability (Fig. 1) and evaluate for the presence of pulmonary metastasis. MRI angiography is frequently helpful preoperatively to determine resectability because it delineates the vascular anatomy more precisely. Local radiological availability, expertise extent, and multiplicity of the lesions and to detect metastases may facilitate surgical planning and may determine resectability, however, definitive diagnosis can be proven only through biopsy findings [25, 26, 27].

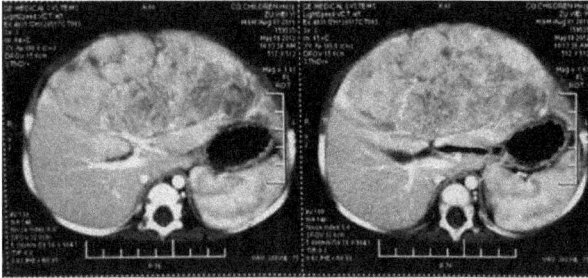

Figure 1. CT scan of a hepatoblastoma amenable to surgical resection.

Any child with a suspected liver tumor should also have AFP and ß-HCG serum assays. The alpha-fetoprotein (AFP) and beta-hCG tumor markers are very helpful in diagnosis and management of liver tumors. Alttough elevation of AFP levels is not diagnostic of hepatic malignancy. AFP is markedly elevated in90% of hepatoblastoma cases and in many cases of hepatocellular carcinoma, and it returns to normal with effective therapy. The level of AFP at diagnosis and rate of decrease in AFP during treatment should be compared to the age-adjusted normal range. Caution should be taken in normal term infants who can have AFP levels in excess of 100,000 ng/ml, however, with a half-life of approximately 1 week, the AFP level normalizes to 10 ng/ml over the first few months of life. Absence of elevated AFP levels at diagnosis occurs in a few percentage of children with hepatoblastoma and appears to be associated with poor prognosis, as well as with the small cell undifferentiated variant of hepatoblastoma. Lack of a significant decrease of AFP levels with treatment may predict a poor response to therapy.

Beta-hCG is a hormone commonly produced by liver tumors and, in excess, can result in precocious puberty. It's levels may also be elevated in children with hepatoblastoma or hepatocellular carcinoma, which may result in isosexual precocity in boys. Extremely high levels of beta-hCG are associated with infantile choriocarcinoma of the liver [28, 29].

Because of the association between familial adenomatous polyposis and hepatoblastoma, obtaining a thorough family history is an important aspect of the management of a child with a liver tumor and his family, with particular attention to any family history of colon cancer or colonic polyps.

A chest CT is an important aspect of the workup because the lung parenchyma is the most common distant site for metastasis. A CBC typically displays mild normocytic and normochromic anemia with thrombocytosis.

Tissue diagnosis of the tumor is essential, although some advocate that in the presence of very high AFP in a young child (6 months to 3 years). The practice in the United States is not to treat without a tissue sample except under the most urgent life-threatening circumstances, such as tumor growth into the right atrium. But this may not be necessary, as avoiding the biopsy theoretically reduces the risks of the tumor seeding. In Europe, The Childhood

Liver Tumor Study Group of the Inter-national Society of Pediatric Oncology (SIOPEL) has developed a preoperative evaluation of the tumor extent (PRETEXT) grading system. The rationale for this recommendation is provided in the section on pathology. Segmental assessment of the extent of the tumor and its relation with the main hepatic vessels is of foremost importance for planning the intensity of chemotherapy and eventual surgery., which could provide a valuable tool for the risk stratification. Formal staging of the tumor should include chest and brain CT and bone scanning [30, 31].

Benign hepatic tumors are usually diagnosed incidentally. Some children may develop the Kasabach-Merritt phenomenon, a triad of coagulopathy, hemolytic anemia and thrombocytopenia due to intralesional pooling of the blood. IHE can have an acute presentation, typically within the first couple of weeks or months of life. Dramatic abdominal distension can lead to major respiratory distress, prompting the need for assisted ventilation and intensive care support. Nowadays some IHEs may be detected on routine antenatal ultrasonography, due to their characteristic vascular multichannel appearance. A proportion of children develop a bizarre secondary hypothyroidism that is thought to be secondary to tumor production of the enzyme iodothyronine deiodinase, which stimulates the conversion of thyroxine to reverse triiodothyronine and of triiodothyronine to 3,3'-diio-dothyronine, leading to a biochemical picture of hypothyroidism, requiring thyroxin supplementation. This phenomenon resolves once the tumor is removed or significantly decreases in size, usually within the first 2 years of life.

3.1. Risk factors

Similar to other embryonal tumors, altered imprinting at the 11–15 locus has been observed in hepatoblastoma. Rearrangements involving the pericentric region of chromosome 1 also appear to be important in hepatoblastoma, with roughly 18% of hepatoblastomas displaying an imbalanced translocation involving this region. Hepatoblastoma is associated with several genetic syndromes and familial cancer predisposition conditions, such as familial adenomatous polyposis and Beckwith-Wiedemann syndrome in addition to several other rare syndromes. Other compelling evidence suggests that acquired aberrations in the ß-catenin/Wnt pathways are important in the pathogenesis of hepatoblastoma. Acquired chromosomal changes in tumors include numerical chromosomal changes, most commonly trisomies of chromosomes 2, 8, and 20. Finally, epigenetic changes in methylation patterns of DNA may be altered in hepatoblastoma.

There is limited but compelling evidence that parental exposures are associated with a higher incidence of liver tumors and, more specifically, hepatoblastoma. Children from parents who have been exposed to metals used in soldering and welding, petroleum, or paints are at a higher risk for hepatoblastoma. Recent reports have also implicated parental smoking as a risk factor for hepatoblastoma [32, 33].

3.2. Beckwith-Wiedemann syndrome

The incidence of hepatoblastoma is increased 1,000 to 10,000-fold in infants and children with Beckwith-Wiedemann syndrome (BWS). BWS can be caused by either genetic mutations and be familial, or much more commonly, by epigenetic changes and be sporadic. Hepatoblastoma is also increased in hemihypertrophy, an overgrowth syndrome caused by the same epigenetic changes in chromosome 11p15.5 that cause many cases of BWS, but in a genetically mosaic fashion. Either mechanism can be associated with an increased incidence of embryonal tumors including Wilms tumor and hepatoblastoma. The gene dosage and ensuing increase in expression of insulin-like growth factor 2 (IGF 2) has been implicated in the macrosomia and embryonal tumors in BWS and hemihypertrophy. When sporadic, the types of embryonal tumors associated with BWS have frequently also undergone somatic changes in the BWS locus and IGF 2. All children with BWS or isolated hemihypertrophy should be screened regularly by ultrasound to detect abdominal malignancies at an early stage. Screening using AFP levels has helped in the early detection of hepatoblastoma in children with BWS or hemihypertrophy. Other somatic overgrowth syndromes, such as Simpson-Golabi-Behmel syndrome, may also be associated with hepatoblastoma.

3.3. Familial adenomatous polyposis

There is an association between hepatoblastoma and familial adenomatous polyposis (FAP); children in families that carry the APC gene are at an 800-fold increased risk for hepatoblastoma. However, hepatoblastoma occurs in less than 1% of FAP family members, so ultrasound and AFP screening for hepatoblastoma in members of families with FAP is controversial. The predisposition to hepatoblastoma may be limited to a specific subset of APC mutations. It has been recommended that all children with hepatoblastoma be examined for congenital hypertrophy of the retinal pigment epithelium, a marker of APC mutation carriers in 70% of polyposis families. In the absence of APC germline mutations, childhood hepatoblastomas do not have somatic mutations in the APC gene; however, they frequently have mutations in the beta-catenin gene, the function of which is closely related to APC.

3.4. Hepatitis B and hepatitis C infection

Hepatocellular carcinoma is associated with hepatitis B and hepatitis C infection, especially in children with perinatally acquired hepatitis B virus [33]. Compared with adults, the incubation period from hepatitis virus infection to the genesis of hepatocellular carcinoma is extremely short in a small subset of children with perinatally acquired virus. Widespread hepatitis B immunization has decreased the incidence of hepatocellular carcinoma in Asia. Mutations in the met/hepatocyte growth factor receptor gene occur in childhood hepatocellular carcinoma, and this could be the mechanism that results in a shortened incubation period.Hepatocellular carcinoma may also arise in very young children with mutations in the bile salt export pump ABCB11, which causes progressive familial hepatic cholestasis. Several specific types of nonviral liver injury and cirrhosis are associated with hepatocellular carcinoma in children including tyrosinemia and biliary cirrhosis.

3.5. Undifferentiated Embryonal Sarcoma of the Liver

Undifferentiated embryonal sarcoma of the liver (UESL) is the third most common liver malignancy in children and adolescents, comprising 9% to 13% of liver tumors. Widespread infiltration throughout the liver and pulmonary metastasis are common, usually between the ages of 5 and 10 years. It could also presents as an abdominal mass, often with pain or malaise. It may appear solid or cystic on imaging, frequently with central necrosis. Distinctive features are characteristic intracellular hyaline globules and marked anaplasia on a mesenchymal background. Many UESL contain diverse elements of mesenchymal cell maturation, such as smooth muscle and fat.

Strong clinical and histological evidence suggest that some UESLs arise from mesenchymal hamartomas of the liver (MHL), which are large benign multicystic masses that present in the first 2 years of life. Many MHLs have a characteristic translocation with a breakpoint at 19q13.4 and several UESLs have the same translocation. In a report of 11 cases of UESL, five arose in association with MHL, and transition zones between the histologies were noted. Some UESLs arising from MHLs may have complex karyotypes not involving 19q13.4.

3.6. Infantile Choriocarcinoma of the Liver

Choriocarcinoma of the liver is a very rare tumor that appears to originate in the placenta and presents with a liver mass in the first few months of life. Infants are often unstable due to hemorrhage from the tumor. Clinical diagnosis may be made without biopsy based on extremely high serum beta-hCG levels and normal AFP levels for age.

3.7. Epithelioid Hemangioendothelioma

Epithelioid hemangioendothelioma (EHE) is a rare vascular cancer that occurs in the liver and other organs.

Generally, children with liver masses display normal growth and development unless they show the phenotypes associated with Beckwith-Wiedemann syndrome or the other genetic cancer predisposition syndromes associated with liver tumors.

4. Screening

Hepatic neoplasms develop in a myriad of chronic liver disorders of childhood, often without or with minimal symptoms. Therefore, regular screening with abdominal ultrasound and serum AFP measurement should be in place for all children with CLD at least annually. Therefore, awareness of antecedent conditions that permit screening is essential. Detection of a liver tumor prior to dissemination and/or massive growth is the single most important management tool for all tumor types at all ages. Children with chronic hepatitis B should be also regularly checked, but because communities in which immunization has yet to be provided are typically impoverished and medically underserved, recommendations for screening have not yet been implemented. Some of the conditions with known increased propensity to develop malignancies such as tyrosinemia type 1 (even on nitizinone treatment) or bile salt export pump (BSEP) deficiency should be assessed every 6 months. However, there is no formal guideline for the frequency and manner of screening at this time [34, 35].

Extraordinary advances in neonatal care in the past 25 years have led to a wholly new population of children, the long-term survivors of birth as early as 22 to 23 weeks of gestation with a weight less than 1000 g. In addition to many other chronic problems, they have extraordinary susceptibility to HB. HB is dramatically more common in expremature babies but arranging effective screening programs could prove to be difficult because of their increasing numbers and fact that their long term care is typically provided outside hepatological clinics. Monitoring much smaller cohorts of children with Beckwith-Wiedemann Syndrome for HB is more feasible, and one study has suggested abdominal ultrasonography and serum AFP every 3 months until 4 years of age.

There are several conditions for which screening of children for primary liver cancer is recommended by virtue of the attendant risk. Hepatitis B virus can cause HCC as early as age 4 following perinatal transmission from infected carrier mothers. Vaccination and perinatal administration of hepatitis B immunoglobulin have already reduced the incidence dramatically. A relative risk for such prematures versus term babies of 16- to 52-fold is recognized around the world. HB occurs at the same age as HB in term babies or later. Screening of infants with hemihypertrophy or hemiaplasia, as part of the Beckwith-Wiedemann over-growth syndrome, has been carried out for many years via ultrasound to detect intraabdominal malignancies. These include Wilms' tumor and adreno cortical carcinoma, in addition to the less common HB, which has a relative risk of 2280. HB is not the only proliferative lesion of the Beckwith-Wiedemann syndrome liver, as hemangioendothelioma and mesenchymal hamartoma have also been observed, either con-currently or sequentially [37, 38].

In familial adenomatous polyposis (FAP), the first manifestation of an autosomal dominant mutation in a family may be HB in a baby, with the colonic polyps detected only afterwards in a parent. The relative risk for children in such cohorts is 800-fold, but many examples are due to new germ-line mutations at 5q21,22 or only in the tumor.

A series from the Children's Oncology Group focused primarily on known FAP families but raised the issue of de novo cases or the potential for infants of parents too young to be aware of the symptoms of FAP themselves.

The largest report of sporadic cases looked at 50 patients and found 5 germline antigen-presenting cell (APC) mutations. This led the authors to recommend routine screening for APC mutations in all cases of sporadic HB, including both a screen for APC deletion or duplication and sequencing through the gene itself. In the only prospective screening study to date, 20 children with confirmed or suspected FAP were followed for 10 years by ultrasonography, and no tumors were detected. In FAP, other forms of hepatocellular neoplasia are also observed, including adenoma and HCC, as well as biliary adenomas.

The timelines of the development of these various cancers in distinct tissues are not linked, and therefore, surveillance for these cancers needs to continue throughout the patient's life

[39]. Chronic cholestatic syndromes may be the substrate for liver cancers, with HB, cholangiocarcinoma, and in the Alagille syndrome of a paucity of intrahepatic bile ducts due to Jagged 1 or NOTCH mutations. Also, we have observed HB in three 2-year olds with congenital hepatic fibrosis and autosomal recessive polycystic disease. HB and HCC have been seen in the explants of infants with cirrhosis due to biliary atresia as early as 1 year. On the basis of the growth rate of HCC and with the aim of detecting tumors when they are 3 cm in diameter, the American Association for the Study of Liver Disease and the European Association for the Study of the Liver recommend screening ultrasound examinations at 6-month intervals, and some institutions shorten this interval to 3 months when the patient is on a transplant waiting list. These organizations have also published diagnostic criteria for liver nodules detected during the screening process.

HCC can be diagnosed noninvasively by computed tomography (CT) or magnetic resonance imaging (MRI) if a lesion 2cm in diameter within a cirrhotic liver demonstrates rapid contrast enhancement during the arterial phase and washout on the delayed venous phase. These guidelines were developed for cirrhotic adults, and there are no validated evidence-based guidelines for screening for tumors in children and adolescents with chronic liver disease.

According to adult data, ultrasound is insensitive for the diagnosis of HCC in the cirrhotic liver and should not be used for the detection of focal liver lesions in this setting. MRI is more sensitive than multidetector 3-phase CT for the diagnosis of regenerative and dysplastic nodules and is comparable to CT for the detection of HCC. There is a lower false-positive rate with MRI. Interval growth is probably the best indicator of malignancy, and there is a definite need for the establishment of protocols for follow-up imaging in centers that care for children with diffuse liver disease.

In the case of hereditary tyrosinemia type 1 due to fumaryl acetoacetate hydrolase deficiency, prompt medical management, by blocking an enzyme upstream in the tyrosine catabolic pathway, can avert the injury that otherwise leads to HCC more often than any other metabolic defect. However, a low risk of developing HCC remains even with adequate medical management, so these children require life-long surveillance. Therefore, for the conditions listed, periodic abdominal ultrasonography and serum alpha fetoprotein measurements, at 3-month intervals in the case of Beck-with-Wiedemann syndrome and similarly for the first 3 years of life for others and then every 6 months thereafter, are advocated [40, 41]. In addition, recognition of the rare sequential occurrences of mesenchymal hamartoma and sarcoma and of hemangioendothelioma with angiosarcoma indicates the need for surveillance ultrasonography whenever a complete resection or transplant has not taken place [42, 43].

5. Staging

The process used to find out if cancer has spread within the liver or to other parts of the body is called staging. The staging system would be useful in determining treatment plans and offers good prognostic value for overall and disease-free survival outcome. Historically, north Americans have staged liver tumors similar to other solid tumors, with surgical resectability and the presence of metastases as the primary criteria. The European staging system considers only the pretreatment extent of disease, and was developed by the Childhood Liver Tumor Strategy Group. After childhood liver cancer has been diagnosed, tests are done to find out if cancer cells have spread within the liver or to other parts of the body. The PRETEXT staging system divides the liver into four sectors, and the number of segments involved by tumor indicates stage. A lettering system further indicates extrahepatic involvement.The information gathered from the staging process determines the stage of the disease [44, 45].

The following tests and procedures may be used in the staging process: -CT scan (CAT scan): This procedure is also called computed tomography, computerized tomography, or computerized axial tomography. The pictures are made by a computer linked to an x-ray machine. A procedure that makes a series of detailed pictures of areas inside the body, taken from different angles. A dye may be injected into a vein or swallowed to help the organs or tissues show up more clearly.

-MRI (magnetic resonance imaging): Also called nuclear magnetic resonance imaging (NMRI), a procedure that uses a magnet, radio waves, and a computer to make a series of detailed pictures of areas inside the body.

-Ultrasound exam: A procedure in which high-energy sound waves (ultrasound) are bounced off internal tissues or organs and make echoes. The echoes form a picture of body tissues called a sonogram. The picture can be printed to be looked at later.

-Surgery: An operation will be done to look at or remove the tumor. Tissues removed during surgery will be checked by a pathologist.

There are 2 staging systems for childhood liver cancer.

-Presurgical (before surgery) staging: This staging system is called PRETEXT, based on imaging procedures such as MRI or CT, where the tumor has shown within the four parts (sections) of the liver.

The liver is divided into 4 vertical sections.

In PRETEXT stage 1(Fig. 2A), the cancer is found in one section of the liver. Three sections of the liver that are next to each other do not have cancer in them.

In PRETEXT stage 2 (Fig. 2B), cancer is found in one or two sections of the liver. Two sections of the liver that are next to each other do not have cancer in them.

In PRETEXT stage 3(Fig. 2C), the cancer is found in three sections of the liver and one section does not have cancer. OR, cancer is found in two sections of the liver and two sections that are not next to each other do not have cancer in them.

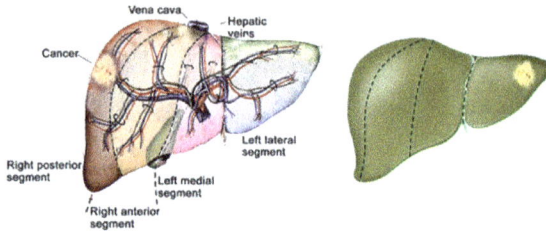

Figure 2.

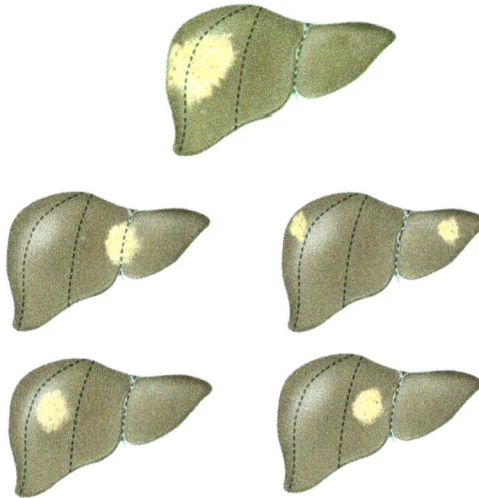

Figure 3.

Postsurgical (after surgery) staging: The stage is based on the amount of tumor that remains after the patient has had surgery to look at or remove the tumor.

Stage I

In stage I, all of the cancer was removed by surgery in the liver.

Stage II

In stage II, a small amount of cancer remains in the liver, but it can be seen only with a microscope, or the tumor cells may have spilled into the abdomen before surgery or during surgery.

Stage III

In stage III:

In stage III, the tumor cannot be removed by surgery; orcancer that can be seen without a microscope remains after surgery; or the cancer has spread to nearby lymph nodes.

Stage IV

In stage IV, the cancer has spread to other parts of the body. Cancer invades the surrounding normal tissue. Cancer invades the lymph system and travels through the lymph vessels to other places in the body. Cancer invades the veins and capillaries and travels through the blood to other places in the body.

The metastasis is described as when cancer cells break away from the primary (original) tumor and travel through the lymph or blood to other places in the body, another (secondary) tumor may form [46]. The secondary (metastatic) tumor is the same type of cancer as the primary tumor. For example, if breast cancer spreads to the bones, the cancer cells in the bones are actually breast cancer cells. The disease is metastatic breast cancer, not bone cancer.

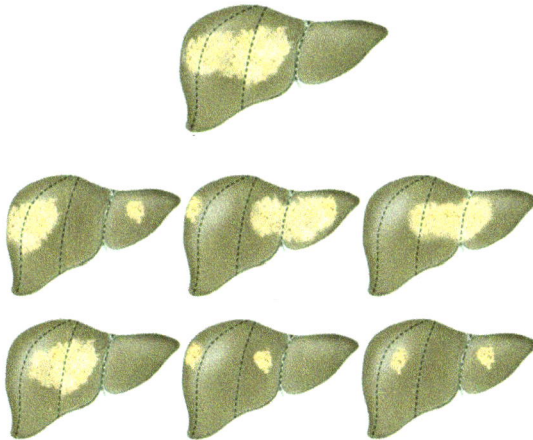

Figure 4.

In PRETEXT stage 4(Fig. 2D), cancer is found in all four sections of the liver.

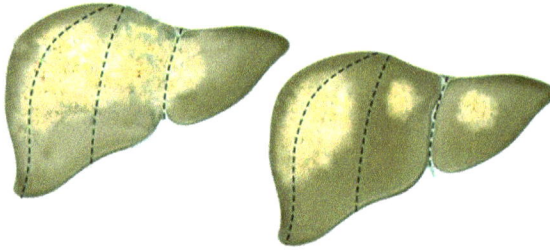

Figure 5.

6. Management

The key to successful treatment of malignant liver tumors in children is surgical removal, either by tumor resection/partial hepatectomy or Live Transplantation. Historically, complete surgical resection of the primary tumor has been required to cure malignant liver tumors in children. Complete surgical resection of the primary tumor continues to be the goal of definitive surgical procedures, but surgical resection is often combined with other treatment modalities (e.g., chemotherapy) to achieve this goal. SIOPEL recommends initial chemotherapy, while the American guidelines from COG require primary resection if possible, followed by chemotherapy, unless the tumor is pure fetal type HB stage 1, when the chemotherapy is not given. Both strategies have been successful in increasing the 5-year survival rates in HB to approximately 80% due to effective chemotherapy (cisplatinum in combination with doxorubicin or vincristine). Moreover, the timing and nature of surgical interventions are better defined for HB, and they are well-placed within the management protocols. For HCC, however, complete surgical excision or transplantation are essential for cure, and chemotherapy is not effective. On the whole, treatment planning by a multidisciplinary team of cancer specialists with experience treating tumors of childhood is required to determine and implement optimum treatment [47, 48].

The most important step in the management of benign tumors in children is confirmation of their genuine benign nature. Multiphase contrast CT imaging and, less frequently, direct angiography are required for the radiological diagnosis. Some of the benign tumors, including IHE, mesenchymal hamartoma, and FNH, would have characteristic radiological features, not always requiring a tissue diagnosis.

Many of the improvements in survival in childhood cancer have been made using new therapies that have attempted to improve on the best available, accepted therapy. Clinical trials in pediatrics are designed to compare potentially better therapy with therapy that is currently accepted as standard.Because of the relative rarity of cancer in children, all children with liver cancer should be considered for entry into a clinical trial. This comparison may be done in a randomized study of two treatment arms or by evaluating a single new treatment, comparing the results with those previously obtained with standard therapy [49].

6.1. Surgical approaches

The timing of the surgical approach is critical. For this reason, surgeons with experience in pediatric liver resection and transplantation should be involved early in the decision-making process for determining optimal timing and extent of resection.There are three ways in which surgery is used to treat primary pediatric liver cancer, including initial surgical resection (alone or followed by chemotherapy), delayed surgical resection (chemotherapy followed by surgery) and orthotopic liver transplantation [50].

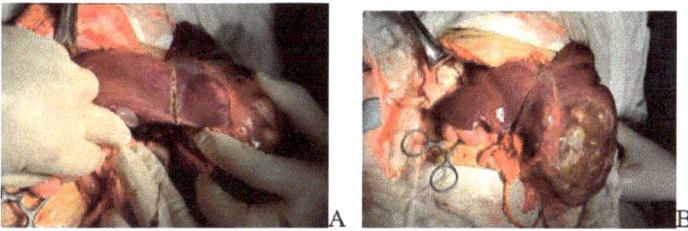

Figure 6. The lesion to resect is marked out.

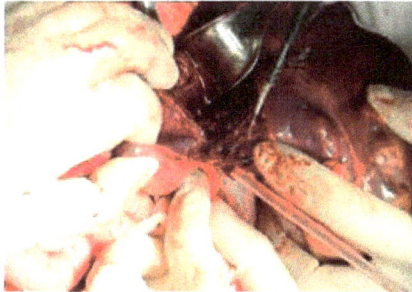

Figure 7. Electrocautery is useful for dissecting through the liver capsule and parenchyma.

Resection is typically performed through a bilateral subcostal incision, and, occasionally, a right thoracoabdominal approach is necessary for large lesions arising high in the right lobe. Surgical resection has seen applications of newer technology. Intraoperative ultrasonography has been widely applied to determine the exact location of the tumor relative to the vessels. Once deemed resectable, the resection is marked out (Fig. 3, 4), and various tools may then be used to perform the resection; electrocautery, bipolar devices such as LigaSure, and argon beam coagulation for hemostasis have been used.

The most frequently performed procedure is a right hepatectomy (60%) because hepatoblastomas (HBs) occur 3 times more often in the right lobe than in the left. The hilar plate is divided, exposing the bifurcation of the hepatic artery and portal vein. These structures are ligated (Fig. 5).

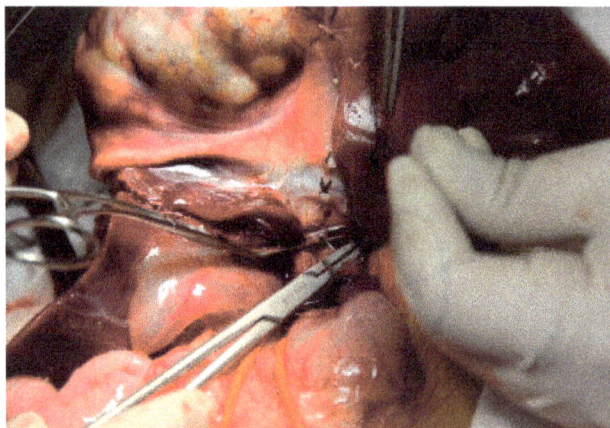

Figure 8. Suture and ligation may be useful in sealing blood vessels and hepatic ducts.

In an extended right hepatectomy, the middle hepatic vein is ligated and segment 4 is resected. The right hepatic vein is identified and ligated before any division of the hepatic parenchyma. At completion, only segments 2 and 3 and the caudate lobe remain.

Left hepatic lobectomy begins the same way right hepatectomy, with division of the left hepatic artery and left branch of the portal vein. The left and middle hepatic veins are identified after dissection through the sinus venosus. The liver is then transected after vascular isolation of the resected segments. An extended left hepatectomy includes removal of all or most of segments 5 and 8. Unresectability is usually determined by involvement of hilar structures or all hepatic veins, multicentricity, and invasion of inferior vena cava (IVC) or portal vein. Centrally located tumors are, by definition, more likely unresectable.

Laparoscopic and robotic resections of both benign and malignant liver tumors have been described. Their role in standard practice is still being defined.

If preoperative chemotherapy is to be administered, it is very important to consult frequently with the surgical team concerning the timing of resection, as prolonged chemotherapy can lead to unnecessary delays and in rare cases, tumor progression. If the tumor can be completely excised by an experienced surgical team, less postoperative chemotherapy may be needed.

In PRETEXT stage 3 or 4 disease patients with involvement of major liver vessels, early involvement with an experienced pediatric liver surgeon is especially important, patients with. Although initially thought to be a contraindication to resection, experienced liver surgeons could also perform aggressive approaches avoiding transplantation for vascular involvement patients. Accomplishing a complete resection is imperative since rescue transplant of incompletely resected patients has an inferior outcome compared to patients who are transplanted as the primary surgical therapy.

Surgical resection of distant disease has also contributed to the cure of children with hepatoblastoma and is often performed at the same time as resection of the primary tumor. Resection of pulmonary metastases is recommended when the number of metastases is limited. When possible, resection of areas of locally invasive disease, such as in the diaphragm, and of isolated brain metastasis is recommended. Second resection of positive margins and/or radiation therapy may not be necessary in patients with incompletely resected hepatoblastoma whose residual tumor is microscopic and who receive subsequent chemotherapy.

Major intraoperative complications include hemorrhage, air embolism, tumor embolus, and bile duct injury. Only 20% of the liver is necessary to maintain hepatic function; thus, postoperative insufficiency is rare. Postoperative complications include hemorrhage, bile leak, abscess formation, pulmonary complications, and wound problems. Postoperative care consists of adequate fluid replacement, intravenous albumin supplementation, vitamin K, and clotting factors for the first 3-4 days. The liver function test results generally normalize within the first 2 weeks, and hepatic insufficiency is reasonably rare. Postoperative monitoring consists of frequent ultrasonography, chest radiography, and serial α -fetoprotein (AFP) level measurements, generally at 3-month to 6-month intervals.

Tumor rupture at presentation, resulting in major hemorrhage that can be controlled by transcatheter arterial embolization or partial resection to stabilize the patient, does not preclude a favorable outcome when followed by chemotherapy and definitive surgery. The decision as to which surgical approach to use depends on many factors including: PRETEXT stage, size of the primary tumor, presence of multifocal hepatic disease, AFP levels, Vascular involvement, preoperative chemotherapy as well as orthotopic liver transplantation criteria.

In North American clinical trials, the Children's Oncology Group (COG) has recommended that surgery be performed initially if a complete resection can be accomplished. COG is investigating the use of PRETEXT stage at diagnosis and after chemotherapy to determine the optimal surgical approach and its timing. In European clinical trials, only patients with PRETEXT stage 1 receive resection surgery and all other patients are biopsied [51, 52, 53].

It is difficult to compare the North American and European approaches. Somewhat comparable results for children with PRETEXT stage 1 and 2 tumors were obtained in two international studies. The 5-year survival of PRETEXT stage 1 and 2 patients(chemotherapy prior to attempted surgical resection of the primary liver tumor) is 90% to 100% on the European studies and seems to be similar to that of children treated on North American studies where surgery was performed before chemotherapy. In comparison, a survey of children with liver tumors who were treated prior to the consistent use of combination chemotherapy found that 45 of 78 patients (57%) with hepatoblastoma who had complete excision of the tumor survived while no children with positive margins or gross disease following resection survived.

6.2. Orthotopic liver transplantation

Orthotopic liver transplantation was first described in 1968 by Starzl. Liver transplantation has recently been associated with significant success in the treatment of children with unresectable hepatic tumors. The criteria currently used to evaluate adult transplant candidates may not be applicable for pediatric patients. The main indication for transplantation is nonmetastatic, unresectable lesions. Extrahepatic disease and lymph node involvement did not prove to be contraindications. Hepatoblastoma (HB) now constitutes an indication for 3% of all pediatric liver transplantations, whereas the role of liver transplantation for HCC is more controversial. In hepatocellular carcinoma, vascular invasion, distant metastases, lymph node involvement, tumor size, and male gender were significant risk factors for recurrence. Because of the poor prognosis in patients with hepatocellular carcinoma, liver transplant should be considered for disorders such as tyrosinemia and familial intrahepatic cholestasis early in the course, prior to the development of liver failure and malignancy. Because no good medical therapy for pediatric HCC has been identified, liver transplantation should be carefully evaluated as front-line therapy. Additionally, successful transplantation has been used benign lesions such as diffuse hepatic hemangiomas. In addition, liver transplantation may be an option in children with unresectable primary tumors, without metastatic disease, after neoadjuvant chemotherapy and pulmonary metastasectomy, if necessary. It has been suggested that adjuvant chemotherapy following transplant may decrease the risk of tumor recurrence. Generally, preoperative and postoperative chemotherapy are recommended, in addition to postoperative immunosuppression [54, 55, 56].

Transplantation may also be used in selected cases of tumor recurrence but is much less successful when used for salvage therapy. There are discrepant results on the outcomes for patients with lung metastases at diagnosis who undergo orthotopic liver transplantation following complete resolution of lung disease in response to pretransplant chemotherapy. Some studies have reported favorable outcomes for this group of patients, while others have noted high rates of hepatoblastoma recurrence. All of these studies are limited by small patient numbers; further study is needed to better define outcomes for this subset of patients [57, 58].

A review of the world experience has documented a posttransplant survival rate of 70% to 80% for children with hepatoblastomas. Intravenous invasion, positive lymph nodes, and contiguous spread did not have a significant adverse effect on outcome.

The primary cause of death for both HB and HCC was metastatic disease. Generally, the 5-year survival rate for patients transplanted for HB is 70%.

A study of the United Network for Organ Sharing (UNOS) database reported 135 patients undergoing 135 transplants for HB and 43 transplants for HCC with 1-year, 5-year, and 10-year survival of 79%, 69%, and 66% for HB, respectively, and 86%, 63%, and 58% for HCC, respectively [59, 60]. Liver transplantation for hepatic hemangioma has been studied in 59 patients in Europe with 1-year, 5-year, and 10-year patient survival rates of 93%, 83%, and 72%, respectively.

The availability of donor organs has increased with the use of split-liver grafting and other "technical variant" techniques, along with living-related liver transplant techniques. Prognosis in terms of graft and patient survival appear to be the same between full-size liver and technical variant liver transplants; however, morbidity following transplant appears to be higher in those patients who receive technical variant grafts [61, 62, 63, 64].

Early failure of liver transplant (< 30 d) is usually due to vascular complications or primary nonfunction. Late failure is usually more a result of infection, posttransplant lymphoproliferative disease, chronic rejection, biliary complications, or recurrence of malignant disease. These failures may warrant retransplantation. The predictors of success after retransplantation remain unknown. The United Network for Organ Sharing (UNOS) Standard Transplant and Research Files registry reported all children younger than 18 years listed for a liver transplant in the United that the 5-year survival rates of 69% for hepatoblastoma and 63% for hepatocellular carcinoma and the 10-year survival rates were similar to the 5-year rates. Application of the Milan criteria for UNOS selection of recipients of deceased donor livers is controversial. However, living donor liver transplants are more common with children and the outcome is similar [65, 66, 67, 68, 69].

6.3. Chemotherapy

In recent years, virtually all children with hepatoblastoma have been treated with chemotherapy, which may reduce the incidence of surgical complications at the time of resection, and in some centers, even children with resectable hepatoblastoma are treated with preoperative chemotherapy. For PRETEXT stage 1 hepatoblastoma, it was resected and treated with doxorubicin and cisplatin chemotherapy. The pre-resection neoadjuvant chemotherapy (doxorubicin and cisplatin) was given to all children with PRETEXT stage 2, 3, or 4 hepatoblastoma with or without metastases. The chemotherapy was well tolerated. This strategy resulted in an OS of 75% at 5 years after diagnosis. Identical overall results were seen in a follow-up international study. Following chemotherapy, and excluding those who received liver transplant (less than 5% of patients), complete resection was obtained in 87% of children. In contrast, an American Intergroup protocol for treatment of children with hepatoblastoma, encouraged resection at the time of diagnosis for all tumors amenable to resection without undue risk. The protocol did not treat children with stage I tumors of purely fetal histology with preoperative or postoperative chemotherapy unless they developed progressive disease. Further study will be needed to determine whether presurgical chemotherapy is preferable to resection followed by chemotherapy for children with PRETEXT stage 2, 3, and 4 hepatoblastoma [70, 71].

Routine assessment of hearing, renal, and cardiac function is standard during treatment for pediatric malignancies. Post-chemotherapy neutropenia rarely represents additional concerns during the surgical treatment. Platinum compounds (cisplatin and carboplatin), which have been a backbone of the successful treatment for pediatric liver tumors, are also quite ototoxic. Around 40% of children develop significant hearing loss, which typically affects high-register tones, and could be delayed. Chronic dose-related nephrotoxicity remains a significant long-term issue for both chemotherapy for malignant liver tumors and calcineurin inhibitor-based immunosuppression. Therefore, early use of calcineurin inhibitor-sparing agents, such as mycophenolate mofetil or sirolimus, is recommended for children after LT for liver tumors. Nevertheless, it is prudent not to give chemotherapy 2 weeks before or after resection or LT.

In rare cases, intensive platinum- and doxorubicin-based multidrug chemotherapy can induce complete regressions in approximately 50% of patients, with subsequent 3-year event-free survival of 56% for pulmonary metastases and eliminated multinodular tumor foci in the liver. Chemotherapy has been much more successful in the treatment of hepatoblastoma than in hepatocellular carcinoma.

6.4. Other Treatment Approaches

Other treatment approaches such as transarterial chemoembolization, have been used for patients with postsurgically-staged stage III hepatoblastoma. Transarterial chemoembolization has been used in a few children to successfully shrink tumor size to permit resection.Cryosurgery, intratumoral injection of alcohol, and radiofrequency ablation can successfully treat small (<5 cm) tumors in adults with cirrhotic livers. Some local approaches such as cryosurgery, radiofrequency ablation, and transarterial chemoembolization that suppress hepatocellular carcinoma tumor progression are used as bridging therapy in adults to delay tumor growth while on a waiting list for cadaveric liver transplant [72].

7. Medical issues related to current chemotherapy

It is no surprise that most of the toxicity data stem from HB treatment survivors, while information from the HCC setting is lacking.

7.1. Recurrent hepatic tumors

The prognosis for a patient with recurrent or progressive hepatoblastoma depends on many factors, including the site of recurrence, prior treatment, and individual patient considerations. If possible, isolated metastases should be resected completely in patients whose primary tumor is controlled. For example, in patients with stage I hepatoblastoma at initial diagnosis, aggressive surgical treatment of isolated pulmonary metastases that develop in the course of the disease may make extended disease-free survival possible. Liver transplant should be considered for patients with isolated recurrence in the liver. Combined vincristine/irinotecan has been used with some success. Some patients treated with cisplatin/vincristine/fluorouracil could be salvaged with doxorubicin-containing regimens, but patients treated with doxorubicin/cisplatin could not be salvaged with vincristine/fluorouracil. Treatment in a clinical trial should be considered if all of the recurrent disease cannot be surgically removed. Phase I and phase II clinical trials may be appropriate and should be considered [73, 74].

The prognosis for a patient with recurrent or progressive hepatocellular carcinoma is poor. Chemoembolization or liver transplant should be considered for those with isolated recurrence in the liver. Phase I and phase II clinical trials may be appropriate and should be considered [75, 76].

8. Summary and future issues

Management of pediatric liver tumors has significantly improved over the last 2 decades. The principal reasons are that efficient chemotherapy and established medico-surgical treatment algorithms for HB have now integrated LT as a very valuable complementary treatment option. The management options for HCC are less effective and not well defined, broadly mirroring the therapeutic guidelines in adults except for a more cautionary approach to neoadjuvant and loco-regional methods. In the pediatric context the main clinical aims are to reduce chemotherapy toxicity (predominantly ototoxicity and nephrotoxicity) in children treated for HB and to investigate additional modes of treatment for HCC.

Improved understanding of HB and HCC biology may improve risk stratification a presentation and direct the treatment at specific molecular targets in the future. Management of less common benign and malignant tumors should benefit from establishing international collaborative pediatric networks such as the Pediatric Liver Unresectable Tumor Observatory (PLUTO).

Author details

Chunbao Guo* and Mingman Zhang*

*Address all correspondence to:

*Address all correspondence to:

Dept. of hepatobiliary Surgery, Children's Hospital, Chongqing Medical University, ChongqingP.R. China, P.R. China

References

[1] Smith, N. L., Altekruse, S. F., Ries, L. A., Melbert, D. L., O'Leary, M., Smith, F. O., & Reaman, G. H. (2010). Outcomes for children and adolescents with cancer: challenges for the twenty-first century. *J Clin Oncol.*, 28(15), 2625-34.

[2] Guidelines for the pediatric cancer center and role of such centers in diagnosis and treatment. (1997). *American Academy of Pediatrics Section Statement Section on Hematology/Oncology. Pediatrics*, 99(1), 139-41.

[3] Eheman, C., Henley, S. J., Ballard-Barbash, R., Jacobs, E. J., Schymura, Noone. A. M., Pan, L., Anderson, Fulton. J. E., Kohler, J. A., Ward, E., Plescia, M., Ries, L. A., & Edwards, B. K. (2012). Annual Report to the Nation on the status of cancer, 1975-2008, featuring cancers associated with excess weight and lack of sufficient physical activity. *Cancer.*, 118(9), 2338-66.

[4] Darbari, A., Sabin, K. M., Shapiro, C. N., & Schwarz, K. B. (2003). Epidemiology of primary hepatic malignancies in U.S. children. *Hepatology*, 38(3), 560-6.

[5] Czauderna, P., Otte, J. B., Aronson, D. C., Gauthier, F., Mackinlay, G., Roebuck, D., Plaschkes, J., & Perilongo, G. (2005). Childhood Liver Tumour Strategy Group of the International Society of Paediatric Oncology (SIOPEL). Guidelines for surgical treatment of hepatoblastoma in the modern era--recommendations from the Childhood Liver Tumour Strategy Group of the International Society of Paediatric Oncology (SIOPEL). *Eur J Cancer*, 41(7), 1031-6.

[6] Exelby, P. R., Filler, R. M., & Grosfeld, J. L. (1975). Liver tumors in children in the particular reference to hepatoblastoma and hepatocellular carcinoma: American Academy of Pediatrics Surgical Section Survey--1974. *J Pediatr Surg.*, 10(3), 329-37.

[7] Katzenstein, H. M., Krailo, Malogolowkin. M. H., Ortega, J. A., Liu-Mares, W., Douglass, E. C., Feusner, J. H., Reynolds, M., Quinn, J. J., Newman, K., Finegold, Haas. J. E., Sensel, M. G., Castleberry, R. P., & Bowman, L. C. (2002). Hepatocellular carcinoma in children and adolescents: results from the Pediatric Oncology Group and the Children's Cancer Group intergroup study. *J Clin Oncol.*, 20(12), 2789-97.

[8] Czauderna, P., Mackinlay, G., Perilongo, G., Brown, J., Shafford, E., Aronson, D., Pritchard, J., Chapchap, P., Keeling, J., Plaschkes, J., & Otte, J. B. (2002). Liver Tumors Study Group of the International Society of Pediatric Oncology. Hepatocellular carcinoma in children: results of the first prospective study of the International Society of Pediatric Oncology group. *J Clin Oncol.*, 20(12), 2798-804.

[9] Ortega, J. A., Douglass, E. C., Feusner, J. H., Reynolds, M., Quinn, J. J., King, D. R., Liu-Mares, W., & Sensel, M. G. (2000). Randomized comparison of cisplatin/vincristine/fluorouracil and cisplatin/continuous infusion doxorubicin for treatment of pediatric hepatoblastoma: A report from the Children's Cancer Group and the Pediatric Oncology Group. *J Clin Oncol.*, 18(14), 2665-75.

[10] Katzenstein, H. M., Krailo, Malogolowkin. M. H., Ortega, J. A., Liu-Mares, W., Douglass, E. C., Feusner, J. H., Reynolds, M., Quinn, J. J., Newman, K., Sensel, M. G., Castleberry, R. P., & Bowman, L. C. (2002). Hepatocellular carcinoma in children and adolescents: results from the Pediatric Oncology Group and the Children's Cancer Group intergroup study. *J Clin Oncol.*, 20(12), 2789-97.

[11] Andres, A. M., Hernandez, F., Lopez-Santamaría, M., Gámez, M., Murcia, J., Leal, N., López, Gutierrez. J. C., Frauca, E., Sastre, A., & Tovar, J. A. (2007). Surgery of liver tumors in children in the last 15 years. *Eur J Pediatr Surg.*, 17(6), 387-92.

[12] D'Antiga, L., Vallortigara, F., Cillo, U., Talenti, E., Rugge, M., Zancan, L., Dall'Igna, P., De Salvo, G. L., & Perilongo, G. (2007). Features predicting unresectability in hepatoblastoma. *Cancer.*, 110(5), 1050-8.

[13] Hemming, A. W., Reed, A. I., Fujita, S., Zendejas, I., Howard, R. J., & Kim, R. D. (2008). Role for extending hepatic resection using an aggressive approach to liver surgery. *J Am Coll Surg.*, 206(5), 870-5.

[14] Czauderna, P., Mackinlay, G., Perilongo, G., Brown, J., Shafford, E., Aronson, D., Pritchard, J., Chapchap, P., Keeling, J., Plaschkes, J., Otte, J. B., Liver, Tumors., Study, Group., of, the., International, Society., & of, Pediatric. (2002). Hepatocellular carcinoma in children: results of the first prospective study of the International Society of Pediatric Oncology group. *J Clin Oncol.*, 20(12), 2798-804.

[15] Otte, J. B., Pritchard, J., Aronson, D. C., Brown, J., Czauderna, P., Maibach, R., Perilongo, G., Shafford, E., Plaschkes, J., International, Society., of, Pediatric., & Oncology, . S. I. O. P. (2004). Liver transplantation for hepatoblastoma: results from the International Society of Pediatric Oncology (SIOP) study SIOPEL-1 and review of the world experience. *Pediatr Blood Cancer.*, 42(1), 74-83.

[16] Austin, M. T., Leys, C. M., Feurer, I. D., Lovvorn, H. N., O'Neill, J. A., Pinson, C. W., & Pietsch, J. B. (2006). Liver transplantation for childhood hepatic malignancy: a review of the United Network for Organ Sharing (UNOS) database. *J Pediatr Surg.*, 41(1), 182-6.

[17] Czauderna, P., Otte, J. B., Aronson, D. C., Gauthier, F., Mackinlay, G., Roebuck, D., Plaschkes, J., & Perilongo, G. (2005). Childhood Liver Tumour Strategy Group of the International Society of Paediatric Oncology (SIOPEL).Guidelines for surgical treatment of hepatoblastoma in the modern era--recommendations from the Childhood Liver Tumour Strategy Group of the International Society of Paediatric Oncology (SIOPEL). *Eur J Cancer.*, 41(7), 1031-6.

[18] Tsukuma, H., Hiyama, T., Tanaka, S., Nakao, M., Yabuuchi, T., Kitamura, T., Nakanishi, K., Fujimoto, I., Inoue, A., Yamazaki, H., et al. (1993). Risk factors for hepatocellular carcinoma among patients with chronic liver disease. *N Engl J Med.*, 328(25), 1797-801.

[19] González-Peralta, R. P., Langham, M. R., Jr Andres, J. M., Mohan, P., Colombani, P. M., Alford, M. K., & Schwarz, K. B. (2009). Hepatocellular carcinoma in 2 young adolescents with chronic hepatitis C. *J Pediatr Gastroenterol Nutr.*, 48(5), 630-5.

[20] Ni, Y. H., Chang, M. H., Hsu, H. Y., Hsu, H. C., Chen, C. C., Chen, W. J., & Lee, C. Y. (1991). Hepatocellular carcinoma in childhood. Clinical manifestations and prognosis. *Cancer*, 68(8), 1737-41.

[21] Stocker JT.Hepatic tumors in children. Clin Liver Dis. (2001). , 5(1), 259-81.

[22] De Ioris, M., Brugieres, L., Zimmermann, A., Keeling, J., Brock, P., Maibach, R., Pritchard, J., Shafford, L., Zsiros, J., Czaudzerna, P., & Perilongo, G. (2008). Hepatoblastoma with a low serum alpha-fetoprotein level at diagnosis: the SIOPEL group experience. *Eur J Cancer.*, 44(4), 545-50.

[23] Meyers, R. L., Rowland, J. R., Krailo, M., Chen, Z., Katzenstein, H. M., & Malogolowkin, M. H. (2009). Predictive power of pretreatment prognostic factors in children with hepatoblastoma: a report from the Children's Oncology Group. *Pediatr Blood Cancer*, 53(6), 1016-22.

[24] Schneider, D. T., Calaminus, G., & Göbel, U. (2001). Diagnostic value of alpha 1-fetoprotein and beta-human chorionic gonadotropin in infancy and childhood. *Pediatr Hematol Oncol.*, 18(1), 11-26.

[25] Nicol, K., Savell, V., Moore, J., Teot, L., Spunt, S. L., Qualman, S., Children's, Oncology., Group, Soft., & Tissue, Sarcoma. (2007). Distinguishing undifferentiated embryonal sarcoma of the liver from biliary tract rhabdomyosarcoma: a Children's Oncology Group study. *Pediatr Dev Pathol.*, 10(2), 89-97.

[26] Katzenstein, H. M., Steelman, C. K., Wulkan, M. L., Gow, K. W., Bridge, J. A., Kenney, Thompson. K., de Chadarévian, J. P., & Abramowsky, C. R. (2011). Undifferentiated embryonal sarcoma of the liver is associated with mesenchymal hamartoma and multiple chromosomal abnormalities: a review of eleven cases. *Pediatr Dev Pathol.*, 14(2), 111-6.

[27] Stringer, M. D., & Alizai, N. K. (2005). Mesenchymal hamartoma of the liver: a systematic review. *J Pediatr Surg.*, 40(11), 1681-90.

[28] Malogolowkin, M. H., Stanley, P., Steele, D. A., & Ortega, J. A. (2000). Feasibility and toxicity of chemoembolization for children with liver tumors. *J Clin Oncol.*, 18(6), 1279-84.

[29] Zsíros, J., Maibach, R., Shafford, E., Brugieres, L., Brock, P., Czauderna, P., Roebuck, D., Childs, M., Zimmermann, A., Laithier, V., Otte, J. B., de Camargo, B., Mac, Kinlay. G., Scopinaro, M., Aronson, D., Plaschkes, J., & Perilongo, G. (2010). Successful treatment of childhood high-risk hepatoblastoma with dose-intensive multiagent chemotherapy and surgery: final results of the SIOPEL-3HR study. *J Clin Oncol.*, 28(15), 2584-90.

[30] Clericuzio, C. L., Chen, E., Mc Neil, D. E., O'Connor, T., Zackai, E. H., Medne, L., Tomlinson, G., & De Baun, M. (2003). Serum alpha-fetoprotein screening for hepatoblastoma in children with Beckwith-Wiedemann syndrome or isolated hemihyperplasia. *J Pediatr.*, 143(2), 270-2.

[31] Malogolowkin, M. H., Stanley, P., Steele, D. A., & Ortega, J. A. (2000). Feasibility and toxicity of chemoembolization for children with liver tumors. *J Clin Oncol.*, 18(6), 1279-84.

[32] Tanimura, M., Matsui, I., Abe, J., Ikeda, H., Kobayashi, N., Ohira, M., Yokoyama, M., & Kaneko, M. (1998). Increased risk of hepatoblastoma among immature children with a lower birth weight. *Cancer Res.*, 58(14), 3032-5.

[33] Mc Laughlin, C. C., Baptiste, M. S., Schymura, M. J., Nasca, P. C., & Zdeb, M. S. (2006). Maternal and infant birth characteristics and hepatoblastoma. *Am J Epidemiol.*, 163(9), 818-28.

[34] Chang, M. H., Chen, T. H., Hsu, H. M., Wu, T. C., Kong, M. S., Liang, D. C., Ni, Y. H., Chen, C. J., & Chen, D. S. (2005). Taiwan Childhood HCC Study Group. Prevention of hepatocellular carcinoma by universal vaccination against hepatitis B virus: the effect and problems. *Clin Cancer Res.*, 11(21), 7953-7.

[35] Zsíros, J., Maibach, R., Shafford, E., Brugieres, L., Brock, P., Czauderna, P., Roebuck, D., Childs, M., Zimmermann, A., Laithier, V., Otte, J. B., de Camargo, B., Mac, Kinlay. G., Scopinaro, M., Aronson, D., Plaschkes, J., & Perilongo, G. (2010). Successful treatment of childhood high-risk hepatoblastoma with dose-intensive multiagent chemotherapy and surgery: final results of the SIOPEL-3HR study. *J Clin Oncol.*, 28(15), 2584-90.

[36] Schnater, J. M., Aronson, D. C., Plaschkes, J., Perilongo, G., Brown, J., Otte, J. B., Brugieres, L., Czauderna, P., Mac, Kinlay. G., & Vos, A. (2002). Surgical view of the treatment of patients with hepatoblastoma: results from the first prospective trial of the International Society of Pediatric Oncology Liver Tumor Study Group. *Cancer*, 94(4), 1111-20.

[37] Yoon, J. M., Burns, R. C., Malogolowkin, M. H., & Mascarenhas, L. (2007). Treatment of infantile choriocarcinoma of the liver. *Pediatr Blood Cancer.*, 49(1), 99-102.

[38] Brown, J., Perilongo, G., Shafford, E., Keeling, J., Pritchard, J., Brock, P., Dicks-Mireaux, C., Phillips, A., Vos, A., & Plaschkes, J. (2000). Pretreatment prognostic factors for children with hepatoblastoma-- results from the International Society of Paediatric Oncology (SIOP) study SIOPEL 1. *Eur J Cancer*, 36(11), 1418-25.

[39] Perilongo, G., Shafford, E., Maibach, R., Aronson, D., Brugières, L., Brock, P., Childs, M., Czauderna, P., Mac, Kinlay. G., Otte, J. B., Pritchard, J., Rondelli, R., Scopinaro, M., Staalman, C., Plaschkes, J., International, Society., of, Paediatric., & Oncology-S, I. O. P. E. L. . (2004). Risk-adapted treatment for childhood hepatoblastoma. final report of the second study of the International Society of Paediatric Oncology--SIOPEL 2. *Eur J Cancer.*, 40(3), 411-21.

[40] DeBaun, M.R., & Tucker, M.A. (1998). Risk of cancer during the first four years of life in children from The Beckwith-Wiedemann Syndrome Registry. *J Pediatr.*, 132, (3 Pt 1):398-400.

[41] Sparago, A., Russo, S., Cerrato, F., Ferraiuolo, S., Castorina, P., Selicorni, A., Schwienbacher, C., Negrini, M., Ferrero, G. B., Silengo, M. C., Anichini, C., Larizza, L., & Riccio, A. (2007). Mechanisms causing imprinting defects in familial Beckwith-Wiedemann syndrome with Wilms' tumour. *Hum Mol Genet*, 16(3), 254-64.

[42] Algar, E. M., St, Heaps. L., Darmanian, A., Dagar, V., Prawitt, D., Peters, G. B., & Collins, F. (2007). Paternally inherited submicroscopic duplication at 1115 implicates insulin-like growth factor II in overgrowth and Wilms' tumorigenesis. *Cancer Res.*

[43] Steenman, M., Westerveld, A., & Mannens, M. (2000). Genetics of Beckwith-Wiedemann syndrome-associated tumors: common genetic pathways. *Genes Chromosomes Cancer.*, 28(1), 1-13.

[44] Roebuck, D. J., Olsen, Ø., & Pariente, D. (2006). Radiological staging in children with hepatoblastoma. *Pediatr Radiol.*, 36(3), 176-82.

[45] Tiao, G. M., Bobey, N., Allen, S., Nieves, N., Alonso, M., Bucuvalas, J., Wells, R., & Ryckman, F. (2005). The current management of hepatoblastoma: a combination of chemotherapy, conventional resection, and liver transplantation. *J Pediatr.*, 146(2), 204-11.

[46] Atri, P., Paredes, J. L., Di Cicco, L. A., Sindhi, R., Soltys, K. A., Mazariegos, G. V., & Kane, T. D. (2010). Review of outcomes of primary liver cancers in children: our institutional experience with resection and transplantation. *Surgery*, 148(4), 778-82.

[47] Otte, J. B., Pritchard, J., Aronson, D. C., Brown, J., Czauderna, P., Maibach, R., Perilongo, G., Shafford, E., & Plaschkes, J. (2004). International Society of Pediatric Oncology (SIOP). Liver transplantation for hepatoblastoma: results from the International Society of Pediatric Oncology (SIOP) study SIOPEL-1 and review of the world experience. *Pediatr Blood Cancer*, 42(1), 74-83.

[48] Douglass, E. C., Reynolds, M., Finegold, M., Cantor, A. B., & Glicksman, A. (1993). Cisplatin, vincristine, and fluorouracil therapy for hepatoblastoma: a Pediatric Oncology Group study. *J Clin Oncol.*, 11(1), 96-9.

[49] Pritchard, J., Brown, J., Shafford, E., Perilongo, G., Brock, P., Dicks-Mireaux, C., Keeling, J., Phillips, A., Vos, A., & Plaschkes, J. (2000). Cisplatin, doxorubicin, and delayed surgery for childhood hepatoblastoma: a successful approach--results of the first prospective study of the International Society of Pediatric Oncology. *J Clin Oncol.*, 18(22), 3819-28.

[50] Perilongo, G., Shafford, E., Maibach, R., Aronson, D., Brugières, L., Brock, P., Childs, M., Czauderna, P., Mac, Kinlay. G., Otte, J. B., Pritchard, J., Rondelli, R., Scopinaro, M., Staalman, C., & Plaschkes, J. (2004). International Society of Paediatric Oncology-SIOPEL 2.Risk-adapted treatment for childhood hepatoblastoma. final report of the second study of the International Society of Paediatric Oncology--SIOPEL 2. *Eur J Cancer*, 40(3), 411-21.

[51] Feusner, J. H., Krailo, M. D., Haas, J. E., Campbell, J. R., Lloyd, D. A., & Ablin, A. R. (1993). Treatment of pulmonary metastases of initial stage I hepatoblastoma in childhood. *Report from the Childrens Cancer Group. Cancer*, 71(3), 859-64.

[52] Perilongo, G., Brown, J., Shafford, E., Brock, P., De Camargo, B., Keeling, J. W., Vos, A., Philips, A., Pritchard, J., & Plaschkes, J. (2000). Hepatoblastoma presenting with

lung metastases: treatment results of the first cooperative, prospective study of the International Society of Paediatric Oncology on childhood liver tumors. *Cancer*, 89(8), 1845-53.

[53] Malogolowkin, M. H., Katzenstein, H. M., Krailo, M., Chen, Z., Quinn, J. J., Reynolds, M., & Ortega, J. A. (2008). Redefining the role of doxorubicin for the treatment of children with hepatoblastoma. *J Clin Oncol.*, 26(14), 2379-83.

[54] Lubienski, A. Hepatocellular carcinoma: interventional bridging to liver transplantation. *Transplantation*, 2005. 80(1 Suppl):S113-9.

[55] Otte, J. B., Pritchard, J., Aronson, D. C., Brown, J., Czauderna, P., Maibach, R., Perilongo, G., Shafford, E., Plaschkes, J., International, Society., of, Pediatric., & Oncology, . S. I. O. P. (2004). Liver transplantation for hepatoblastoma: results from the International Society of Pediatric Oncology (SIOP) study SIOPEL-1 and review of the world experience. *Pediatr Blood Cancer*, 42(1), 74-83.

[56] Reyes, Carr. B., Dvorchik, I., Kocoshis, S., Jaffe, R., Gerber, D., Mazariegos, G. V., Bueno, J., & Selby, R. (2000). Liver transplantation and chemotherapy for hepatoblastoma and hepatocellular cancer in childhood and adolescence. *J Pediatr.*, 136(6), 795-804.

[57] Austin, M. T., Leys, C. M., Feurer, I. D., Lovvorn, H. N., O'Neill, J. A., Pinson, C. W., & Pietsch, J. B. (2006). Liver transplantation for childhood hepatic malignancy: a review of the United Network for Organ Sharing (UNOS) database. *J Pediatr Surg.*, 41(1), 182-6.

[58] Beaunoyer, M., Vanatta, J. M., Ogihara, M., Strichartz, D., Dahl, G., Berquist, W. E., Castillo, R. O., Cox, K. L., & Esquivel, C. O. (2007). Outcomes of transplantation in children with primary hepatic malignancy. *Pediatr Transplant.*, 11(6), 655-60.

[59] Guiteau, J. J., Cotton, R. T., Karpen, S. J., O'Mahony, C. A., & Goss, J. A. (2010). Pediatric liver transplantation for primary malignant liver tumors with a focus on hepatic epithelioid hemangioendothelioma: the UNOS experience. *Pediatr Transplant.*, 14(3), 326-31.

[60] Suh, M. Y., Wang, K., Gutweiler, J. R., Misra, M. V., Krawczuk, L. E., Jenkins, R. L., & Lillehei, C. W. (2008). Safety of minimal immunosuppression in liver transplantation for hepatoblastoma. *J Pediatr Surg.*, 43(6), 1148-52.

[61] Browne, M., Sher, D., Grant, D., Deluca, E., Alonso, E., Whitington, P. F., & Superina, R. A. (2008). Survival after liver transplantation for hepatoblastoma: a 2-center experience. *J Pediatr Surg.*, 43(11), 1973-81.

[62] Faraj, W., Dar, F., Marangoni, G., Bartlett, A., Melendez, H. V., Hadzic, D., Dhawan, A., Mieli-Vergani, G., Rela, M., & Heaton, N. (2008). Liver transplantation for hepatoblastoma. *Liver Transpl.*, 14(11), 1614-9.

[63] Austin, M. T., Leys, C. M., Feurer, I. D., Lovvorn, H. N., 3rd O'Neill, J. A., Pinson, C. W., & Pietsch, J. B. (2006). Liver transplantation for childhood hepatic malignancy: a

review of the United Network for Organ Sharing (UNOS) database. *J Pediatr Surg.*, 41(1), 182-6.

[64] Heaton, N., Faraj, W., Melendez, H. V., Jassem, W., Muiesan, P., Mieli-Vergani, G., Dhawan, A., & Rela, M. (2008). Living related liver transplantation in children. *Br J Surg.*, 95(7), 919-24.

[65] Reyes, Carr. B., Dvorchik, I., Kocoshis, S., Jaffe, R., Gerber, D., Mazariegos, G. V., Bueno, J., & Selby, R. (2000). Liver transplantation and chemotherapy for hepatoblastoma and hepatocellular cancer in childhood and adolescence. *J Pediatr.*, 136(6), 795-804.

[66] Sevmis, S., Karakayali, H., Ozçay, F., Canan, O., Bilezikci, B., Torgay, A., & Haberal, M. (2008). Liver transplantation for hepatocellular carcinoma in children. *Pediatr Transplant.*, 12(1), 52-6.

[67] Madanur, Battula. N., Davenport, M., Dhawan, A., & Rela, M. (2007). Staged resection for a ruptured hepatoblastoma: a 6-year follow-up. *Pediatr Surg Int.*, 23(6), 609-11.

[68] Schnater, J. M., Aronson, D. C., Plaschkes, J., Perilongo, G., Brown, J., Otte, J. B., Brugieres, L., Czauderna, P., Mac, Kinlay. G., & Vos, A. (2002). Surgical view of the treatment of patients with hepatoblastoma: results from the first prospective trial of the International Society of Pediatric Oncology Liver Tumor Study Group. *Cancer*, 94(4), 1111-20.

[69] Otte, J.B. (2008). Should the selection of children with hepatocellular carcinoma be based on Milan criteria? *Pediatr Transplant.*, 12(1), 1-3.

[70] Douglass, E. C., Reynolds, M., Finegold, M., Cantor, A. B., & Glicksman, A. (1993). Cisplatin, vincristine, and fluorouracil therapy for hepatoblastoma: a Pediatric Oncology Group study. *J Clin Oncol.*, 11(1), 96-9.

[71] Ortega, J. A., Douglass, E. C., Feusner, J. H., Reynolds, M., Quinn, J. J., Finegold, Haas. J. E., King, D. R., Liu-Mares, W., Sensel, M. G., & Krailo, M.D. (2000). Randomized comparison of cisplatin/vincristine/fluorouracil and cisplatin/continuous infusion doxorubicin for treatment of pediatric hepatoblastoma: A report from the Children's Cancer Group and the Pediatric Oncology Group. *J Clin Oncol.*, 18(14), 2665-75.

[72] Habrand, J. L., Nehme, D., Kalifa, C., Gauthier, F., Gruner, M., Sarrazin, D., & Terrier-Lacombe, Lemerle. J. (1992). Is there a place for radiation therapy in the management of hepatoblastomas and hepatocellular carcinomas in children? *Int J Radiat Oncol Biol Phys.*, 23(3), 525-31.

[73] Feusner, J. H., Krailo, M. D., Haas, J. E., Campbell, J. R., Lloyd, D. A., & Ablin, A. R. (1993). Treatment of pulmonary metastases of initial stage I hepatoblastoma in childhood. *Report from the Childrens Cancer Group. Cancer*, 71(3), 859-64.

[74] Perilongo, G., Brown, J., Shafford, E., Brock, P., De Camargo, B., Keeling, J. W., Vos, A., Philips, A., Pritchard, J., & Plaschkes, J. (2000). Hepatoblastoma presenting with lung metastases: treatment results of the first cooperative, prospective study of the International Society of Paediatric Oncology on childhood liver tumors. *Cancer.*, 89(8), 1845-53.

[75] Robertson, P. L., Muraszko, K. M., & Axtell, R. A. (1997). Hepatoblastoma metastatic to brain: prolonged survival after multiple surgical resections of a solitary brain lesion. *J Pediatr Hematol Oncol.*, 19(2), 168-71.

[76] Perilongo, G., Maibach, R., Shafford, E., Brugieres, L., Brock, P., Morland, B., de Camargo, B., Zsiros, J., Roebuck, D., Zimmermann, A., Aronson, D., Childs, M., Widing, E., Laithier, V., Plaschkes, J., Pritchard, J., Scopinaro, M., Mac, Kinlay. G., & Czauderna, P. (2009). Cisplatin versus cisplatin plus doxorubicin for standard-risk hepatoblastoma. *N Engl J Med.*, 361(17), 1662-70.

Chapter 6

Surgical Management in Portal Hypertension

Hiroshi Yoshida, Yasuhiro Mamada,
Nobuhiko Taniai, Takashi Tajiri and Eiji Uchida

Additional information is available at the end of the chapter

1. Introduction

Bleeding from esophagogastricvarices is a catastrophic complication of chronic liver disease. There are various treatments for esophagogastricvarices, such as endoscopic treatment, interventional radioligy, and surgical procedure [1-3]. Recently, "General Rules for Recording Endoscopic Findings of EsophagogastricVarices [4]" were establised and endoscopic treatment further improved survival rates [5].

Many years ago, operation was the only treatment available. A number of surgical procedures have been developed to manage esophagogastricvarices [6]. Broadly, these can be classified as shunting and nonshunting procedures.

We showed the surgical procedures for the treatment of esophagogastricvarices.

2. Operation technique

2.1. Shunting procedures

There are various shunting procedures for the treatment of esophagogastricvarices [7-25]. There are two types of shunting procedures, nonselective shunt and selective shunt. Nonselective shunts, such as portacaval or mesocaval shunts, reduce portal venous pressure and improve esophagogastricvarices. While nonselective shunt is associated with a high risk of hepatic encephalopathy secondary to the hyperammonemia that is caused by impaired protein metabolism in the liver [26-28].

Selective shunts, such as distal splenorenal shunt (DSRS) or left gastric venous caval shunt (Inokuchi shunt), maintain portal pressure and selectively reduce esophagogastricvariceal pressure. Shunt surgery is the best procedure in terms of preventing recurrent bleeding [20-22], but carries a high risk of postoperative encephalopathy, especially after nonselective shunt [26-28]. Even in selective shunt, loss of shunt selectivity occurs occasionally, leading to postoperative encephalopathy [8, 14].

2.1.1. Nonselective shunt

2.1.1.1. Portacaval and mesocaval shunt

The mesocaval shunt was initially used to control bleeding from esophageal varices in children with congenital abnormalities of the hepatobiliary system. The procedure consisted of transposition of the divided inferior vena cava and the divided superior mesenteric vein, hence its name, mesocaval shunt. This operation was modified, and some reports have described a portacaval or mesocaval interposition shunt with a graft (H-graft mesocaval shunt) [9, 10, 29-33]. Millikan et al. [26] have reported that the incidence of hyperammonemia after nonselective shunt procedures was as high as 75%.

2.1.2. Selective shunt

2.1.2.1. Left gastric venous caval shunt (Inokuchi shunt)

To assure postoperative portal perfusion and to prevent Eck's syndrome, in 1967 Inokuchi designed a selective shunt, called the left gastric venous caval shunt [7, 19, 23-25].

After dilatation, and engorgement of the left gastric vein is confirmed by splenoportography, the gastrohepatic ligament is opened and the left gastric vein is identified, and dissected 2 cm towards its junction with the portal system or splenic vein. The vein dissection must be done carefully to avoid hemorrhage, since the wall of the left gastric vein is weak due to increased portal vein pressure. The anastomosis is then performed between the distal end of the transected left gastric vein and the inferior vena cava. The autograft, the great saphenous vein, is anastomosed to the inferior vena cava in an end-to-side fashion, and opposite end is pulled through the suprapancreatic space. After the anastomosis is completed, a splenectomysi done. If splenectomy is not indicated, short gastric vein ligation is necessary in order to decrease the collateral circulation from the greater curvature of the stomach. The selection of a caval anastomosis procedure depends upon anatomical individuality or operative difficulty or both. The left gastric venous-caval shunt can be modified in three ways, left gastric-spermatic (ovarian) shunt, left gastric-adrenal shunt, or left gastric-renal shunt.

Postoperative mean portal pressure was 335 mm of water, and although it is decreased whe compared to 363 mm water at laparotomy, this may be the result of solenectomy. On the other hand, left gastric venous pressure decreased from 316 mm of water to 211 mm of water postoperatively [7].

2.1.2.2. DSRS

Original DSRS: The DSRS is a selective shunt that was developed by Warren (original DSRS) in 1967 [12] to preserve portal blood flow through the liver while lowering variceal pressure. The hope was that both bleeding and hyperammonemia would be prevented. DSRS effectively prevents rebleeding, but still carries a risk of hyperammonemia [14].

The procedure for DSRS consists of anastomosis of the distal end of the splenic vein to the left renal vein, and devascularization of left gastric artery and vein. The specific objectives of DSRS as stated in the original publication [12] were : 1) selective reduction of pressure and volume of flow through gastroesophageal veins; 2) maintaining portal venous perfusion of the liver; and 3) maintaining continual venous hypertension in the intestinal bed. These three objectives formed a basis for much subsequent work.

Henderson et al. [34]compared hemodynamics between alcoholic and nonalcoholic cirrhotic patients after DSRS. Portal perfusion and liver blood flow are maintained, both quantitatively and qualitatively, in nonalcoholic patients with cirrhosis, resulting in better hepatocyte function and improved survival.

Stenosis of a DSRS shunt may lead to inadequate variceal decompression, accompanied by a risk of rebleeding. Henderson et al. [35]reported that the patients with stenosis of a DSRS were successfully managed by balloon dilation. All of the shunts were patent, but showed a mean pressure gradient of 15 millimeters of mercury, which was reduced to a mean of 7 millimeters of mercury by dilation. Although, repeat angiography should be performed in patients with rebleeding or reappearance of varices after DSRS to determine the cause.

DSRS + splenopancreatic disconnection (SPD): Belghiti et al. [8] reported loss of shunt selectivity during long-term follow-up in patients who underwent original DSRS, confirmed via the pancreatic vein. Warren et al. [36] subsequently improved the DSRS procedure by adding SPD, i.e., skeletonization of the splenic vein from the pancreas to its bifurcation at the splenic hilum. The operation technique is as follows: The pancreas is approached through the lesser sac, with the additional takedown of the splenic flexure to improve access to the retropancreatic plane. The whole pancreas is mobilized along its inferior border from the superior mesenteric vein to the splenic hilus. The pancreatic perforating veins are ligated as they enter the splenic vein. It is imperative to sufficiently dissect the splenic vein from the pancreas and to carefully manipulate the junction between the splenic and superior mesenteric vein to ensure that skeletonization proceeds to the renal vein without kinking. The key to the entire procedure lies in accurate identification and ligation of the pancreatic perforating veins as they enter the splenic vein. The anastomosis should also be performed without tension or kinking of the splenic vein. Typically, the anastomosis lies just in front of the ligated adrenal vein on the left renal vein with continuous suture.

Moon et al. [37] examined the outcomes of DSRS+SPD in children to evaluate the usefulness of this operation. The platelet count and white cell count increased significantly after DSRS +SPD. Spleen size decreased significantly. No patient underwent subsequent transplantation or endoscopic treatment for esophagogastricvarices after DSRS+SPD.

DSRS + SPD + gastric transection (GT): Loss of shunt selectivity was still observed via collateral pathways through the stomach [20]. We therefore modified DSRS by additionally performing SPD and GT to prevent loss of shunt selectivity. GT involved transection and anastomosis of the upper stomach with an autosuture instrument. The short gastric arteries and veins were spared. Katoh et al. [38] performed transection and re-suture of the seromuscular layer of the upper stomach to prevent loss of selectivity after DSRS + SPD. They called this procedure "superselective DSRS." We performed transection of all layers, whereas Katoh et al. transected only the seromuscular layer of the upper stomach.

We compared long-term results for three types of DSRS for the treatment of esophageal varices. Additional treatment for recurrent varices was required in the original DSRS group (9.1%), DSRS with SPD group (18.2%), and DSRS with SPD plus GT group (4.3%). All of the patients with recurrent varices had shunt stenosis within the first year after DSRS. The prevalence of hyperammonemia in the DSRS with SPD plus GT group was significantly lower than that in the original DSRS group and the DSRS with SPD group (P<0.01). There were no significant differences in survival among the three groups. DSRS with SPD plus GT may reduce the incidence of postoperative hyperammonemia [14]. Kanaya et al. [39] have reported that the incidence of hyperammonemia after DSRS with SPD plus gastric disconnection (transection of only the seromuscular layer of the upper stomach) was 3.2%. We found that the prevalence of hyperammonemia after DSRS with SPD plus GT was 0% at 1 year, 9.1% at 5 years, and 9.1% at 10 years [14]. The loss of shunt selectivity promotes hyperammonemia and decreases portal blood flow. High serum ammonia concentrations result in encephalopathy. We previously reported that obliteration of portosystemic shunts followed by partial splenic embolization is beneficial in patients with portosystemic encephalopathy. Portal venous pressures were similar before and after treatment in patients who underwent embolization of portosystemic shunts followed by partial splenic embolization [40, 41]. In patients who had portosystemic encephalopathy after DSRS, however, elevated portal venous pressures after embolization of portosystemic shunts can notreduced by partial splenic embolization. Fisher et al. [42] have reported normalization of hyperammonemia after administration of a solution enriched with branched chain amino acids. All patients with hyperammonemia in our study should received branched chain amino acids [14]. However, patients with hyperammonemia require long-term nutritional support, negatively affecting their quality of life. Liver dysfunction was controlled with good nutritional support. We found no significant differences in cumulative survival among the original DSRS group, DSRS with SPD group, and DSRS with SPD plus GT group [14]. Kanaya et al. [39] have reported better 5- and 7-year survival rates after DSRS with SPD plus gastric disconnection than after standard DSRS.

Santambrogio et al. [43] compared endoscopic injection sclerotherapy (EIS) with DSRS for the prevention of recurrent variceal bleeding in cirrhotic patients who underwent long-term follow-up. They concluded that DSRS with a correct portal-azygos disconnection more effectively prevents varicealrebleeding than EIS in a subgroup of patients with good liver function. However, this positive effect did not influence long-term survival because other factors (e.g., hepatocellular carcinoma) were more important determinants of the outcomes of the cirrhotic patients with portal hypertension.

Rikkers et al. (13)performed a prospective, randomized trial to evaluate the effectiveness of DSRS for the treatment of cirrhotic patients who previously had bleeding from esophageal varices. A total of 55 patients were randomly assined to receive a DSRS (26 patients) or a nonselective shunt (29 patients). Three operative deaths occurred in each group. Early post-operative angiography revealed preservation of hepatic portal perfusion in 14 of 16 selective patients (88%), but in only 1 of 20 nonselective patients (p<0.001). Quantitative measures of hepatic function (maximal rate of urea synthesis and Child's score) were similar to preoperative values in the selective shunt, but had significantly decreased in the nonselective shunt on the first postoperative evaluation. Encephalopathy has not developed in any patient with continued portal perfusion, as compared with 45% of patients without portal flow (p<0.05). No significant differences the between selective and nonselective shunt have been detected with respect to total cumulative mortality (10 selective, 38%; 8 nonselective, 28%), shunt occlusion (2 selective, 10%; 5 nonselective, 18%), or recurrent variceal hemorrhage (1 selective, 4%; 2 nonselective, 8%). Overall, postoperative encephalopathy has developed in significantly fewer selective patients (3 selective, 12%; 15 nonselective, 52%; p<0.001). Therefore, they conclude that the DSRS, especially when its objective of maintaining hepatic portal perfusion is achieved, results in significantly less morbidity than nonselective shunt.

Warren et al. (44) reported the metabolic basis of portosystemic encephalopathy and compared the effects of selective vs. nonselective shunts. Metabolic studies were done in the Clinical Research Unit during a 14-day stay under carefully controlled dietary conditions. Maximal rate of urea systhesis did not change in patients with DSRS, but decreased significantly in those with nonselective shunt. Likewise, ammonium chloride tolerance, defined as the smallest dose required to produce a 40-μg/dL rise in the plasma ammonia concentration, was unchanged in the DSRS group, but significantly worsened in the nonselective shunt group.

Galambos et al. [45]compared nonselective shunt with selective shunt for the treatment of bleeding esophageal varices in a randomized controlled trial. A total of 48 patients were randomly assigned to receive a nonselective shunt (24 patients) or a selective shunt (24 patients). Mortality rates, the frequencies of shunt occlusion, and the frequencies of recurrent gastrointestinal bleeding were similar. Encephalopathy developed more often after a nonselective shunt than after a selective shunt. Nonselective shunts consistently diverted the hepatopetal mesenteric-portal flow from the liver. Deterioration of hepatic function was greater after nonselective than selective shunt.

2.2. Nonshunting procedures

Historically, nonshunting procedures were developed in an attempt to decrease the high rates of encephalopathy associated with portosystemic anastomoses. An alternative to total shunt was developed by Sugiura and Futagawa in 1973 [46]. Esophageal transection (ET) disrupts the blood supply to esophagogastricvarices. ET solves the problem of hepatic encephalopathy; unfortunately, however, varices can recur because portal pressure remains high.

Various nonshunting procedures, such as the Hassab operation, ET, splenectomy, or terminal esophago-proximal gastrectomy, have been developed to treat esophagogastricvarices

[46-49]. All nonshunting procedures performesplenectomy. Portal vein thrombosis is not a rare complication of splenectomy and can be fatal in patients with hypersplenism. Kawana- ka et al. reported that low antithrombin 3 activity and futher decreases in this activity are associated with portal vein thrombosis after splenectomy in cirrhotic patients, and that treat- ment with antithrombin 3 concentrates is likely to prevent the development of portal vein thrombosis in thease patients [50].

2.2.1. Splenectomy

Splenectomy was one of the earliest nonshunting procedures. It was found to be generally ineffective for preventing recurrent variceal bleeding [51]. Despite elimination of the splenic component of the portal circulation, portal hypertension is maintained after simple splenec- tomy, and the risk of continued bleeding via the splenic venous branches is high.

Recently, laparosopicsplenectomy is wadely accepted as a standard treatment for hemato- logic disorders such as idiopathic thrombocytopenic purpura. Laparoscopic splenectomy is improved safty in liver cirrhosis patients with portal hypertension [52].

2.2.2. Hassab operation

In 1967, Hassab [47] reported a successful technique for gastroesophageal decongestion and splenectomy, developed in Egypt. Most of his patients had schistosomiasis. The operation entailed removal of the spleen as well as devascularization of the cardiac portion of the stomach and abdominal portion of the esophagus, including the supraphrenic veins. By li- gating the left gastric artery and splenic artery, portal blood flow was also decreased, there- by decompressing the portal system. Recently, the Hassab operation has been employed in patients with varices limited to the stomach.

2.2.3. Terminal esophago-proximal gastrectomy

Terminal esophago-proximal gastrectomy involves proximal gastric transection and autosuture proximal gastrectomy in association with extensive devascularization and splenectomy [49].

2.2.4. ET

Among non-shunting procedures for the treatment of esophagogastricvarices, ET has been the most popular operation. ET in Japan was first performed in 1967 [53], using a modifica- tion of Walker's procedure for transthoracic ET [54]. The procedure was then refined by Su- giura and Futagawa in 1973 [46]. ET consists of paraesophagealdevascularization, esophageal transection and reanastomosis, splenectomy, and pyloroplasty. First, splenecto- my with devascularization of the greater curvature was performed. Devascularization of the lesser curvature was done from the angle to the esophagogastric junction, and the left gas- tric artery was ligated and divided. The esophagus and cardia were devascularized from the lesser to the greater curvature. Then, the vagal nerve and paraesophageal vessels were ligat- ed and divided. The esophagus was completely transected above the esophagogastric junc- tion, and the mucosa was anastomosed with interrupted sutures, performed recently with an autosuture instrument. ET was done using three different approaches, transthoracic, thoracoabdominal, and transabdominal. Devascularization of the esophagus and the stomach is most extensive and complete in the thoracoabdominal approach; however, this is the most drastic procedure.

Sugiura et al. [55] reported on 636 patients with portal hypertension in whom ETs with paraesophagogastricdevascularization were performed to manage esophageal varices. The operative mortality rates were as follows: emergency cases 13.7%, elective cases 3.2%, prophylactic cases 4.3%, and overall 5.2%. There were no deaths among the 233 patients in Child's class A; the 232 patients in class B had a 2% mortality rate, and the 171 patients in class C had a 17% mortality rate. The 10-year actuarial survival rates in patients with cirrhosis were 55% in emergency cases, 72% in prophylactic cases, and 72% in elective cases. In patients without cirrhosis, the corresponding survival rates were 90%, 96%, and 95%, respectively. The recurrence rate of variceal bleeding or varices was less than 5%. They concluded that the Sugiura procedure is safe and effective for controlling esophageal varices and prolongs the long-term survival of patients with portal hypertension.

In our study, however, the recurrence rate of varices after ET was high [21]. We examined hemodynamic changes associated with recurrent esophageal varices after ET and evaluated the effectiveness of EIS for their treatment. Nineteen patients with recurrent esophageal varices after ET were treated by EIS. Endoscopic varicealography during injection sclerotherapy (EVIS), following oral blockage of flow by a balloon, identified three patterns: type 1 (common type), continuous filling by the feeder vessel of the varix; type 2 (retrograde disappearing type), confirmed hepatofugal flow; and type 3 (immediate washout type), immediate washout of contrast medium. Angiography showed that the hepatofugal feeder vessel was the right gastric vein in all cases. Recurrent esophageal varices were classified as type 1 in 14 patients (73.7%), type 2 in 4 (21.1%), and type 3 in 1 (5.3%). Fewer treatment sessions were required in type 1 than in type 2 varices (p<0.005). Recurrent varices were completely eradicated in all patients except the patient with type 3 disease. Cumulative re-recurrence rates at 5 and 10 years were higher in type 1 than in type 2 varices without significance (28.6% and 71.4% vs. 25.0% and 25.0%, respectively). Cumulative survival rates after EIS at 5 and 10 years also were similar for type 1 and type 2 varices (77.1% and 66.1% vs. 66.7% and 66.7%). EIS was thus effective for the management of recurrent esophageal varices after ET, excluding type 3 disease [56].

Cleva et al. [57] compared the systemic hemodynamic effects of DSRS with those of esophagogastricdevascularization and splenectomy in patients treated for schistosomal portal hypertension. The hyperdynamic circulatory state observed in Manson's schistosomiasis was corrected by esophagogastricdevascularization and splenectomy, but persisted in patients who underwent DSRS. Similarly, the elevated mean pulmonary artery pressure resolved after esophagogastricdevascularization and splenectomy, but persisted after DSRS. They concluded that esophagogastricdevascularization and splenectomy seems to be the most physiologic operation for patients with schistosomal portal hypertension.

We compared the long-term results of DSRS and ET in cirrhotic patients with complete variceal eradication who were followed up for at least 3 years. There was no recurrent varix in the DSRS group. The cumulative recurrence rates of varices in the ET group were 31.6% and

52.5% at 5 and 10 years, respectively. The cumulative rates of hyperammonemia at 5 and 10 years were significantly higher in the DSRS group (30.4%, 30.4%) than in the ET group (0%, 5.6%) (p=0.009). The cumulative survival rates in the DSRS group vs. the ET group were 90.9% vs. 94.7% at 5 years and 85.2% vs. 81.7% at 10 years (NS). These results suggest that DSRS is more effective than ET in preventing recurrence of esophageal varices, but is associated with a higher incidence of hyperammonemia [21]. In that study, no patient who underwent DSRS with complete eradication had recurrent varices. When collateral pathways to the esophagus develop after DSRS, flow is via the short gastric veins, the splenic vein, and the left renal vein. After ET, collateral pathways to the esophagus develop across the transection site and generate new varices. Most of the recurrent varices in the ET group were supplied by the right gastric vein across the transection site [56]. However, collateral flow in the DSRS group decreased hepatic blood flow and led to the development of postoperative hyperammonemia. Rikkers et al. [58] reported that patients with no hepatic portal perfusion had the worst survival and greatest morbidity after DSRS.

Idiopathic portal hypertension (IPH) is a disease of unknown etiology characterized by splenomegaly, anemia, and portal hypertension. This disorder develops in the absence of liver cirrhosis, extrahepatic portal vein occlusion, schistosomiasis, or any other identifiable cause [59, 60]. We evaluated the results of shunting and nonshunting procedures for the treatment of esophagogastricvarices in patients with IPH. Esophagogastricvarices were completely eradicated in 3 (75.0%) patients in the shunting group and 4 (80.0%) in the nonshunting group. Additional endoscopic treatment (one session) was performed in 2 patients with incompletely eradicated varices. There was no recurrence in the shunting group. In the nonshunting group, esophagogastricvarices recurred in all 4 patients with completely eradicated varices. All recurrent esophageal varices were completely eradicated. Postoperative platelet counts ($\times 10^4/\mu L$) were significantly lower in the shunting group (10.0±2.6) than in the nonshunting group (42.0±14.0) (p=0.0029). The increase in the platelet count after operation was significantly lower in the shunting group (1.7±0.2 times) than in the nonshunting group (5.8±2.9 times) (p=0.0267). No patient received anticoagulants postoperatively. Portal venous thrombus did not develop in the shunting group, but appeared in 4 patients (80.0%) in the nonshunting group. No patient had loss of shunt selectivity or portal-systemic encephalopathy. One patient in the nonshunting group died of cerebral hemorrhage; all others are alive. Shunting procedure, DSRS, was suggested to be useful for the management of esophagogastricvarices in patients with IPH [61].

Author details

Hiroshi Yoshida[1*], Yasuhiro Mamada[2], Nobuhiko Taniai[2], Takashi Tajiri[2] and Eiji Uchida[2]

*Address all correspondence to: hiroshiy@nms.ac.jp

1 Department of Surgery, Nippon Medical School Tama Nagayama Hospital, Japan

2 Department of Surgery, Nippon Medical School, Japan

References

[1] Yoshida H, Mamada Y, Taniai N, Tajiri T. New methods for the management of esophageal varices. World J Gastroenterol. 2007 Mar 21;13(11):1641-5.

[2] Yoshida H, Mamada Y, Taniai N, Tajiri T. New methods for the management of gastric varices. World J Gastroenterol. 2006 Oct 7;12(37):5926-31.

[3] Yoshida H, Mamada Y, Taniai N, Yoshioka M, Hirakata A, Kawano Y, et al. Treatment modalities for bleeding esophagogastricvarices. J Nippon Med Sch. 2012;79(1): 19-30.

[4] Tajiri T, Yoshida H, Obara K, Onji M, Kage M, Kitano S, et al. General rules for recording endoscopic findings of esophagogastricvarices (2nd edition). Dig Endosc. 2010 Jan;22(1):1-9.

[5] Yoshida H, Mamada Y, Taniai N, Yamamoto K, Kawano Y, Mizuguchi Y, et al. A randomized control trial of bi-monthly versus bi-weekly endoscopic variceal ligation of esophageal varices. Am J Gastroenterol. 2005 Sep;100(9):2005-9.

[6] Yoshida H, Mamada Y, Taniai N, Tajiri T. New trends in surgical treatment for portal hypertension. Hepatol Res. 2009 Oct;39(10):1044-51.

[7] Inokuchi K, Kobayashi M, Kusaba A, Ogawa Y, Saku M, Shiizaki T. New selective decompression of esophageal varices. By a left gastric venous-caval shunt. Arch Surg. 1970 Feb;100(2):157-62.

[8] Belghiti J, Grenier P, Nouel O, Nahum H, Fekete F. Long-term loss of Warren's shunt selectivity. Angiographic demonstration. Arch Surg. 1981 Sep;116(9):1121-4.

[9] Shields R. Small-diameter PTFE portosystemic shunts: portocavalvsmesocaval. HPB Surg. 1998;10(6):413-4.

[10] Mercado MA, Morales-Linares JC, Granados-Garcia J, Gomez-Mendez TJ, Chan C, Orozco H. Distal splenorenal shunt versus 10-mm low-diameter mesocaval shunt for variceal hemorrhage. Am J Surg. 1996 Jun;171(6):591-5.

[11] Paquet KJ, Lazar A, Koussouris P, Hotzel B, Gad HA, Kuhn R, et al. Mesocaval interposition shunt with small-diameter polytetrafluoroethylene grafts in sclerotherapy failure. Br J Surg. 1995 Feb;82(2):199-203.

[12] Warren WD, Zeppa R, Fomon JJ. Selective trans-splenic decompression of gastroesophagealvarices by distal splenorenal shunt. Ann Surg. 1967 Sep;166(3):437-55.

[13] Rikkers LF, Rudman D, Galambos JT, Fulenwider JT, Millikan WJ, Kutner M, et al. A randomized, controlled trial of the distal splenorenal shunt. Ann Surg. 1978 Sep; 188(3):271-82.

[14] Tajiri T, Onda M, Yoshida H, Mamada Y, Taniai N, Umehara M, et al. Long-term results of modified distal splenorenal shunts for the treatment of esophageal varices.
Hepatogastroenterology. 2000 May-Jun;47(33):720-3.

[15] Stipa S, Balducci G, Ziparo V, Stipa F, Lucandri G. Total shunting and elective management of variceal bleeding. World J Surg. 1994 Mar-Apr;18(2):200-4.

[16] Klein AS, Fair JH, Cameron JL. Suprarenal mesocaval shunt. SurgGynecol Obstet.
1991 Oct;173(4):319-22.

[17] Sato Y, Hatakeyama K. Left gastric venous caval direct shunt in esophagogastricvarices. Hepatogastroenterology. 2002 Sep-Oct;49(47):1251-2.

[18] Inokuchi K, Beppu K, Koyanagi N, Nagamine K, Hashizume M, Sugimachi K. Exclusion of nonisolated splenic vein in distal splenorenal shunt for prevention of portal
malcirculation. Ann Surg. 1984 Dec;200(6):711-7.

[19] Inokuchi K. Selective decompression of esophageal varices by a left gastric venacaval
shunt. SurgAnnu. 1978;10:215-36.

[20] Henderson JM, Warren WD, Millikan WJ, Galloway JR, Kawasaki S, Kutner MH.
Distal splenorenal shunt with splenopancreatic disconnection. A 4-year assessment.
Ann Surg. 1989 Sep;210(3):332-9; discussion 9-41.

[21] Tajiri T, Onda M, Yoshida H, Mamada Y, Taniai N, Yamashita K. Comparison of the
long-term results of distal splenorenal shunt and esophageal transection for the treatment of esophageal varices. Hepatogastroenterology. 2000 Nov-Dec;47(36):1619-21.

[22] Rikkers LF. Definitive therapy for variceal bleeding: a personal view. Am J Surg.
1990 Jul;160(1):80-5.

[23] Inokuchi K, Beppu K, Koyanagi N, Nagamine K, Hashizume M, Iwanaga T, et al. Fifteen years' experience with left gastric venous caval shunt for esophageal varices.
World J Surg. 1984 Oct;8(5):716-21.

[24] Inokuchi K, Kobayashi M, Ogawa Y, Saku M, Nagasue N. Results of left gastric vena
caval shunt for esophageal varices: Analysis of one hundred clinical cases. Surgery.
1975 Nov;78(5):628-36.

[25] Inokuchi K. A selective portacaval shunt. Lancet. 1968 Jul 6;2(7558):51-2.

[26] Millikan WJ, Jr., Warren WD, Henderson JM, Smith RB, 3rd, Salam AA, Galambos JT,
et al. The Emory prospective randomized trial: selective versus nonselective shunt to
control variceal bleeding. Ten year follow-up. Ann Surg. 1985 Jun;201(6):712-22.

[27] Rikkers LF, Jin G. Variceal hemorrhage: surgical therapy. GastroenterolClin North
Am. 1993 Dec;22(4):821-42.

[28] Rikkers LF, Sorrell WT, Jin G. Which portosystemic shunt is best? GastroenterolClin
North Am. 1992 Mar;21(1):179-96.

[29] Smith RB, 3rd, Warren WD, Salam AA, Millikan WJ, Ansley JD, Galambos JT, et al. Dacron interposition shunts for portal hypertension. An analysis of morbidity correlates. Ann Surg. 1980 Jul;192(1):9-17.

[30] Sarfeh IJ, Rypins EB. The emergency portacaval H graft in alcoholic cirrhotic patients: influence of shunt diameter on clinical outcome. Am J Surg. 1986 Sep;152(3): 290-3.

[31] Sarfeh IJ, Rypins EB, Fardi M, Conroy RM, Mason GR, Lyons KP. Clinical implications of portal hemodynamics after small-diameter portacaval H graft. Surgery. 1984 Aug;96(2):223-9.

[32] Sarfeh IJ, Rypins EB, Mason GR. A systematic appraisal of portacaval H-graft diameters. Clinical and hemodynamic perspectives. Ann Surg. 1986 Oct;204(4):356-63.

[33] Sarfeh IJ, Rypins EB, Raiszadeh M, Milne N, Conroy RM, Lyons KP. Serial measurement of portal hemodynamics after partial portal decompression. Surgery. 1986 Jul; 100(1):52-8.

[34] Henderson JM, Millikan WJ, Jr., Wright-Bacon L, Kutner MH, Warren WD. Hemodynamic differences between alcoholic and nonalcoholic cirrhotics following distal splenorenal shunt--effect on survival? Ann Surg. 1983 Sep;198(3):325-34.

[35] Henderson JM, El Khishen MA, Millikan WJ, Jr., Sones PJ, Warren WD. Management of stenosis of distal splenorenal shunt by balloon dilation. SurgGynecol Obstet. 1983 Jul;157(1):43-8.

[36] Warren WD, Millikan WJ, Jr., Henderson JM, Abu-Elmagd KM, Galloway JR, Shires GT, 3rd, et al. Splenopancreatic disconnection. Improved selectivity of distal splenorenal shunt. Ann Surg. 1986 Oct;204(4):346-55.

[37] Moon SB, Jung SE, Ha JW, Park KW, Seo JK, Kim WK. The usefulness of distal splenorenal shunt in children with portal hypertension for the treatment of severe thrombocytopenia and leukopenia. World J Surg. 2008 Mar;32(3):483-7.

[38] Katoh H, Shimozawa E, Kojima T, Tanabe T. Modified splenorenal shunt with splenopancreatic disconnection. Surgery. 1989 Nov;106(5):920-4.

[39] Kanaya S, Katoh H. Long-term evaluation of distal splenorenal shunt with splenopancreatic and gastric disconnection. Surgery. 1995 Jul;118(1):29-35.

[40] Yoshida H, Mamada Y, Taniai N, Yamamoto K, Kaneko M, Kawano Y, et al. Long-term results of partial splenic artery embolization as supplemental treatment for portal-systemic encephalopathy. Am J Gastroenterol. 2005 Jan;100(1):43-7.

[41] Yoshida H, Mamada Y, Taniai N, Tajiri T. Partial splenic embolization. Hepatol Res. 2008 Mar;38(3):225-33.

[42] Fischer JE, Rosen HM, Ebeid AM, James JH, Keane JM, Soeters PB. The effect of normalization of plasma amino acids on hepatic encephalopathy in man. Surgery. 1976 Jul;80(1):77-91.

[43] Santambrogio R, Opocher E, Costa M, Bruno S, Ceretti AP, Spina GP. Natural history of a randomized trial comparing distal spleno-renal shunt with endoscopic sclerotherapy in the prevention of varicealrebleeding: a lesson from the past. World J Gastroenterol. 2006 Oct 21;12(39):6331-8.

[44] Warren WD, Rudman D, Millikan W, Galambos JT, Salam AA, Smith RB, 3rd. The metabolic basis of portasystemic encephalopathy and the effect of selective vs nonselective shunts. Ann Surg. 1974 Oct;180(4):573-9.

[45] Galambos JT, Warren WD, Rudman D, Smith RB, 3rd, Salam AA. Selective and total shunts in the treatment of bleeding varices. A randomized controlled trial. N Engl J Med. 1976 Nov 11;295(20):1089-95.

[46] Sugiura M, Futagawa S. A new technique for treating esophageal varices. J Thorac-Cardiovasc Surg. 1973 Nov;66(5):677-85.

[47] Hassab MA. Gastroesophageal decongestion and splenectomy in the treatment of esophageal varices in bilharzial cirrhosis: further studies with a report on 355 operations. Surgery. 1967 Feb;61(2):169-76.

[48] Hassab MA. Gastro-esophageal decongestion and splenectomy GEDS (Hassab), in the management of bleeding varices. Review of literature. Int Surg. 1998 Jan-Mar; 83(1):38-41.

[49] Yamamoto S, Hidemura R, Sawada M, Takeshige K, Iwatsuki S. The late results of terminal esophagoproximalgastrectomy (TEPG) with intensive devascularization and splenectomy for bleeding esophageal varices in cirrhosis. Surgery. 1976 Jul;80(1): 106-14.

[50] Kawanaka H, Akahoshi T, Kinjo N, Konishi K, Yoshida D, Anegawa G, et al. Impact of antithrombin III concentrates on portal vein thrombosis after splenectomy in patients with liver cirrhosis and hypersplenism. Ann Surg. 2010 Jan;251(1):76-83.

[51] Smith GW. Splenectomy and coronary vein ligation for the control of bleeding esophageal varices. Am J Surg. 1970 Feb;119(2):122-31.

[52] Kawanaka H, Akahoshi T, Kinjo N, Konishi K, Yoshida D, Anegawa G, et al. Technical standardization of laparoscopic splenectomy harmonized with hand-assisted laparoscopic surgery for patients with liver cirrhosis and hypersplenism. J HepatobiliaryPancreat Surg. 2009;16(6):749-57.

[53] Idezuki Y, Sugiura M, Sakamoto K, Abe H, Miura T, Hatano S, et al. Rationale for transthoracic esophageal transection for bleeding varices. Dis Chest. 1967 Nov;52(5): 621-31.

[54] Walker RM. Transection operations for portal hypertension. Thorax. 1960 Sep; 15:218-24.

[55] Sugiura M, Futagawa S. Results of six hundred thirty-six esophageal transections with paraesophagogastricdevascularization in the treatment of esophageal varices. J Vasc Surg. 1984 Mar;1(2):254-60.

[56] Yoshida H, Onda M, Tajiri T, Toba M, Umehara M, Mamada Y, et al. Endoscopic injection sclerotherapy for the treatment of reccurent esophageal varices after esophageal transection.. Dig Endosc. [original]. 2002;14:93-8.

[57] de Cleva R, Herman P, D'Albuquerque L A, Pugliese V, Santarem OL, Saad WA. Pre- and postoperative systemic hemodynamic evaluation in patients subjected to esophagogastricdevascularization plus splenectomy and distal splenorenal shunt: a comparative study in schistomomal portal hypertension. World J Gastroenterol. 2007 Nov 7;13(41):5471-5.

[58] Rikkers LF, Cormier RA, Vo NM. Effects of altered portal hemodynamics after distal splenorenal shunts. Am J Surg. 1987 Jan;153(1):80-5.

[59] Boyer JL, Sen Gupta KP, Biswas SK, Pal NC, BasuMallick KC, Iber FL, et al. Idiopathic portal hypertension. Comparison with the portal hypertension of cirrhosis and extrahepatic portal vein obstruction. Ann Intern Med. 1967 Jan;66(1):41-68.

[60] Okuda K, Kono K, Ohnishi K, Kimura K, Omata M, Koen H, et al. Clinical study of eighty-six cases of idiopathic portal hypertension and comparison with cirrhosis with splenomegaly. Gastroenterology. 1984 Apr;86(4):600-10.

[61] Yoshida H, Mamada Y, Taniai N, Mineta S, Kawano Y, Mizuguchi Y, et al. Shunting and nonshunting procedures for the treatment of esophageal varices in patients with idiopathic portal hypertension. Hepatogastroenterology. 2010 Sep-Oct;57(102-103): 1139-44.

Chapter 7

Vasoactive Substances and Inflammatory Factors in Progression of Liver Cirrhosis with Portal Hypertension

Hao Lu, Guoqiang Li, Ling Lu, Ye Fan,
Xiaofeng Qian, Ke Wang and Feng Zhang

Additional information is available at the end of the chapter

1. Introduction

Portal hypertension (PH), a detrimental complication of many diseases, is abnormalities in pre-, intra- or post-hepatic portal venous system. Intrahepatic PH is the most common type, which is mainly cause by liver cirrhosis [1], liver cancer, and sometimes intrahepatic vascular abnormalities [2].

Hepatic venous pressure gradient (HVPG) is the difference between wedged hepatic venous pressure and infra vena cava pressure. PH is defined as an HVPG higher than 5 mmHg [3]. According to absence or presence of complications (splenomegaly and hypersplenism, esophageal varices and ascites), PH can be classified into compensated or decompensated phase. Meanwhile, an HVPG higher than 10 mmHg has been considered as a direct predictor of decompensation and a 10-year-follow-up study showed the significant worse long-term survival when HVPG > 10 mmHg [4-6].

In cirrhotic PH, increased intrahepatic vascular resistance (IHVR) is the primary factor [7, 8] and subsequently increased portal vein inflow (PVI) worsens the situation of PH patients. This review will focus on the physiopathological changes happened in PH.

2. Correlation between vasoactive substances and IHVR/PVI

2.1. Nitric oxide

Nitric oxide (NO) is a potential vasodilator, produced by NO synthase (NOS). In a rat PH model induced by Thioacetamide, contraction of hepatic stellate cells, which resulting the increase of intrahepatic vascular tone, was inhibited by incubated with nitroflurbiprofen *in vitro*, a nitric oxide-releasing cyclooxygenase inhibitor in a dose-dependent manner. In wild-type BDL mice, expression of NOS, especially eNOS was down-regulated [9]. Moreover, the significantly elevated total intrahepatic resistance was reduced significantly *in vivo* by the drug, indicating a potential role of NO on portal pressure [10]. In another rat PH model induced by bile-duct-ligation, intrahepatic vascular resistance increased significantly. Besides, relative level of phos-NOS decreased compared with sham group, leading to an inhibition of intrahepatic NO, although the relative mRNA level was increased [11]. Intrahepatic NO production is largely mediated by endothelial NO synthase (eNOS) and impaired when cirrhosis and secondary endothelial dysfunction existed, leading to the increase of intrahepatic vascular resistance. But the inhibition of NO might be the result of up-regulation of caveolin-1, a down-regulator of eNOS [12].

Contrastingly, extrahepatic NO is increased in PH patients. A clinical trial has shown that serum nitrate level was positively correlated with clinical presentation, (e.g. pulse rate, jaundice, hepatic encephalopathy, lower limb edema) and esophageal varices [13]. It is well established that NO results in dilation of splanchnic and systemic circulation as a powerful vasodilator and blood level of NO is increased as PH progresses [14-16]. Administration of CCl4 to eNOS(-/-) mice also led to an elevated NO production, which is eNOS independent [17]. Another study suggested that iNOS might be involved [18].

2.2. Carbon monoxide

Carbon monoxide (CO), a vasodilator producing by heme oxygenases (HOs) from heme [19], changes as HO-1 expression altered in PH patients [20, 21], which shares the same characters with NO [12]. Expression of intrahepatic HO-1 and -2 decreased in cirrhotic rats than that in normal ones. In situ perfusion with CO-releasing molecule-2, which leads to relaxation of hepatic stellate cells, and HO-1 inducer hemin could attenuated increased IHVR. ZnPP caused a higher IHVR attributing to inhibition of intrahepatic HO-1 in cirrhotic liver[22].

But things are different in splanchnic and systemic circulation. Reportedly, portal vein pressure (PVP) was significantly higher in bile-duct-ligated rats than that in sham group. Meanwhile, mRNA and protein level of HO-1 was also elevated significantly in lung [23].A clinical study has shown an activated HO/CO system in cirrhotic patients while the HO-1 activity and plasma level of CO were related with the severity of PH [20]. Arterial blood gas analysis showed an increase of COHb in bile-duct-ligated rats which could be reversed by ZnPP [23]. HO-1 could promote expression of VEGF and thereafter lead to formation of collateral vessels and higher splanchnic circulation [24].

2.3. Endothelin

Endothelin-1 (ET-1) is the most powerful vasoconstrictor in ETs family [25], which is primarily synthesized and acts in liver mainly in a paracrine fashion via ET A receptor causing vessel constriction [26]. In liver cirrhotic rats induced by carbon tetrachloride, both plasma

ET-1 level and PVP elevated dramatically while the mean hepatic tissue portal inflow reduced. And, perfusion with an antagonist of ET A receptor led to a reduction of plasma ET-1 level and PVP but did not improve the hepatic infusion suggesting that ET-1 was involved in development of PH [26]. It is consistent with a previous study which had demonstrated that liver blood inflow fluctuated in ET A and B receptors antagonist infusion groups and control group [27]. ET A and B receptors play different roles in CCl4-induced portal hypertensive rats. Antagonism of ET A or B receptor led to a reduced or increased of PVP and sinusoidal area in the cirrhotic rats respectively [28]. However, activation of ET B receptor leads to production of other vasoactive molecules, e.g. TXA_2 [29]. Besides, antagonism of ET A receptor alone cannot improve splanchnic circulation indicating ET B receptor plays a role on regulation in PH [30].

2.4. RAAS

It is well established that renin -angiotensin II (Ang II) -aldosterone -system (RAAS) plays an important role on body circulation. Ang II promotes proliferation and contraction of HSC and formation of collagen, leading to liver fibrosis [31]. In hepatorenal syndrome, a severe complication of cirrhotic portal hypertension with hyperdynamic circulation, systemic resistance, circulatory renin activity and plasma aldosterone were significantly increased [32]. Besides, angiotensin converting enzyme (ACE) and Ang II elevated in liver cirrhosis [33, 34]. Role of RAAS on portal pressure provides a new therapeutic alternative [35]. Animal model studies and clinical trials have shown that blockade of Ang II type 1 receptor (AT1R) significantly reduced portal perfusion pressure and HVPG [36-39]. ACE inhibitor also effects to reduce portal pressure in cirrhotic patients [40]. Inhibition of RAAS by losartan could also lead to a reduction of eNOS and ROS level in BDL rats [41].

2.5. Catecholamines

Catecholamines (CA) cause general physiological changes including increases in heart rate, blood pressure, blood glucose levels, and a general reaction of the sympathetic nervous system. In BDL cirrhotic rats, noradrenaline correlated with perfusion pressure dose-dependently, and this constrictive effect might be normalized by phentolamine but not propranolol, indicating that noradrenaline influences PVP through α-receptor on portal-systemic collaterals [42]. In short-term PH induced by partial portal vein ligation (PVL), antagonism of phentolamine on α-receptor was reduced; meanwhile, release of noradrenaline was down-regulated as NO up-regulated, indicating a potential role of CA, together with NO, on hyperhemodynamics and increased PVI [43]. Besides, expressions of tyrosine hydroxylase and dopamine β-hydroxylase were down-regulated in superior mesenteric artery revealing genetic regulation of adrenergic neurotransmitter system participating in the splanchnic vasodilation in PH [44]. Nevertheless, protein level of α-receptor was higher in cirrhotic livers than in normal livers; activation of these α-receptors located on HSC induced calcium spikes and HSC constriction through MAPK, NK-κB and AP-1 pathways, resulting in increased intrahepatic resistance [45]. When response to β-blockers was defined as a reduction > 10% in HVPG from baseline, the proportion of non-responsers decreased, the rate of first-bleeding among them increased and the diagnostic acuracy improved significantly contrasting with a 20% cut-off value.[46] Also, acute responsers to β-blockers have a better long-term outcome.[47]

2.6. Cannabinoid

Correlation between Cannabinoid and portal hypertension was paid attention in the last decades. Administration of anandamide, an endogenous cannabinoid, resulted in a drop of systemic circulation, mainly mean arterial pressure, although venous pressure changes verified, because of its effect on heart rate. Contrastingly, PVI and PVP increased in a dose-dependent fashion [48]. Treatment with antagonist of cannabinoid CB1 receptor in rats might lead to an elevation of blood pressure and a reduction of PVI and PVP, indicating cannabinoid is responsible for the dilation of systemic circulation [49]. It is in agreement with human. In cirrhotic patients, plasma level of cannabinoid was increased regardless of well-compensated or not [50]. But things are different in liver. Expression of CB1 receptor was dramatically down-regulated in both wild-type and eNOS knock-out group mice [9]. However, more researches are needed.

2.7. Cyclooxygenase, prostanoids and TXA_2

Activation of COX-2/prostanoid pathway promotes production of TXA_2 and PGE_2 [51]. In BDL rats, TXB_2, a stable metabolic of TXA_2 in isolated liver perfusate and PVP were increased in a time-dependent manner. Both inhibition of Kuffer cells and COX attenuate these changes. Further results indicated that COX-2 interact with Kuffer cells-derived TXA_2 was involved and its expression increased significantly [52]. Another group reported that COX-1 and PGI2 were responsible for decreased splanchnic resistance and increased PVI [53, 54]. However, elevated PVP of intrahepatic or pre-hepatic hypertension rats might be reduced by short- or long-term administration of COX inhibitor [18]. It is consistent with Graupera M et. al. [55]. In BDL portal hypertensive rats, elevated ET-1 interacted with Kuffer cells, increasing the responsiveness of p38MAPK through ET B receptor, activating $cPLA_2$ and promoting production of TXA_2, contributing to progression of portal hypertension [29].

2.8. Reactive oxygen species

Reactive oxygen species (ROS) is involved in many pathologic processes. In the case of PH, ROS level increases when circulatory NO decreases [56]. Administration of tempol, a type of superoxide dismutase, normalizes these changes with statistical significance in endothelial cells and cirrhotic liver, reduces intrahepatic vessel resistance and consequently increases PVI [57]. ROS also takes part in oxidative stress [58], lipid peroxidation, apoptosis and dysfunction of endothelial cells [41]. Reportedly, carvedilol, a β-blocker might ameliorate oxidative stress as well as inflammation and fibrosis in a CCl4-induced liver damage model, by reducing depletion of antioxidant enzyme, formation of collagen, and activation of NF-κB pathway, indicating a relationship between ROS and liver damage and fibrosis [59].

3. Cytokines and liver fibrosis

Cytokine is a group of soluble protein or polypeptide, regulating immunologic response and hematopoiesis, participating inflammatory damage and repair. It consists of interleukins (IL), interferons (IFN), tumor necrosis factors (TNF), colony stimulating factors (CSF), chemokines, and growth factors. It has been reported that serum levels IL-6, TNF-α [60 61], and IL-1β [62] were elevated in hepatoportal sclerosis, and plasma IL-6 level was correlated with the deterioration of liver function [63]. Although IL-6 was increased, expression of IL-6 receptor in cirrhotic liver was decreased, leading to a reduction of hepatocyte response to IL-6, accompanied by an increase of gp130, indicating gp130 might be the potential negative regulator of liver IL-6 signal pathway [64]. In chronic patients with hepatitis C and/or schistosomal, plasma IL-4 level, as well as ROS, was increased and correlated with portal vein diameter, suggesting IL-4 might plays a role on PVI [65]. A clinical trial has shown that administration of probiotic led to a trend to reduction of plasma endotoxin, a mild but significant increase of TNF-α and a significant reduction of aldosterone [66]. Besides, increased PVP induced a up-regulation of α-smooth muscle actin and collagen ● and ethanol exposure enhanced expression of TGF-β and production of extracellular matrix via ERK1/2-JNK and p38MAPK pathway respectively, leading to fibrosis of liver [67]. Reportedly, IL-18 gene knock-out mice fed with methionine-choline-deficient diet (MCDD) showed significant exacerbated inflammation, revealing IL-18 was a negative regulator of non-alcoholic fatty liver disease and non-alcoholic steatohepatitis. Tnf mRNA, but not il-6 or il-1b levelm was higher in db/db (Asc-/-) group than db/db (wt) group, indicating TNF-α expression drove the progression of non-alcoholic steatohepatitis [68]. In another type of liver cirrhosis caused by chronic infection of schistosomiasis, inflammation and following tissue repair led to obstruction of intrahepatic vessels and increased intrahepatic resistance. These defenses in liver was mediated by IL-10. But surprisingly, blockade of IL-10R resulted in an elevation of PH and a reduction of parasitic antigen specific B cells, but worsened pulmonary accumulation of eggs without an increase of PVP [69]. Co-infection of bacteria led to production of IL-17 [70]. Consistently, knock-out of IL-10, IL-12p40, and IL-13Rα2 contributed to a progressive and lethal liver fibrosis, showing the anti-fibrosis effects of these Th2-derived interleukins in schistosomiasis mansoni treated mice [71]. As demonstrated by Pinter M et. Al. [72], responders to sorafenib showed a decreased HVPG and VEGF, PDGF, PlGF, RhoA kinase, and TNF-α expression, revealed a potential effect of these growth factors and TNF-α on HVPG. And level of soluble TNF-α receptor in portal vein and hepatic vein was correlated with model for end-stage liver disease score, in accordance with previous studies [73]. However, intrahepatic TNF-α, IL-1β, IL-4, and IL-10 were down-regulated while splanchnic levels were increased [74]. It is shown that IFN is involved in progression of hypertension, especially in viral infection- associated hepatitis [60, 75, 76]. Nowadays, IFN is usually used as antiviral treatment. Combination of 5-fluorouracil and IFN might reduce the portal hypertension related events [77]. Also, combination with IFN enhanced the viral clearance effect of ribavirin [78]. But IFN alone therapy only led to a temporary reduction of viral DNA load [79]. As documented, TGF-β promotes liver fibrosis in rats with biliary cirrhosis, cooperates with IFN-γ, IL-4, and TNF-α, etc [80]. More studies are needed to illustrate the detail effects of cytokines network on portal hypertension and liver fibrosis.

4. Molecules in further physiopathological progression

4.1. Splenomegaly and hypersplenism

Volume of spleen or splenomegaly in cirrhotic hypertension patients is primarily attributed to increased splanchnic circulation and congestion, in which vasoactive substances play important roles. And the main pathologic changes are lower counts of red blood cells, white blood cells, and platelets. Compared to normal spleen, lymphocytes in PH spleen were relatively reduced with a similar distribution; but total number of lymphocytes was increased due to the increase of spleen weight, with an elevated proliferation [81, 82]. MicroRNAome analysis showed that microRNA, expecially miR-615-3p was up-regulated in PH spleen significantly [83, 84]. It targeted on ligand-dependent nuclear receptor corepressor (LCoR), promoted the phagocytic capacity of macrophages through PPARγ pathway [84]. On the other hand, phagocytic capacity of macrophages might be inhibit by Phosphatidylinositol 3-kinase regulatory subunit 1 (PI3KR1) knock-down, accompanied by down-regulation of IL-1β and TNF-α [85]. Similarly, expressions of IL-1β and NALP3, a potential NF-κB activator participating in inflammation and immunologic response were up-regulated significantly in CCl$_4$-induced cirrhotic PH group compared to control group, together with typical splenomegaly histopathological changes [86]. In cirrhotic spleen, different from extrahepatic portal vein obstruction, thromopoietin (TPO) was reduced and this reduction is positively correlated with exacerbation of liver function, leading to a decrease of platelet counts [87].

4.2. Esophageal varices

Cirrhotic hypertension is characterized by hyperdynamic circulation and increased intrahepatic resistance as discussed before in this review. Splanchnic vasodilation results in increasing in HVPG. When HVPG is higher than 12 mmHg, risk of esophageal varices dramatically increased [88, 89]. Generally speaking, esophageal varices, as well as development of other collateral vessels, occur after HVPG and is followed by variceal bleeding [90]. Angiogenesis is associated with esophageal varices and portal hypertension, and expressions of VEGF are up-regulated, alone or together with TNF-α or PEGF[91-93]. Inhibition of VEGF/VEGF receptor pathway led to a decrease in hyperdynamic splanchnic circulation and collateral vessels [94]. Besides, metabolic disturbances occurred in cirrhotic PH lead to an elevation of glucagon [95]. The ratio of glycated albumin (GA) to glycated hemoglobin (HbA1c) was associated positively with the progression of liver cirrhosis, and patients with elevated GA/HbA1c ratio have severer esophageal variceal and higher risk of bleeding in HCV-related cirrhotic patients. This parameter might become a potential biomarker to predict the prognosis of these patients [96].

4.3. Ascites

Portal hypertension in cirrhotic liver diseases is a main cause of ascites. As discussed before, vasoactive substances lead to an elevation of intrahepatic vessels resistance and a relative decrease of blood back-flow to liver. Besides, mechanisms below are involved: 1) hyperdynamic circulation. Hyperdynamic circulation is associated with disturbance of vasoactive substances. It is characterized by increased cardiac index and plasma volume and decreased systemic and splanchnic resistance [90]. 2) hypoalbuminemia following damage of liver function. One of the hyperalbuminemia occurred in cirrhotic PH is dysfunction of hepatocytes. In is shown that hypertension is a negative regulator to the number and structure of hepatocytes [97]. Poor blood supply induced by liver fibrosis and disturbance of hemodynamics results in intrahepatic hypoxia and damage of hepatocytes. Besides, primary liver diseases also cause inflammation and damage in liver. 3) renal function changes. This part will be discussed below.

4.4. Hepatorenal syndrome

It is well established that main cause of hepatorenal syndrome (HRS) is constriction of vessels in kidney induced by reduction of effective circulating blood volume (ECBV). As discussed previously, ECBV is reduced by systemic and splanchnic vasodilation induced by changes of NO, ET, PGs and TXA_2. Besides, some localized physiopathologic should be paid attention on. Expression of HO-1 in kidney was significantly reduced in BDL-induced cirrhotic rats [98]. Cyctatin C was increased in decompensated liver cirrhosis and HRS, thus it could be used as a predictor of HRS [99, 100]. Additionally, plasma level of ADAMTS13 was decreased and supplemental therapy might improve prognosis of patients with severe liver cirrhosis and HRS [101, 102].

4.5. Hepatic encephalopathy

Hepatic encephalopathy (HE) in portal hypertension is defined as C type HE. In PVL-induced PH rats, chemokine changes in splanchnic system, liver, and central nervous system (CNS) are different [103]. As reported, in CNS, CX3CL1/CX3CR1 and SDF1-α/CXCR4 were increased. The former one promotes inflammation in CNS while the latter one modulates neuron activity through inhibitory neurotransmitters, e.g. gamma-amino butyric acid (GABA) [104]. ROS also participates in pre-hepatic portal hypertension [105, 106]. GABA level is also negatively regulated by dehydroepiandrosterone sulfate (DHEAS), which reduced in cirrhotic HE [107]. Besides, IL-6 has synergistic effect with ammonia in cirrotic HE patients [108]. Ammonia impairs brain eNOS activity, leading to significant abnormality of NO regulation and disturbance of blood supply [109]. Due to liver dysfunction in HE patients, elevated plasma manganese also indicates a bad prognosis [110].

5. Conclusion

Portal hypertension concerns a great number of molecules and complicated physiopathologic mechanisms. It can be classified into pre-, intra-, and post-hepatic PH according to the primary disease, with similar but not same involvement of molecules and mechanisms. However, we can still conclude that: 1) vasoactive substances play an important in systemic, splanchnic, hepatic, and even neurologic circulations which are closely related to blood supply, affecting the development, progression, and outcome of PH; 2) imbalance of pro-/anti-inflammatory cytokines lead to a systemic and/or localized regulation of signal pathways and modulate gene expression and silencing, cell proliferation and apoptosis, tissue damage and repair, and eventually life and death; 3) accumulating research advancements provide us new targets for treatment of PH, but it has a long way to go from bench to bedside.

Acknowledgements

This study was supported by the International Collaboration Foundation of Jiangsu Province (BZ2011041, BK2009439, ZX05 200904, WS2011106), Development of Innovative Research Team in the First Affiliated Hospital of NJMU and the National Nature Science Foundation of China (81210108017, 81100270, 81070380). First Innovation Team Foundation of Jiangsu province Hospital (for Sun BC).

Author details

Hao Lu, Guoqiang Li, Ling Lu, Ye Fan, Xiaofeng Qian, Ke Wang and Feng Zhang[*]

*Address all correspondence to: zhangf@njmu.edu.cn

Liver Transplantation Center, First Affiliated Hospital of Nanjing Medical Univerisity, Nanjing, China

Hao Lu and Guoqiang Li contribute equally to this work.

References

[1] Bari K,Garcia-Tsao G. Treatment of portal hypertension. World J Gastroenterol 2012;18:1166-1175. PMID: 22468079

[2] Arya A, Kakani N, Hussain N, Chandok N. Massive avascular malformations causing life threatening portal hypertension. Ann Hepatol 2012;11:552-553. PMID: 22700638

[3] Bosch J. Vascular deterioration in cirrhosis: the big picture. J Clin Gastroenterol 2007;41 Suppl 3:S247-253. PMID: 17975472

[4] Bruix J, Castells A, Bosch J, Feu F, Fuster J, Garcia-Pagan JC, et al. Surgical resection of hepatocellular carcinoma in cirrhotic patients: prognostic value of preoperative portal pressure. Gastroenterology 1996;111:1018-1022. PMID: 8831597

[5] Llovet JM, Fuster J, Bruix J. Intention-to-treat analysis of surgical treatment for early hepatocellular carcinoma: resection versus transplantation. Hepatology 1999;30:1434-1440. PMID: 10573522

[6] Zipprich A, Garcia-Tsao G, Rogowski S, Fleig WE, Seufferlein T, Dollinger MM. Prognostic indicators of survival in patients with compensated and decompensated cirrhosis. Liver Int 2012. PMID: 22679906

[7] Bosch J,Garcia-Pagan JC. Complications of cirrhosis. I. Portal hypertension. J Hepatol 2000;32:141-156. PMID: 10728801

[8] Rodriguez-Vilarrupla A, Fernandez M, Bosch J, Garcia-Pagan JC. Current concepts on the pathophysiology of portal hypertension. Ann Hepatol 2007;6:28-36. PMID: 17297426

[9] Biecker E, Sagesser H, Reichen J. Vasodilator mRNA levels are increased in the livers of portal hypertensive NO-synthase 3-deficient mice. Eur J Clin Invest 2004;34:283-289. PMID: 15086360

[10] Laleman W, Van Landeghem L, Van der Elst I, Zeegers M, Fevery J, Nevens F. Nitro-flurbiprofen, a nitric oxide-releasing cyclooxygenase inhibitor, improves cirrhotic portal hypertension in rats. Gastroenterology 2007;132:709-719. PMID: 17258737

[11] Luo W, Meng Y, Ji HL, Pan CQ, Huang S, Yu CH, et al. Spironolactone Lowers Portal Hypertension by Inhibiting Liver Fibrosis, ROCK-2 Activity and Activating NO/PKG Pathway in the Bile-Duct-Ligated Rat. PLoS One 2012;7:e34230. PMID: 22479572

[12] Goh BJ, Tan BT, Hon WM, Lee KH, Khoo HE. Nitric oxide synthase and heme oxy-genase expressions in human liver cirrhosis. World J Gastroenterol 2006;12:588-594. PMID: 16489673

[13] El-Sherif AM, Abou-Shady MA, Al-Bahrawy AM, Bakr RM, Hosny AM. Nitric oxide levels in chronic liver disease patients with and without oesophageal varices. Hepatol Int 2008;2:341-345. PMID: 19669263

[14] Bories PN, Campillo B, Azaou L, Scherman E. Long-lasting NO overproduction in cirrhotic patients with spontaneous bacterial peritonitis. Hepatology 1997;25:1328-1333. PMID: 9185747

[15] Arkenau HT, Stichtenoth DO, Frolich JC, Manns MP, Boker KH. Elevated nitric oxide levels in patients with chronic liver disease and cirrhosis correlate with disease stage and parameters of hyperdynamic circulation. Z Gastroenterol 2002;40:907-913. PMID: 12436367

[16] Moriyama A, Masumoto A, Nanri H, Tabaru A, Unoki H, Imoto I, et al. High plasma concentrations of nitrite/nitrate in patients with hepatocellular carcinoma. Am J Gastroenterol 1997;92:1520-1523. PMID: 9317076

[17] Theodorakis NG, Wang YN, Wu JM, Maluccio MA, Sitzmann JV, Skill NJ. Role of endothelial nitric oxide synthase in the development of portal hypertension in the carbon tetrachloride-induced liver fibrosis model. Am J Physiol Gastrointest Liver Physiol 2009;297:G792-799. PMID: 19628654

[18] Xu J, Cao H, Liu H, Wu ZY. Role of nitric oxide synthase and cyclooxygenase in hyperdynamic splanchnic circulation of portal hypertension. Hepatobiliary Pancreat Dis Int 2008;7:503-508. PMID: 18842497

[19] Pannen BH, Kohler N, Hole B, Bauer M, Clemens MG, Geiger KK. Protective role of endogenous carbon monoxide in hepatic microcirculatory dysfunction after hemorrhagic shock in rats. J Clin Invest 1998;102:1220-1228. PMID: 9739056

[20] Tarquini R, Masini E, La Villa G, Barletta G, Novelli M, Mastroianni R, et al. Increased plasma carbon monoxide in patients with viral cirrhosis and hyperdynamic circulation. Am J Gastroenterol 2009;104:891-897. PMID: 19277027

[21] Makino N, Suematsu M, Sugiura Y, Morikawa H, Shiomi S, Goda N, et al. Altered expression of heme oxygenase-1 in the livers of patients with portal hypertensive diseases. Hepatology 2001;33:32-42. PMID: 11124818

[22] Van Landeghem L, Laleman W, Vander Elst I, Zeegers M, van Pelt J, Cassiman D, et al. Carbon monoxide produced by intrasinusoidally located haem-oxygenase-1 regulates the vascular tone in cirrhotic rat liver. Liver Int 2009;29:650-660. PMID: 18795901

[23] Guo SB, Duan ZJ, Li Q, Sun XY. Effects of heme oxygenase-1 on pulmonary function and structure in rats with liver cirrhosis. Chin Med J (Engl) 2011;124:918-922. PMID: 21518603

[24] Angermayr B, Mejias M, Gracia-Sancho J, Garcia-Pagan JC, Bosch J, Fernandez M. Heme oxygenase attenuates oxidative stress and inflammation, and increases VEGF expression in portal hypertensive rats. J Hepatol 2006;44:1033-1039. PMID: 16458992

[25] Giaid A. Nitric oxide and endothelin-1 in pulmonary hypertension. Chest 1998;114:208S-212S. PMID: 9741571

[26] Takashimizu S, Kojima S, Nishizaki Y, Kagawa T, Shiraishi K, Mine T, et al. Effect of endothelin A receptor antagonist on hepatic hemodynamics in cirrhotic rats. Implications for endothelin-1 in portal hypertension. Tokai J Exp Clin Med 2011;36:37-43. PMID: 21769771

[27] Watanabe N, Takashimizu S, Nishizaki Y, Kojima S, Kagawa T, Matsuzaki S. An endothelin A receptor antagonist induces dilatation of sinusoidal endothelial fenestrae: implications for endothelin-1 in hepatic microcirculation. J Gastroenterol 2007;42:775-782. PMID: 17876548

[28] Feng HQ, Weymouth ND, Rockey DC. Endothelin antagonism in portal hypertensive mice: implications for endothelin receptor-specific signaling in liver disease. Am J Physiol Gastrointest Liver Physiol 2009;297:G27-33. PMID: 19299580

[29] Miller AM,Zhang JX. Altered endothelin-1 signaling in production of thromboxane A2 in kupffer cells from bile duct ligated rats. Cell Mol Immunol 2009;6:441-452. PMID: 20003820

[30] Andersson A, Fenhammar J, Weitzberg E, Sollevi A, Hjelmqvist H, Frithiof R. Endo-thelin-mediated gut microcirculatory dysfunction during porcine endotoxaemia. Br J Anaesth 2010;105:640-647. PMID: 20710019

[31] Liu J, Gong H, Zhang ZT, Wang Y. Effect of angiotensin II and angiotensin II type 1 receptor antagonist on the proliferation, contraction and collagen synthesis in rat hepatic stellate cells. Chin Med J (Engl) 2008;121:161-165. PMID: 18272044

[32] Umgelter A, Wagner KS, Reindl W, Luppa PB, Geisler F, Huber W, et al. Renal and circulatory effects of large volume plasma expansion in patients with hepatorenal syndrome type 1. Ann Hepatol 2012;11:232-239. PMID: 22345341

[33] Lotfy M, El-Kenawy Ael M, Abdel-Aziz MM, El-Kady I, Talaat A. Elevated renin lev-els in patients with liver cirrhosis and hepatocellular carcinoma. Asian Pac J Cancer Prev 2010;11:1263-1266. PMID: 21198274

[34] Beyazit Y, Ibis M, Purnak T, Turhan T, Kekilli M, Kurt M, et al. Elevated levels of cir-culating angiotensin converting enzyme in patients with hepatoportal sclerosis. Dig Dis Sci 2011;56:2160-2165. PMID: 21290180

[35] Hidaka H, Kokubu S, Nakazawa T, Okuwaki Y, Ono K, Watanabe M, et al. New an-giotensin II type 1 receptor blocker olmesartan improves portal hypertension in pa-tients with cirrhosis. Hepatol Res 2007;37:1011-1017. PMID: 17608670

[36] Huang HC, Chang CC, Wang SS, Lee FY, Teng TH, Lee JY, et al. The roles of angio-tensin II receptors in the portosystemic collaterals of portal hypertensive and cirrhot-ic rats. J Vasc Res 2012;49:160-168. PMID: 22285953

[37] Loiola RA, Fernandes L, Eichler R, Passaglia Rde C, Fortes ZB, de Carvalho MH. Vas-cular mechanisms involved in angiotensin II-induced venoconstriction in hyperten-sive rats. Peptides 2011;32:2116-2121. PMID: 21945423

[38] Hidaka H, Nakazawa T, Shibuya A, Minamino T, Takada J, Tanaka Y, et al. Effects of 1-year administration of olmesartan on portal pressure and TGF-beta1 in selected pa-tients with cirrhosis: a randomized controlled trial. J Gastroenterol 2011;46:1316-1323. PMID: 21850387

[39] Debernardi-Venon W, Martini S, Biasi F, Vizio B, Termine A, Poli G, et al. AT1 recep-tor antagonist Candesartan in selected cirrhotic patients: effect on portal pressure and liver fibrosis markers. J Hepatol 2007;46:1026-1033. PMID: 17336417

[40] Tandon P, Abraldes JG, Berzigotti A, Garcia-Pagan JC, Bosch J. Renin-angiotensin-aldosterone inhibitors in the reduction of portal pressure: a systematic review and meta-analysis. J Hepatol 2010;53:273-282. PMID: 20570385

[41] Dal-Ros S, Oswald-Mammosser M, Pestrikova T, Schott C, Boehm N, Bronner C, et al. Losartan prevents portal hypertension-induced, redox-mediated endothelial dysfunction in the mesenteric artery in rats. Gastroenterology 2010;138:1574-1584. PMID: 19879274

[42] Chan CC, Chang CC, Huang HC, Wang SS, Lee FY, Chang FY, et al. Effects of norepinephrine and acetylcholine on portal-systemic collaterals of common bile duct-ligated cirrhotic rat. J Gastroenterol Hepatol 2005;20:1867-1872. PMID: 16336446

[43] Sastre E, Balfagon G, Revuelta-Lopez E, Aller MA, Nava MP, Arias J, et al. Effect of short- and long-term portal hypertension on adrenergic, nitrergic and sensory functioning in rat mesenteric artery. Clin Sci (Lond) 2012;122:337-348. PMID: 21999248

[44] Coll M, Genesca J, Raurell I, Rodriguez-Vilarrupla A, Mejias M, Otero T, et al. Downregulation of genes related to the adrenergic system may contribute to splanchnic vasodilation in rat portal hypertension. J Hepatol 2008;49:43-51. PMID: 18457899

[45] Sancho-Bru P, Bataller R, Colmenero J, Gasull X, Moreno M, Arroyo V, et al. Norepinephrine induces calcium spikes and proinflammatory actions in human hepatic stellate cells. Am J Physiol Gastrointest Liver Physiol 2006;291:G877-884. PMID: 16782692

[46] Villanueva C, Aracil C, Colomo A, Hernandez-Gea V, Lopez-Balaguer JM, Alvarez-Urturi C, et al. Acute hemodynamic response to beta-blockers and prediction of long-term outcome in primary prophylaxis of variceal bleeding. Gastroenterology 2009;137:119-128. PMID: 19344721

[47] La Mura V, Abraldes JG, Raffa S, Retto O, Berzigotti A, Garcia-Pagan JC, et al. Prognostic value of acute hemodynamic response to i.v. propranolol in patients with cirrhosis and portal hypertension. J Hepatol 2009;51:279-287. PMID: 19501930

[48] Garcia N, Jr., Jarai Z, Mirshahi F, Kunos G, Sanyal AJ. Systemic and portal hemodynamic effects of anandamide. Am J Physiol Gastrointest Liver Physiol 2001;280:G14-20. PMID: 11123193

[49] Shah V. Portal hypertension and the hyperdynamic circulation: nitric oxide in a haze of cannabinoid smoke. Hepatology 2001;34:1060-1061. PMID: 11679979

[50] Fernandez-Rodriguez CM, Romero J, Petros TJ, Bradshaw H, Gasalla JM, Gutierrez ML, et al. Circulating endogenous cannabinoid anandamide and portal, systemic and renal hemodynamics in cirrhosis. Liver Int 2004;24:477-483. PMID: 15482346

[51] Piston D, Wang S, Feng Y, Ye YJ, Zhou J, Jiang KW, et al. The role of cyclooxygenase-2/prostanoid pathway in visceral pain induced liver stress response in rats. Chin Med J (Engl) 2007;120:1813-1819. PMID: 18028778

[52] Yokoyama Y, Xu H, Kresge N, Keller S, Sarmadi AH, Baveja R, et al. Role of throm-
     boxane A2 in early BDL-induced portal hypertension. Am J Physiol Gastrointest Liv-
     er Physiol 2003;284:G453-460. PMID: 12431905

[53] Cao H, Xu J, Liu H, Meng FB, Qiu JF, Wu ZY. Influence of nitric oxide synthase and
     cyclooxygenase blockade on expression of cyclooxygenase and hemodynamics in
     rats with portal hypertension. Hepatobiliary Pancreat Dis Int 2006;5:564-569. PMID:
     17085343

[54] Cao H, Xu J, Hua R, Meng FB, Qiu JF, Wu ZY. Expression of cyclooxygenase in hy-
     perdynamic portal hypertensive rats. Hepatobiliary Pancreat Dis Int 2006;5:252-256.
     PMID: 16698586

[55] Graupera M, Garcia-Pagan JC, Abraldes JG, Peralta C, Bragulat M, Corominola H, et
     al. Cyclooxygenase-derived products modulate the increased intrahepatic resistance
     of cirrhotic rat livers. Hepatology 2003;37:172-181. PMID: 12500202

[56] Vujanac A, Jakovljevic V, Djordjevic D, Zivkovic V, Stojkovic M, Celikovic D, et al.
     Nitroglycerine effects on portal vein mechanics and oxidative stress in portal hyper-
     tension. World J Gastroenterol 2012;18:331-339. PMID: 22294839

[57] Garcia-Caldero H, Rodriguez-Vilarrupla A, Gracia-Sancho J, Divi M, Lavina B, Bosch
     J, et al. Tempol administration, a superoxide dismutase mimetic, reduces hepatic vas-
     cular resistance and portal pressure in cirrhotic rats. J Hepatol 2011;54:660-665.
     PMID: 21159403

[58] Huang YT, Hsu YC, Chen CJ, Liu CT, Wei YH. Oxidative-stress-related changes in
     the livers of bile-duct-ligated rats. J Biomed Sci 2003;10:170-178. PMID: 12595753

[59] Hamdy N,El-Demerdash E. New therapeutic aspect for carvedilol: Antifibrotic ef-
     fects of carvedilol in chronic carbon tetrachloride-induced liver damage. Toxicol
     Appl Pharmacol 2012. PMID: 22543095

[60] Koksal AS, Koklu S, Ibis M, Balci M, Cicek B, Sasmaz N, et al. Clinical features, se-
     rum interleukin-6, and interferon-gamma levels of 34 turkish patients with hepato-
     portal sclerosis. Dig Dis Sci 2007;52:3493-3498. PMID: 17404864

[61] Cariello R, Federico A, Sapone A, Tuccillo C, Scialdone VR, Tiso A, et al. Intestinal
     permeability in patients with chronic liver diseases: Its relationship with the aetiolo-
     gy and the entity of liver damage. Dig Liver Dis 2010;42:200-204. PMID: 19502117

[62] Tan G, Pan S, Li J, Dong X, Kang K, Zhao M, et al. Hydrogen sulfide attenuates car-
     bon tetrachloride-induced hepatotoxicity, liver cirrhosis and portal hypertension in
     rats. PLoS One 2011;6:e25943. PMID: 22022478

[63] [The role of interleukin-6 and nitric oxide in pathogenesis of portal hypertension and
     decompensation of liver cirrhosis]. Klin Med (Mosk) 2012;90:47-49. PMID: 22567940

[64] Lemmers A, Gustot T, Durnez A, Evrard S, Moreno C, Quertinmont E, et al. An in-
     hibitor of interleukin-6 trans-signalling, sgp130, contributes to impaired acute phase

response in human chronic liver disease. Clin Exp Immunol 2009;156:518-527. PMID: 19438606

[65] Elsammak MY, Al-Sharkaweey RM, Ragab MS, Amin GA, Kandil MH. IL-4 and reactive oxygen species are elevated in Egyptian patients affected with schistosomal liver disease. Parasite Immunol 2008;30:603-609. PMID: 19067841

[66] Tandon P, Moncrief K, Madsen K, Arrieta MC, Owen RJ, Bain VG, et al. Effects of probiotic therapy on portal pressure in patients with cirrhosis: a pilot study. Liver Int 2009;29:1110-1115. PMID: 19490420

[67] Okada Y, Tsuzuki Y, Hokari R, Miyazaki J, Matsuzaki K, Mataki N, et al. Pressure loading and ethanol exposure differentially modulate rat hepatic stellate cell activation. J Cell Physiol 2008;215:472-480. PMID: 18064666

[68] Henao-Mejia J, Elinav E, Jin C, Hao L, Mehal WZ, Strowig T, et al. Inflammasome-mediated dysbiosis regulates progression of NAFLD and obesity. Nature 2012;482:179-185. PMID: 22297845

[69] Fairfax KC, Amiel E, King IL, Freitas TC, Mohrs M, Pearce EJ. IL-10R blockade during chronic schistosomiasis mansoni results in the loss of B cells from the liver and the development of severe pulmonary disease. PLoS Pathog 2012;8:e1002490. PMID: 22291593

[70] Perona-Wright G, Lundie RJ, Jenkins SJ, Webb LM, Grencis RK, MacDonald AS. Concurrent bacterial stimulation alters the function of helminth-activated dendritic cells, resulting in IL-17 induction. J Immunol 2012;188:2350-2358. PMID: 22287718

[71] Mentink-Kane MM, Cheever AW, Wilson MS, Madala SK, Beers LM, Ramalingam TR, et al. Accelerated and progressive and lethal liver fibrosis in mice that lack interleukin (IL)-10, IL-12p40, and IL-13Ralpha2. Gastroenterology 2011;141:2200-2209. PMID: 21864478

[72] Pinter M, Sieghart W, Reiberger T, Rohr-Udilova N, Ferlitsch A, Peck-Radosavljevic M. The effects of sorafenib on the portal hypertensive syndrome in patients with liver cirrhosis and hepatocellular carcinoma--a pilot study. Aliment Pharmacol Ther 2012;35:83-91. PMID: 22032637

[73] Trebicka J, Krag A, Gansweid S, Appenrodt B, Schiedermaier P, Sauerbruch T, et al. Endotoxin and tumor necrosis factor-receptor levels in portal and hepatic vein of patients with alcoholic liver cirrhosis receiving elective transjugular intrahepatic portosystemic shunt. Eur J Gastroenterol Hepatol 2011;23:1218-1225. PMID: 21971377

[74] Garcia-Dominguez J, Aller MA, Garcia C, de Vicente F, Corcuera MT, Gomez-Aguado F, et al. Splanchnic Th(2) and Th(1) cytokine redistribution in microsurgical cholestatic rats. J Surg Res 2010;162:203-212. PMID: 20031157

[75] Dragoteanu M, Balea IA, Dina LA, Piglesan CD, Grigorescu I, Tamas S, et al. Staging of portal hypertension and portosystemic shunts using dynamic nuclear medicine investigations. World J Gastroenterol 2008;14:3841-3848. PMID: 18609707

[76] Di Marco V, Almasio PL, Ferraro D, Calvaruso V, Alaimo G, Peralta S, et al. Peg-interferon alone or combined with ribavirin in HCV cirrhosis with portal hypertension: a randomized controlled trial. J Hepatol 2007;47:484-491. PMID: 17692985

[77] Katamura Y, Aikata H, Takaki S, Azakami T, Kawaoka T, Waki K, et al. Intra-arterial 5-fluorouracil/interferon combination therapy for advanced hepatocellular carcinoma with or without three-dimensional conformal radiotherapy for portal vein tumor thrombosis. J Gastroenterol 2009;44:492-502. PMID: 19330281

[78] Iacobellis A, Ippolito A, Andriulli A. Antiviral therapy in hepatitis C virus cirrhotic patients in compensated and decompensated condition. World J Gastroenterol 2008;14:6467-6472. PMID: 19030197

[79] Pozzi M, Pizzala DP, Maldini FF, Doretti A, Ratti L. Portal pressure reduction after entecavir treatment in compensated HBV cirrhosis. Hepatogastroenterology 2009;56:231-235. PMID: 19453064

[80] Albillos A, Nieto M, Ubeda M, Munoz L, Fraile B, Reyes E, et al. The biological response modifier AM3 attenuates the inflammatory cell response and hepatic fibrosis in rats with biliary cirrhosis. Gut 2010;59:943-952. PMID: 20442198

[81] Li ZF, Zhang S, Huang Y, Xia XM, Li AM, Pan D, et al. Morphological changes of blood spleen barrier in portal hypertensive spleen. Chin Med J (Engl) 2008;121:561-565. PMID: 18364147

[82] Li ZF, Zhang S, Lv GB, Huang Y, Zhang W, Ren S, et al. Changes in count and function of splenic lymphocytes from patients with portal hypertension. World J Gastroenterol 2008;14:2377-2382. PMID: 18416465

[83] Li Z, Zhang S, Huang C, Zhang W, Hu Y, Wei B. MicroRNAome of splenic macrophages in hypersplenism due to portal hypertension in hepatitis B virus-related cirrhosis. Exp Biol Med (Maywood) 2008;233:1454-1461. PMID: 18791127

[84] Jiang A, Zhang S, Li Z, Liang R, Ren S, Li J, et al. miR-615-3p promotes the phagocytic capacity of splenic macrophages by targeting ligand-dependent nuclear receptor corepressor in cirrhosis-related portal hypertension. Exp Biol Med (Maywood) 2011;236:672-680. PMID: 21565892

[85] Zhang W, Zhang S, Li ZF, Huang C, Ren S, Zhou R, et al. Knockdown of PIK3R1 by shRNA inhibits the activity of the splenic macrophages associated with hypersplenism due to portal hypertension. Pathol Res Pract 2010;206:760-767. PMID: 20846792

[86] Xia Z, Wang G, Wan C, Liu T, Wang S, Wang B, et al. Expression of NALP3 in the spleen of mice with portal hypertension. J Huazhong Univ Sci Technolog Med Sci 2010;30:170-172. PMID: 20407867

[87] El-Sayed R, El-Ela MA, El-Raziky MS, Helmy H, El-Ghaffar AA, El-Karaksy H. Relation of serum levels of thrombopoietin to thrombocytopenia in extrahepatic portal vein obstruction versus cirrhotic children. J Pediatr Hematol Oncol 2011;33:e267-270. PMID: 21941130

[88] Boleslawski E, Petrovai G, Truant S, Dharancy S, Duhamel A, Salleron J, et al. Hepatic venous pressure gradient in the assessment of portal hypertension before liver resection in patients with cirrhosis. Br J Surg 2012;99:855-863. PMID: 22508371

[89] Garcia-Tsao G, Groszmann RJ, Fisher RL, Conn HO, Atterbury CE, Glickman M. Portal pressure, presence of gastroesophageal varices and variceal bleeding. Hepatology 1985;5:419-424. PMID: 3873388

[90] Maruyama H,Yokosuka O. Pathophysiology of portal hypertension and esophageal varices. Int J Hepatol 2012;2012:895787. PMID: 22666604

[91] Yin ZH, Liu XY, Huang RL, Ren SP. Expression of TNF-alpha and VEGF in the esophagus of portal hypertensive rats. World J Gastroenterol 2005;11:1232-1236. PMID: 15754412

[92] Huang HC, Haq O, Utsumi T, Sethasine S, Abraldes JG, Groszmann RJ, et al. Intestinal and plasma VEGF levels in cirrhosis: the role of portal pressure. J Cell Mol Med 2012;16:1125-1133. PMID: 21801303

[93] Pan WD, Liu Y, Lin N, Xu R. The expression of PEDF and VEGF in the gastric wall of prehepatic portal hypertensive rats. Hepatogastroenterology 2011;58:2152-2155. PMID: 22024088

[94] Fernandez M, Mejias M, Angermayr B, Garcia-Pagan JC, Rodes J, Bosch J. Inhibition of VEGF receptor-2 decreases the development of hyperdynamic splanchnic circulation and portal-systemic collateral vessels in portal hypertensive rats. J Hepatol 2005;43:98-103. PMID: 15893841

[95] Tsui CP, Sung JJ, Leung FW. Role of acute elevation of portal venous pressure by exogenous glucagon on gastric mucosal injury in rats with portal hypertension. Life Sci 2003;73:1115-1129. PMID: 12818720

[96] Sakai Y, Enomoto H, Aizawa N, Iwata Y, Tanaka H, Ikeda N, et al. Relationship between Elevation of Glycated Albumin to Glycated Hemoglobin Ratio in Patients with a High Bleeding Risk of Esophageal Varices. Hepatogastroenterology 2012;59. PMID: 22440250

[97] Dursun H, Albayrak F, Uyanik A, Keles NO, Beyzagul P, Bayram E, et al. Effects of hypertension and ovariectomy on rat hepatocytes. Are amlodipine and lacidipine protective? (A stereological and histological study). Turk J Gastroenterol 2010;21:387-395. PMID: 21331992

[98] Guo SB, Duan ZJ, Li Q, Sun XY. Effect of heme oxygenase-1 on renal function in rats with liver cirrhosis. World J Gastroenterol 2011;17:322-328. PMID: 21253390

[99] Sharawey MA, Shawky EM, Ali LH, Mohammed AA, Hassan HA, Fouad YM. Cystatin C: a predictor of hepatorenal syndrome in patients with liver cirrhosis. Hepatol Int 2011. PMID: 21484118

[100] Barakat M,Khalil M. Serum cystatin C in advanced liver cirrhosis and different stages of the hepatorenal syndrome. Arab J Gastroenterol 2011;12:131-135. PMID: 22055590

[101] Uemura M, Fujimura Y, Ko S, Matsumoto M, Nakajima Y, Fukui H. Determination of ADAMTS13 and Its Clinical Significance for ADAMTS13 Supplementation Therapy to Improve the Survival of Patients with Decompensated Liver Cirrhosis. Int J Hepatol 2011;2011:759047. PMID: 21994870

[102] Takaya H, Uemura M, Fujimura Y, Matsumoto M, Matsuyama T, Kato S, et al. ADAMTS13 activity may predict the cumulative survival of patients with liver cirrhosis in comparison with the Child-Turcotte-Pugh score and the Model for End-Stage Liver Disease score. Hepatol Res 2012;42:459-472. PMID: 22292786

[103] Merino J, Aller MA, Rubio S, Arias N, Nava MP, Loscertales M, et al. Gut-brain chemokine changes in portal hypertensive rats. Dig Dis Sci 2011;56:2309-2317. PMID: 21347560

[104] Guyon A,Nahon JL. Multiple actions of the chemokine stromal cell-derived factor-1alpha on neuronal activity. J Mol Endocrinol 2007;38:365-376. PMID: 17339399

[105] Rosello DM, Balestrasse K, Coll C, Coll S, Tallis S, Gurni A, et al. Oxidative stress and hippocampus in a low-grade hepatic encephalopathy model: protective effects of curcumin. Hepatol Res 2008;38:1148-1153. PMID: 19000058

[106] Nikonenko AG, Radenovic L, Andjus PR, Skibo GG. Structural features of ischemic damage in the hippocampus. Anat Rec (Hoboken) 2009;292:1914-1921. PMID: 19943345

[107] Ahboucha S, Talani G, Fanutza T, Sanna E, Biggio G, Gamrani H, et al. Reduced brain levels of DHEAS in hepatic coma patients: Significance for increased GABAergic tone in hepatic encephalopathy. Neurochem Int 2012;61:48-53. PMID: 22490610

[108] Luo M, Li L, Yang EN, Cao WK. Relationship between interleukin-6 and ammonia in patients with minimal hepatic encephalopathy due to liver cirrhosis. Hepatol Res 2012. PMID: 22646055

[109] Balasubramaniyan V, Wright G, Sharma V, Davies NA, Sharifi Y, Habtesion A, et al. Ammonia reduction with ornithine phenylacetate restores brain eNOS activity via the DDAH-ADMA pathway in bile duct-ligated cirrhotic rats. Am J Physiol Gastrointest Liver Physiol 2012;302:G145-152. PMID: 21903766

[110] Zeron HM, Rodriguez MR, Montes S, Castaneda CR. Blood manganese levels in patients with hepatic encephalopathy. J Trace Elem Med Biol 2011;25:225-229. PMID: 21975221

Chapter 8

Laparoscopic Radiofrequency Ablation of Liver Tumors

Mirela Patricia Sîrb Boeti, Răzvan Grigorie and
Irinel Popescu

Additional information is available at the end of the chapter

1. Introduction

The biological effects of radiofrequency (RF) waves were first reported on liver lesions by McGahan et al. in 1990 [1].

The early reports on the efficacy and safety of radiofrequency ablation (RFA) for liver tumors have encouraged rapid spreading of the technique for the treatment of unresectable or even resectable tumors. Nowadays RFA constitutes a wide-range therapeutical option for a variety of tumors. The vast majority of the reports about RFA refer to malignant liver tumors. There are only few authors who attest the efficiency of this in situ ablative method for benign liver tumors (e.g. hepatic cavernous hemangioma, hepatic adenoma). RFA must be integrated in a complex multimodal treatment for patient with liver tumors. Selected patients may also benefit of simultaneous and/or consecutive association of RFA with other treatments like surgery, chemotherapy, and other in situ ablation procedures.

All the authors concur to the fact that RFA is a technology-based treatment. However, the importance of operator experience in this treatment must not be alluded. Not only the complete knowledge of the RF armamentarium but also patient and approach selection for RFA are mandatory to certify this method as an effective and safe technique for treatment of the liver tumors [2].

It must be underscore that RFA is not just a simple technique of inserting a needle to "cook" the tumors but is a new technology in the treatment of liver tumors with a steep learning curve which may offer these patients a 50-95% chance of destroying these lesions [3].

While RFA is most commonly performed in the radiology departments through a percutaneous approach, our experience over 5 years determines us to advocate for the laparoscopic ablation of liver tumor using RF. Even if it is still a debate on the correlation of the different

RFA approaches with the results in terms of recurrence and survival, our recommendation is to use laparoscopic RFA (LRFA) whenever possible.

With this paper we intend to offer a review regarding the laparoscopic ablations with RF for patients suffering from liver tumors. We aim to describe the RF and ultrasound equipment, define the selection criteria of the patients for this kind of approach, present the ablation procedure, and the follow-up criteria, and discuss the LRFA outcomes in terms of procedural-related morbidity and mortality, tumor recurrence, and patient survival.

2. Methods

A review of relevant articles was undertaken based on a Medline search from January 1998 till January 2012.

2.1. Mechanism of RFA

When high-frequency (350-500 kHz) alternating current passes the tissues, polar molecules (e.g. water molecules) are orientated in conformity with the field polarity [4]. With every change of the polarity of the alternating current polar molecules are moving in attempt to follow its direction. Their ionic vibration results in dielectrical losses into tissues because of molecular friction. The dielectric losses generate heat (frictional heating) which causes thermal tissues injuries. The extension and type of the thermal lesions depend on the temperature and duration of current applications. These lesions begin at 42^0C. Above this level the time of lethal exposion drops progressively: 8 min at 46^0C, 4-5 min at 50^0C. At 60^0C the cellular death is inevitable due to irreversible lesions of mitochondrial and cytoplasmatic enzymes secondary to thermal protein denaturation [5]. Tissue desiccation occurs at 100^0C. But quick tissue heating over 100^0C has the disadvantage of fast increasing thetissue impedance due to charring, which consecutively restricts the heat propagation and eventually coagulation necrosis [5]. Malignant cells are more prone to damages due to hyperthermia than normal cells [6].

2.2. Indications of RFA

RFA is now gaining popularity as the preferred modality of local ablation for patients with malignant liver tumors who are not surgical candidates (table 1).

RFA is used to treat liver lesions considered unresectable due to their bulky volume, position near key vessels, multiplicity or insufficiency of remnant liver parenchyma.

In terms of the extend of hepatic disease we consider safe to perform LRFA on patients with total tumor volume less than 20% contrary with opinion of other authors who reported good results in patients with up to 50% total liver replacement [3].

RFA has an important role in converting nonresectable in resectable tumors and also in increasing resectability of multiple liver tumors. Resections of such tumors are feasible d'emblee or in two-stage procedure. RFA of the small and deeply situated tumor(s) in one hepatic lobe can be associated with resection of a large tumor or multiple tumors located in the controlateral lobe or with controlateral portal vein ligation. The procedure can also be performed before liver resection for tumors located in the section plane in order to obtain disease-free margins.

Patients with liver tumor but with general contraindications for hepatic resection or those who refuse the operation are also candidates for RFA.

Moreover, the application of RFA has now expanded to patients as a bridge to liver transplantation. RFA proved benefits for patients with cirrhotic and HCC who are within Milano criteria on the waiting list for liver transplantation. It also have been shown to result in down staging the HCC in cirrhotic patients beyound the Milano criteria and thus in listing these patients for liver transplantation.

Patient with primary or metastatic hepatic tumor(s) which are not candidates for hepatic resection
Tumor characteristics
multiple diffuse bilobar
in association with hepatic resection
in association with transarterial chemoembolization of hepatic artery
deeply situated
near the portal pedicles, hepatic veins, inferior vena cava
recurrence after major hepatectomies
small HCC on cirrhosis in patients (in Milan criteria) on waiting list for LTx
large HCC on cirrhosis in patients (out of Milan criteria) to be included on the waiting list after downstaging
large unresectable tumor for downstaging followed by hepatectomy
number ≤ 5 (14)
maximum diameter ≤ 5 (7, 8) cm
Poor liver parenchyma function
Patient with benign hepatic tumor
Co-morbidities which increase the anesthesia-surgical risk
Patient refusal of hepatic resection
Patient expectation survival ≥ 3 months
Other tumor localizations which can be treated
Written informed consent of the patient

Table 1. Indications of RFA.

Based on some studies there are authors who plead for RFA even as a substitute to hepatic resection for small liver tumors.

Patients with hepatic malignancies, except those with neuroendocrine tumors, should be approached with curative intent and the goal of extending survival. Curative intent means that similar to liver resection the ablation has to completely destroy not only the tumor but also at least 0.5-1 cm zone of normal liver parenchyma.

RFA was successfully used to treat patients with symptomatic and rapid-growth hepatic cavernous hemangioma [7]. Application of LRFA for the treatment of benign tumor proved to be safe and indicated also in patients with liver adenoma [8].

2.2.1. LRFA advantages

We advocate the laparoscopic approach to ablate the liver tumors with RF due to its advantages over the other two methods: percutaneous and open.

Laparoscopy represents a reliable diagnostic tool. Some authors consider that every liver resection must be preceded by abdominal laparoscopic assessment of the disease [9]. By identifying extrahepatic lesions, laparoscopy can up-stage the patients with cancer and can deem these as unresectable or untreatable with in situ ablation procedures (except those with neuroendocrine tumors).

Two third of the patients with advanced liver insufficiency being evaluated for orthotopic liver transplantation are restaged after exploratory laparoscopy, laparoscopic ultrasound (LUS) and Ultrasound-guided biopsy, half being downstaged and half upstaged [10]. This finding determines some authors to indicate laparoscopic staging followed by LRFA for patients with adenocirrhosis evaluated for liver transplantation unless there are unequivocal clinical data supporting the stage of hepatocellular carcinoma [10].

Unsuspected intra-abdominal extrahepatic metastases can be noted in up to 26% of patients with colorectal liver metastases [11].

Moreove laparoscopy either alone or in association with intraoperative ultrasound examination can diagnose other liver lesions missed by the preoperative imaging examinations in up to 38% cases [12]. LUS can detect lesions less than 2 cm in diameter.

The laparoscopic approach proved to be safe for the treatment of subcapsular tumors due to the possibility of direct visualization and active protection of the surrounding structures (gallbladder, stomach, duodenum, colon, diaphragm) and possibility to control the potential bleeding from these lesions.

The pneumoperitoneum creates a working camera which not only removes the surrounding structures from the liver but also reduces the respiratory movements of the liver and thus facilitates the placement of the RF needle.

LRFA is also able to ablate deep-sited lesions difficult or impossible to be visualized by percutaneous US or to be punctured percutaneously. Some authors consider that for lesions located beneath the diaphragm laparoscopic approach can be associated [13] or even replaced with the thoracoscopic one [14, 15].

For treating patients with large or multiple liver tumors LRFA seems to be the first choice. Nevertheless, for tumors larger than 60 mm in diameter, tumors more than 5, and tumors close to the hepatic vein or inferior vena cava, some author consider RFA via laparotomy to be safer than LRFA [16].

During LRFA the Pringle maneuver can be used if it is necessary. Pneumoperitoneum per se has the advantage to decrease the blood flow and increase the area of ablation [17].

In patients with multiple hepatic lesions surgeons with high expertise can performed LRFA in association with laparoscopic hepatic resection.

Comparing with the open technique, LRFA determines less intra-operative blood loss and fewer postoperative complications [16].

Due to its minimal surgical trauma, LRFA determines a fast recovery time and short hospital stay. It is our practice to discharge the patient 24-48 hours after the operation.

The benefits of LRFA in cirrhotic patients are certain when comparing with the open approach. First, preservation of the abdominal wall and lack of the need to mobilize the liver avoid interruption of large collateral veins and perihepatic ligaments, thus decreasing postoperative ascitic syndrome. Second, nonexposure of the viscera restricts the electrolytic and protein losses and hence the fluids requirements which secondary improves absorption of ascitis. Third, the laparoscopic approach is associated with lower intraoperative blood loss due to the haemostatic effect of the positive pressure of peritoneum, meticulous intraoperative manipulations of the tissue under magnification, and smaller abdominal incisions. It was reported that intraoperative blood loss is a major risk factor of postoperative morbidity and death [18].

For liver tumor recurrences, LRFA can be repeated as needed.

It is still not finally settled which is the best RFA approach in terms of recurrence and survival but we favor the laparoscopic one based on literature data and our experience.

2.2.2. Hepatocellular carcinoma (HCC)

Hepatocellular carcinoma (HCC) is the fifth most common malignancy and fourth in annual mortality. Its incidence continues to grow up secondary to the increasing prevalence of viral hepatitis [19]. Hepatic resection and liver transplantation are considered the mainstay of treatment of HCC being proven as the most effective treatments in means of disease-free interval and survival. However, less than 20% of HCC can be treated surgically because of multifocal diseases, proximity of the tumor to key vascular or biliary structures precluding a margin-negative resection, and inadequate functional hepatic reserve with cirrhosis. Usually, noncirrhotic or Child A cirrhotic patients with single small HCC (≤5 cm) or up to three lesions ≤3 cm are indicated for surgery.

2.2.2.1. Bridge to transplantation

The efficacy of RFA in wait-listed transplant candidates has been studied. Johnson et al. reported eight pretransplant patients treated solely by RFA and matched to a similar group by age, sex, Child-Turcotte-Pugh class, and Model for End-Stage Liver Disease (MELD) score who did not undergo treatment prior to transplant.[20] Patients pretreated with RFA were able to remain on the transplant list for longer periods of time than their matched counterparts. Dropout rates without RFA have been shown to be as high as 40%; however, the use of RFA has decreased them to as low as 20%. The use of RFA as a bridge to transplantation has proven to be an effective strategy. Control of tumor size and the theoretical prevention of metastatic disease formation allow patients to remain on the waiting list for longer periods, increasing their likelihood of obtaining a donor organ. RFA remains limited in its ability to provide complete necrosis of large tumors and should not be expected to do so in patients who are near the upper limits of transplant candidacy because of size criteria.

The need for an accurate intrahepatic staging is crucial for patients with HCC candidates to an aggressive surgical or ablative treatment. Combinations of resection and ablation may be required in certain cases, extending the indications for the laparoscopic approach to hepatocellular carcinoma in liver cirrhosis. Laparoscopy with LUS seems to be useful to identify unsuspected new nodules and to help in choosing the most suitable treatment. Laparoscopy with LUS could represent a sound preliminary examination in patients who are candidates to liver transplantation in order to both improve the staging and guide an interstitial therapy as a bridge to the transplantation itself [21].

2.2.2.2. Resection versus RFA

Surgical resection is the gold standard of treatment for HCC in noncirrhotic and cirrhotic patients who can tolerate hepatic resection. Noncirrhotic patients with HCC can usually undergo resection. However, patients with underlying cirrhosis are rarely candidates for resection and often face a dismal prognosis. As a result, prospective studies comparing patients who are surgical candidates and underwent RFA with those who underwent resection are fairly limited.

2.2.2.3. The use of RFA in nonsurgical candidates

The reported rate of resectable HCC is low and ranges from 9% to 27%. It is limited by the proximity of the tumor to major vascular and biliary structures that would preclude negative resection margins, but more importantly by the degree of underlying liver disease and Ability of the patient to tolerate hepatectomy. Small tumors are generally best suited for RFA and provide the best results. However, larger lesions have also been ablated with mixed success, occasionally even providing overall long-term survival of some patients with HCC. Small lesions are generally considered those that are <3–3.5 cm in diameter.

Larger lesions are known to be more difficult to treat using RFA. Tumors >3 cm may require repositioning of the electrode or multiple treatment sessions in order to obtain clear margins. However, even using a more aggressive approach, the efficacy of RFA has been proven to be limited by tumor size. Lesions measuring >5 cm have at best only a 50% chance of being completely ablated.

Therefore, most authors do not recommend the use of RFA for tumors >5–6 cm because of the technical limitations of the current used equipment and their inability to provide complete coagulative necrosis.

Despite the tumor size limitations of RFA, its use in unresectable HCC is significant. Those who are not transplant candidates or are unable to undergo resection face a dismal prognosis, and RFA provides a chance for survival, especially for patients with smaller lesions. However, the use of RFA should be discouraged in patients with large lesions or those who have evidence of metastatic disease, because these groups have such a poor outcome that RFA is unlikely to provide any tangible benefit.

2.2.2.4. Surgical resection in combination with LRFA

Patients with multifocal disease may be treated by a combined approach using both surgical resection and RFA. The bulk of the tumor burden is initially resected, and RFA is then performed on any remaining unresectable lesions. However, there are few data to support this approach, especially in the setting of HCC. Most agree that if HCC has progressed so extensively, the patient is unlikely to be cured even by aggressive combined modalities of this nature. Additionally, although well tolerated intraoperatively, RFA combined with hepatic resection does place the patient at a higher risk for postoperative liver failure and death. This is especially true in the cirrhotic patient with poor hepatic reserve prior to intervention. Therefore, the role of LRFA in conjunction with resection must be used judiciously and mandates further reviews before it can be recommended in the treatment of HCC.

2.2.3. Metastatic colorectal cancer

The liver is the most common site of distant metastases second only to lymph nodes [22]. Initially considered to be a terminal diagnosis, treatment of these lesions has provided significantly better outcomes for many of these patients, in comparision to those untreated.

Akin with the primary liver masses, surgical resection remains the gold standard therapy for liver metastases from colorectal cancer.

Colorectal cancer is the leading cause of cancer death in US. At the time of exploration for their primary tumor 16-25% of patients have liver metastases and about 25% will develop such lesions in the disease course.

Colorectal cancer is responsible for up to 75% of liver metastases that undergo surgical treatment. For those who undergo resection of isolated liver metastases, the 5-year survival rate has recently been shown to be as high as 58% [23]. Prospective studies that compare RFA with Resection in operative candidates are extremely limited.

Unfortunately, up to 80% of the patients diagnosed with stage IV disease are not candidates for resection. For unresectable liver metastases, alternative options, such as RFA alone or in conjunction with other therapeutic modalities, are being explored to further improve survival [24]. Criteria for unresectable metastases include bilobar disease that cannot be completely excised, proximity to major vasculature structures precluding margin-negative resection, and comorbid conditions that preclude surgery [25]. For these untreated patients, survival is <5%–10% at 5 years [26].

Large trials evaluating the combination of RFA and resection are limited, and therefore it is difficult to draw definitive conclusions regarding its efficacy and safety. As larger portions of hepatic parenchyma are resected or ablated, the risk for liver failure increases, making it difficult to support the use of a combined approach without achieving a survival benefit. At this time, there are few data to support combining RFA with surgical resection.

2.2.4. Liver metastasis from neuroendocrine tumors

Liver metastases occur in 5-90% of patients with neuroendocrine tumors and the specific pattern of these is an indolent course, which may be dominated by symptoms related to hormonal secretion.

The goal of surgical resection and RFA in most cases of both primary and metastatic liver disease is curative. However, neuroendocrine tumors represent a unique group of slowly growing, often highly symptomatic tumors that are unlikely to be cured by resection. The untreated patients with unresectable neuroendocrine liver metastases have a 5-year survival rate of 25-38%.[27] In patients with metastatic neuroendocrine tumors who are unlikely to be cured by surgery or unable to tolerate an invasive form of treatment, RFA has been shown to ameliorate the symptoms (95%), significantly or completely control the symptoms (80%), and partially or significantly decrease the circulating hormone levels (65%) [28, 29]. LRFA seems appealing for these patients because the recurrence rate after resection is >80% at 5 years. Moreover, in case of liver recurrence, LRFA can be repeated for maintaining tumor control in the liver without increasing morbidity.

2.2.5. Liver metastasis from nonneuroendocrine and noncolorectal tumors

Regarding the nonneuroendocrine and noncolorectal liver metastases there are few reports on the utility of RFA to treat them. Patients with liver metastases from sarcoma, breast cancer, gastric cancer, pancreatic adenocarcinoma, or malignant melanoma are predicted to have a short survival due to the rapid diffusely disseminated disease. The overall median survival for these patients is 33 months. The aim for these patients is to prolong life with treatments which have low side effects and offer a good quality of life. Notwithstanding the curative intention of the treatments, most of them are ultimately proven to be palliative due to the progression of the disease. For these patients LRFA has not only curative but also debulking target. For the patients with nonresectable liver metastases, LRFA offers an overall median survival of more than 51 months [30].

2.3. Contraindications of LRFA

These contraindication are:

- Patients ≤ 18 years-old or ≥ 80 years-old,
- Sever coagulopathy (PLT <50.000/mm3, PT, APTT >1,5N),
- Renal failure (serum creatinin > 2,5 mg/dl),
- Jaundice (bilirubinemia > 3 mg/dl, bile duct dilatation),
- Acute infection,
- Tumor vascular or organ invasion,

- Patients with cardiac pacemaker, implanted metallic pieces,

- Sever mental disturbances,

- Pregnancy and breast feeding.

2.4. Patient preparation for LRFA

For all patients admitted for LRFA a baseline evaluation has to be done within one week before the procedure. Besides history and clinical examinations, there are some mandatory laboratory tests and imaging examinations.

Laboratory tests consist of complete blood cell counts, coagulation profile, renal and liver panel, and appropriate serum tumor markers.

Imaging examinations include percutaneous abdominal ultrasound, computer tomography, magnetic resonance imaging (MRI), chest Rx, and, in selected cases, positron emission tomography using [18]FDG [12].

The patients known with cardiac problems should have a pretreatment cardiologic assessment in order to prevent the possible arrhythmia due to RFA. Without being an absolute contraindication, patients with implanted cardiac pacemakers need special attention before, during and after the procedure.

Due to the great risk of biliary injury during RFA of the central liver tumors, some authors place preoperative prophylactic biliary stents in patients with such lesions [12].

A dose of intravenous antibiotics is given just before RFA. The duration of administration depends on the various protocol used, being up to 5 days [2].

Informed consent of the patient is obtained before the procedure.

For LRFA the most used is the supine position of the patient. Only when there is a predominance of the disease in the posterior segments of the liver the patient is put on the operating table in left lateral position [31].

The LRFA is performed under general anesthesia.

2.5. The RF-equipment

2.5.1. The RF-equipment

Historically, the major impediment on RFA has been the size of the area to be ablated which could be the explanation of the Achilles' heel of this procedure: local tumor recurrence. In order to improve the results, RF equipments have been continuously perfected.

The rapid increase of temperature (above 100°C) during RFA, leading to charring of the tissue and increase of impedance, was shown to be the main cause of the small coagulation volumes. Many electrodes have been designed to improve energy deposition on tissue and further increase coagulation volume. Nowadays there are various single or combined type of electrodes. The main types are: single, cluster, multitined expandable, spiral expandable, cooled, wet (perfused), monopolar or bipolar electrodes (table 2).[32]

RF system	Rita Model 1500x	Cool –tip	Boston RF 3000	Berchtold	Surtron	Celon Power-Olympus
Power	250 W	200 W	200 W	60 W	200W	250 W
Frequency	460 kHz	480 kHz	480 kHz	375 kHz	480kHz	470 kHz
Ablation control	Impedance and temperature	Impedance	Impedance	Impedance	Impedance	Impedance
Energy delivery	Monopolar bipolar	Monopolar	Monopolar	Monopolar	Monopolar	Bipolar multipolar
Electrode diameter	2.2 mm	1.6mm/ 3x1.6mm	2.5 mm	1.7 mm		1.8 mm
Electrode geometry	"Christmas tree"	Single, Cluster	"Umbrella"	Single, Cluster	Single	Single
Active part of the electrode	5cm/7cm	Single/ Cluster 3cm/2,5cm	4 cm	1.5 cm		4 cm
Electrode	Expended± wet ±flexible	Cooled single/cluster	Expended	Wet		Cooled
MRI	Yes (XL)	Yes (single or cluster)	Yes (3.5cm)	Yes	Yes	Yes (mono/ multipolar)

Table 2. Different characteristics of RF equipments and probes.

2.5.2. The ultrasound equipment

The ultrasound equipment used for ablation must have either a fixed or flexible linear laparoscopic ultrasound probe (figure 1A) or a fixed forward-viewing convex-array transducer (figure 2B) and the possibility of Doppler imaging.

For improvement of tumor visualization and targeting for RFA, a prototype tracked ultrasound-guided laparoscopic surgery system was design and used in clinical practice by some authors [33]. By tracking two-dimensional ultrasound images in physical space, the system generates three-dimensional ultrasound volumes. Once the tumor is manually identified in this volume, a targeting system is used to guide the tip of the RFA probe inside the tumor [33].

A picture-in-picture box with the quarter-size laparoscopic image superimposed over the full-sized ultrasound image is of paramount importance for the coordination of the movement of the instruments.

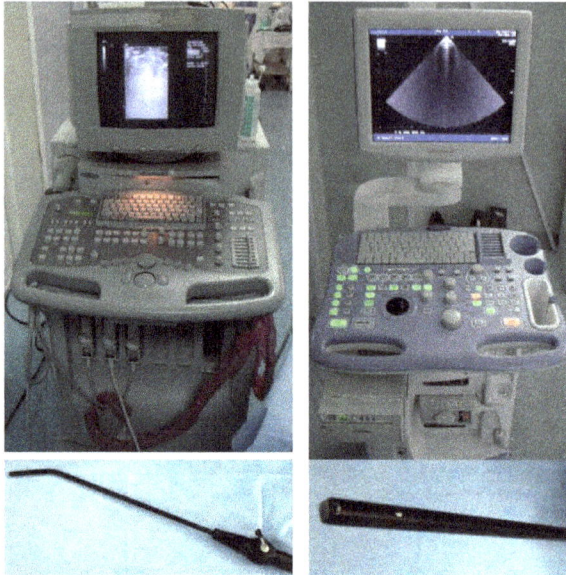

Figure 1. Ultrasound equipment. A. Ultrasound machine with flexible liniar transductor for laparoscopy. B. Ultrasound machine with fixed convex transductor for laparoscopy

2.6. LRFA technique

2.6.1. Pneumoperitoneum induction

In many centers the Veress technique remains the most widespread method of induction of peritoneum. Because the most common complications of laparoscopic surgery are related to insertion of the Veress needle and the first trocar, alternatives such Hasson's open method or optical access trocar-insertion emerged. These alternative methods are especially useful in patients with previous operations and intraabdominal adhesions.

The Hasson's open method implies the transversing of the tissue planes under direct view and carries the disadvantages of continuous air leaks and prolonged operating time. Besides it can be cumbersome in obese patients.

The optical access trocars have been developed as an alternative means of transversing the tissue planes under direct view. We advocate the use of optical access trocar which in our department is the standard device for obtaining abdominal access in laparoscopic practice since 1995 [34]. The method consists in introduction into abdomen of a 12-mm disposable Optiview® trocar (Ethicon Endo-surgery Cincinnati, OH) or a 5-12 mm Visiport™ Plus Optical trocar (Covidien)with an inserted 0⁰ laparoscope.

2.6.2. Trocar insertion

Most of the patients submitted for LRFA can be treated with placement of two right subcostal ports. The umbilical placement of one trocar represents an impediment to reach the dome of the liver from such a location.

Selected patients need insertion of the third or fourth trocar (figure 2). The additional trocars may be needed for dissection of the intra-abdominal adhesions, performing cholecystectomy, retraction of the adjacent organs, or multiple needle insertion for treating multiple tumors.

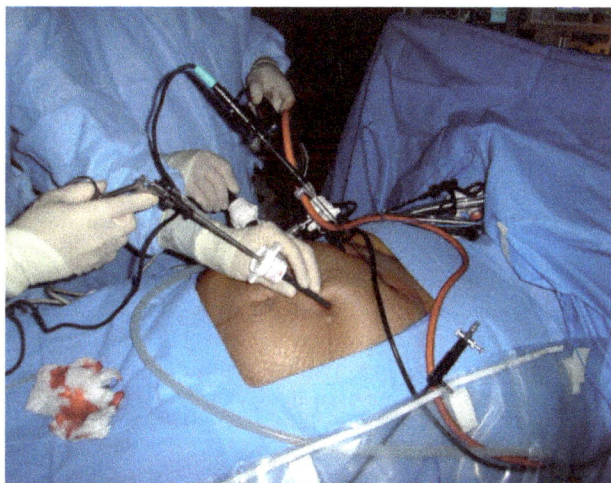

Figure 2. Patient with previous laparotomy, placed in supine position for LRFA of bilateral liver metastases. Three trocars are inserted: one for video, one for ultrasound transductor, and one aditional trocar for forceps. The RF probe is percutaneously introduced.

2.6.3. Abdominal exploration

All adhesions that interfere with proper exploration of the abdomen are taken down. A systematic and thorough visual exploration of the abdominal cavity is performed, and all peritoneal surfaces are carefully examined for possible deposits, paying special attention to the undersurface of the diaphragm, the hepatic round ligament, and the omentum. Lymph nodes in the hepatoduodenal ligament are examined for enlargement. The quality of the liver parenchyma with regard to the degree of cirrhosis or steatosis is also assessed.

Laparoscopic ultrasound is performed systematically in a longitudinal fashion, different from the transverse orientation in intraoperative ultrasound. For laparoscopic ultrasound liver scanning, most authors use the linear probe. For a better visualization of the upper segments or caudate lobe some authors favor the use of others probes. In some cases for a better contact between the convex liver surface and the probe, instillation of normal saline solution

into peritoneum can be very helpful to provide an acoustic window. Sometimes the abdomen need to be desufflated to improve contact with the liver. The laparoscope and LUS probe
can be interchanged between the ports to provide different views of the liver and to enable
varying placements of the probe on the liver surface. Generally it is not needed to take down
the falciform ligament but the creation of a window in the falciform ligament allows the
exploration of the liver in patients with dense midline adhesions. Maintaining visual guidance of the probe's position on the liver with the laparoscope aids in orientation. Scanning is
started with visualization of the point at which the three liver veins drain into the inferior
caval vein. The number and size of hepatic lesions and their segmental locations are carefully documented. The exact location of the liver masses relative to the central vascular structures is aided by color Doppler, and the distance to the vessels is measured in centimeters,
considering a safe margin for ablation of 1 cm. Color Doppler is also used to assess the vascularity
of the hepatic lesions. The distance between hepatic lesion and surrounding viscera is evaluated in order to plan the ablation process.

2.6.4. Tumor biopsy

Once the lesions are mapped in the liver, a core biopsy is performed under ultrasound guidance using an 18-gauge spring-loaded biopsy gun (Microinvasive) and sent for frozen section to confirm malignancy. In some HHC, obtaining of proper amount of tumoral tissue is
difficult due to its inconsistency and repeated biopsy are needed. The tumor biopsy can also
be Obtained after the RFA having the advantage of harvesting a more consistent tissue frag-
ment and avoiding the possible bleeding from liver puncture site. Tissue samples are taken
only from representative tumors and not from all.

2.6.5. RF needle insertion

Laparoscopic introduction of the RF electrodes into the liver tumors are ultrasound guided
and the operator has to plan very carefully the insertions. This represents the most difficult
part of the procedure, and most beginners under treat due to this.

Introduction of the electrodes especially to ablate large tumors, tumors near great vessels or
poor visualized tumor is very demanding using the fix or flexible linear-type ultrasound
probe (figure 1A). Often small and deep-seated tumors necessitate repeated trial-and-error
insertions of the RF electrode. The safety and the complete necrosis of ablation is very much
dependent on the RF electrode positioning.

For ablation of liver tumors under the guidance of a linear-type probe, the RF electrode
must be inserted from the abdominal wall cranially and parallel to the ultrasound probe. For
accurate tumoral insertion of the RF probe operator has to mentally establish in three dimensions the insertion site and angle on the abdominal wall and also on the surface of the
liver. For small and deep-seated tumors, insertion of the electrode can be very difficult due
to the impossibility to observe the needle on a single image. Therefore, the ultrasound probe
has to be moved according to the position of the needle tip.

Continuous monitorization of the position of the needle tip on the ultrasound image immediately after puncturing the liver is possible using the laparoscopic system with a fixed
forward-viewing convex-array transducer, with a guide groove on the back of the shaft
(figure 1B) [35]. Perpendicular direction of scanning of this transducer enable the easy and
accurate puncture of the deep-seated tumors. Unlike with other conventional linear-type, it
is not necessary to consider the insertion site on the abdominal wall and surface of the liver.
This transducer facilitates the needle insertion in tumors situated in segment VII, VIII, for
which scanning by linear-type probes is more difficult [35]. Some authors advocate the use
of the forward-viewing convex-array probe for lesions situated in segment I arguing that
this US-probe makes not only the imaging of the caudate lobe easily but also avoid the
insertion of the needle through segment IV which has the risk to damage major vessels and
biliary ducts [36].

Positioning the needle tip depends on the type of the electrode used. If a straight (nonex-
pendable) electrode is used then it is advanced under US-guidance until its tip reaches and
passes the deep margin of the lesion in order to obtain a safe oncological rim of normal parenchyma. Depending on the tumor size and noninsulated distance of the electrode it might
take more than one application to complete the lesion ablation. Repositioning the electrode
is performed to obtain overlapping spherical or cylindrical ablations.

If the electrode has Christmas tree-type deployment then the tip of the electrode is positioned also in correlation with the tumor diameter and the active size of the electrode. If only one ablation is planned the tip of the electrode is advanced till it reaches the superficial
margin and the prongs are progressively deployed. If more than one ablation is intended
then the tip of the electrode is positioned into the tumor considering the dimension of the
prongs. After completing the first ablation, the prongs are undeployed, the electrode is retracted by 2-2.5 cm, the prongs are again deployed, and ablation reinitiated.

If one considers the use of an umbrella-type expandable electrode, the tip of the electrode
usually targets the center of the tumor. In case of a large tumor, the positioning of the electrode is similar with the previous expandable type.

Using the first-generation RITA Medical System model 30 (4 arrays) or model 70 (7 arrays), a
single ablation cycle is enough to destroy a tumor <3 cm. For tumors >3 cm overlapping
ablations are necessary using these probes. Using the second-generation of probes - RITA
Medical System Starbust XL (9 arrays, 5 cm) - the tumors <3 cm are ablated with a single 3
cm ablation, those of 3-4 cm with a single 4 cm ablation, those of 4-5 cm with one cycle of a 5
cm ablation and those of >5 cm with application of 2-4 cycles of ablation to obtain adequate
margins [29]. The new RITA System Starbust XLi enhanced permits ablation of the 5-7 cm
sized tumors with a single ablation cycle.

In patients with multiple lesions the duration of the ablation process can be shorten using
simultaneously two RF needles. However these simultaneous ablations are very demanding
due to real-time monitorization. In case of performing these, care must be taken to place the
needles apart otherwise much larger ablation area can result.

Withdrawal of the RF needle after the ablation needs some consideration to discuss. RFA of the needle track is needed not only to control the bleeding but also to avoid recurrences along it. Bleeding from the needle track is seldom a problem but it might be cumbersome in cirrhotic patients. Generally RF ablation with application of a 20-30W power suffices. If not, laparoscopy permits us to control the bleeding by other means: electrocautery, haemostatics, argon application.

2.6.6. Real-time monitoring of the ablation process

The ablation process is assessed in three ways:

1.   monitoring the thermocouples temperatures,

2.   observing the ablation effect by ultrasound,

3.   checking the absence of the Doppler signal into the previously vascularized tumors.

Except of RITA generators all the others deliver energy to tissues automatically based on impedance feed-back control. Because the damages of the tissues are well established at certain temperatures, we favor the use of RITA generators which control the ablation process using the thermocouple temperature. The device can be manually preset to the target temperature. We use for ablation a preset 105^0C temperature at thermocouples. During the ablation procedure the temperatures of the thermocouples are monitorized and visualized on the display of the device. The process can also be registered on a notebook connected to the system.

Aiming the enlargement of the ablation area, many authors have developed their own protocol of ablation [37]. Due to animal experimental studies and our clinical experience, LRFA has become a standardized operation. The time of ablation process depends on the tumor volume. The mainstay is to achieve the target temperature progressively till the full deployment appropriate to the tumor diameter. Our protocol is to deploy progressively the prongs of the RF needle. The prongs are deployed at 2 cm and subsequently to 3 cm until target temperature of 105^0C is reached at all thermocouples. Then the catheter is advanced to 4 cm and consecutively to 5 cm and maintain for 7 min at each deployment [37]. If the target temperatures cannot be achieved the prongs are completely retracted and the catheter rotated with 45^0 and then the prongs redeployed. While advancing the deployment of the prongs, the temperature of the thermocouples decreases and then progressively increases. Sometimes the reposition of the needle is needed to avoid the vicinity of the great vessels or to maintain the prongs inside the liver parenchyma. Even when one to three prongs cannot reach the highest temperature, the ablation procedure is continued taking them out of equation.

After the ablation is ceased, the monitoring of the thermocouples temperature is observed and it should be noticed that it drops rapidly over the 10-20 s and slower after. The temperatures higher then $60-70^0$C at 1 min after ablation are considered relevant to a successful ablation. In case of uncertain ablation, the needle is 45^0 rotated and the tines are again fully deployed. If the temperatures are above 60^0C the ablation is well done. If not, the ablation is repeated.

The ultrasound visualization of the tumor ablation is possible due to the microbubbles formation into the tissue. These are caused by out gassing of dissolved nitrogen. The area of the tumor becomes progressively hypoechoic and due to the gas shadow the deep edge of the tumor is obscured (figure 3). This justify the planning of the ablation process from the deepest tumor area to the superficial one. In about 10 min the gas is reabsorbed and the tumor regains the initial aspect with the exception of some amount of gas and the needle track.

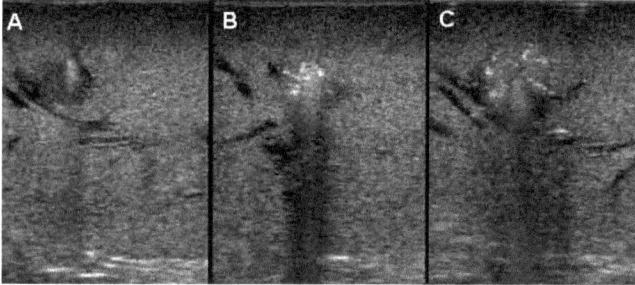

Figure 3. RFA ablation of HCC. A. Positioning the tip of the electrode in the hepatic tumor. B. RFA is started and microbubbles of gas determine appearance of hyperechoic images in the tumor. C. The extension of ablated tissue obscures the deep edge of the tumor. From image collection of Dr. Boros Mirela.

Doppler control of the ablation process is useful in case of vascularized tumors to certify the disappearance of the flow. Usage of the micro bubble contrast agents (e.g. SonoVue ® Bracco International B.V., Holland) can add more help in assessment of the liver blood flow.

Fluorescence spectroscopy was tried in porcine models aiming to detect hepatocellular thermal damage in real time and hence ensure adequate tumor ablation [38].

Due to the skin burn complications reported after RFA, the monitorization of the skin temperature under the grounding pads needs to be mentioned. Especially in patients with large or multiple tumors the position of the grounding pads is essential. The common position is at the same distance on the anterior surface of the tights. These neutral electrodes are needed only when RF monopolar electrodes are used. The bipolar electrodes do not necessitate these pads. It was showed that placing the ground pad over the patient's back resulted in delivering an increased power to the tumor itself and decreasing the time to reach the target temperature [31]. When planning to use two needles two pair of grounding pad are mounted on the patient's back and tight. After completing the ablation the peripheral small tumors become volcanic crater-like and the larger ones appear as a depressed mass.

2.2.7. Useful intraoperative maneuvers

2.6.7.1. Saline-enhanced LRFA

Hypertonic saline injected through a side port on the shaft of the electrode prior to ablation can be uniformly distributed within an encapsulated HCC and thus increase ionicity and conduction within the tumor. The result is an increased volume of ablation up to 6-7 cm diameter. On the contrary, this method is not safe for patients with scirrhous colorectal liver metastases due to the unpredictability distribution of hypertonic saline.

2.6.7.2. Saline infusion systems

The electrodes designed with tiny channels can be used to infuse small volumes of saline into tumor during ablation process in order to prevent desiccation and charring of the tumor that would otherwise prevent conductivity and limit the ablation volume.

2.6.7.3. Vascular occlusion

The application of the Pringle maneuver for limited amounts of time has been shown by some authors [39] to increase ablation volumes but was found inefficient by others [40]. The vascular pedicle occlusion might be justified due to reduction of the heat-sink effect [41]. Total vascular exclusion of the liver was shown to result in the greatest increase in necrosis volume when compared to no occlusion or Pringle maneuver [42].

The possibility of vessel damage or thrombosis secondary to RFA with vascular inflow occlusion was pointed out by some authors [43]. These vascular side effects could be increased in such cases when one or more of electrode prongs are placed in the lumen of a vessel [44]. Moreover, increased ablation secondary to Pringle maneuver carries with it an associated risk of biliary, portal, or parenchymal injury [45].

We consider reasonable not to perform Pringle maneuver also because laparoscopy results in a 30-40% reduction of the blood flow as it was stated by other authors [46].

2.6.7.4. Cooling of the biliary tract

Despite the major vessels, major biliary ducts are deemed to be vulnerable to hyperthermia. Damage of these ducts were reported to occur when the RF needle was located less than 5 mm apart from these [36]. As with the biliary ducts, gallbladder is submitted to damages during and after the ablation process. For tumors situated in segment I, IV, V, in the proximity of the gallbladder cholecystectomy may be recommended before starting the ablation in order to avoid organ perforation or inflammation. The method to prevent the occurrence of biliary system damages is cooling it by pouring cold saline solution onto the surface of the bile duct and gallbladder [36] or by infusing a 4^0 C saline solution quickly through a catheter placed in the bile duct via choledochotomy [47].

3. Results

3.1. Follow-up

Postablation syndrome is a self-limited flu-like syndrome. This systemic inflammatory reaction occurs in one third of patients after RFA and usually depends on the extension of the ablated lesion(s) and ablation time. Its clinical manifestations are milder compared with cryotherapy and consist in transient fever, pain, malaise, myalgia, nausea, and vomiting [48]. The laboratory tests which attest the inflammation are leukocytosis, elevation of serum transaminases, and bilirubin level. The laboratory analysis are performed in the first day after ablation. The WBC count increases more in patients with normal livers and less in patients with previous chemotherapy and cirrhosis [49]. The most dramatic elevations are noticed with AST (14-fold) and ALT (10-fold) but with a fast return to baseline within a week. Serum bilirubin, alkaline phosphatase, and GGT also increase immediately after ablation but with a slower return to baseline up to 3 months. The degree of these elevations is more pronounced in patients with normal hepatic parenchyma than in patients with hepatic steatosis, fibrosis, or cirrhosis [49]. Despite what it would be expected because of the cell death, serum potassium and lactate dehydrogenase levels remain stable after RFA.

To test the tumor markers, blood sample is obtained 1 week after ablation, every 3 months for 2 years, and every 6 months thereafter.

Grayscale ultrasonography of LRFA ablated liver tumor may show hypoechoic, hyperechoic, or mixed appearance. It can be used to early diagnose the hepatic abscess as complication of RFA.

The triphasic (noncontrast, arterial, portal-venous) CT scan is performed to establish a baseline at 1 week postablation and on regular basis every 3 months for 2 years, 6 months for 2 years and yearly thereafter (figure 4).

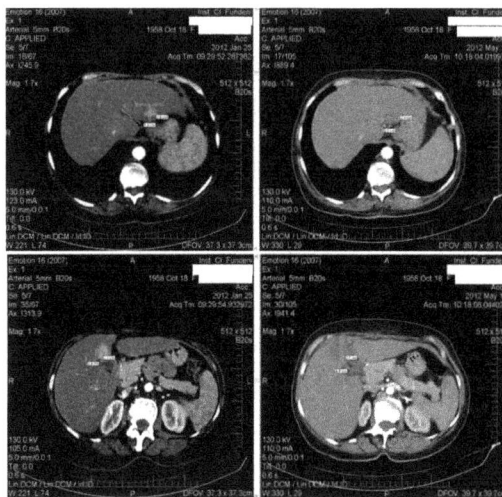

Figure 4. LRFA of a multicentric HCC on cirrhotic liver. The upper images show a hepatic tumor in segment II pre and postablation. The lower images show a hepatic tumor in segment IV pre and postablation. Tactic cholecystectomy was performed during the same operation. There is no tumor recurrence after 3 months postablation.

In the first week postablation, the destroyed tumors appear on contrast-enhanced CT (CECT) with low attenuation when comparing to the normal liver tissue. CECT scan performed in the first 2 weeks postablation may underestimate the actual result due to the presence of granulomatous hypervascularized healing around necrosis which can be misinterpreted as residual viable tumor.

The small ablated lesions have a spherical, "punched out" shape contrary to the large ablated lesions which have a more irregular shape. The success of ablation is announced by CT demonstration of a larger lesion due to the ablation of a rim of nontumoral hepatic parenchyma (figure 5). On further CT scanning the lesion will decrease in size. Any increase in lesion size, irregularity of the edges, or contrast enhancement diagnoses either the incomplete necrosis or local recurrence. Sometimes the appreciation of the contrast enhancement of the lesion might be very difficult especially when comparing the pre- and postablation hypodense liver masses. The assessment of CT Hounsfield unit of the preablated liver lesion was shown to be very reliable in assessment of its evolution. The quantitative measurement of tissue density expressed in Hounsfield unit scale is reproducible over time and is machine independent. In successfully ablated lesions there is a measurable decrease in contrast uptake, which is indicated by the minimal increase in Hounsfield unit density following the administration of contrast in postablation scans [50].

Contrast-enhanced ultrasonography (CEUS) is also useful to provide information regarding ablated lesion but has low sensitivity in identifying the safety margin and incomplete coverage of the liver in patients at high risk of developing new hepatic tumors.

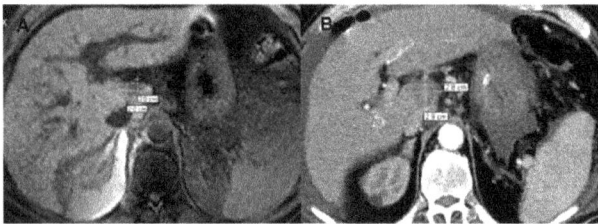

Figure 5. Follow-up of HCC with LFRA. A. RMI is diagnostic for a 2 cm sized tumor situated in caudate lobe. B. Two months after LRFA the tumor is hypodense on CECT and a little larger than prior ablation with a diameter of 2.8 cm. The ablation was successfully completed.

If the CT imaging is doubtful, MRI or PET is indicated. Unenhanced or contrast-enhanced MRI can be used post-LRFA. MRI has a higher sensitivity than CT for detection of recurrences at 2 months (89% vs. 44%) [51] but at 4 months there is no difference between them.

Despite its higher sensitivity for local recurrence comparing with multidetector CT (MDCT), radiolabeled deoxyglucose ([18F]FDG) PET/CT is limited to few centers.

In case of further uncertain imaging results for tumor recurrence, percutaneous biopsy or exploratory laparoscopy with LUS examination and biopsy may be needed [52]. In case of positive malignant fresh sections, the tumor recurrence must be reablated including the whole previous lesion due to the 23% risk of viable tumoral cells in the core of the lesion and respecting 0.5-1 cm edge of oncological safety.[52]

Quality of life is assessed pre- and postablation using different questionnaires.

3.2. Morbidity and mortality

The type of complications after LRFA are mainly the same with those encountered after percutaneous or open approach but with an intermediate rate. The specific complications for the laparoscopic approach are those linked to the introduction of Veress needle and trocars. In LRFA there have not been reported thermal damages of the neighboring organs. The rate of complications seems to be non-related with the histological pattern of the tumor. It has also been proven on large cohort of patients that the rates of complications are comparable if it is the first RFA (5%), repeated RFA (1%), or RFA combined with other procedures (3%) [49].

Hepatic abscess represents the most common complication registered after RFA and is related mostly to large area of necrotic tissue. One explanation for development of hepatic abscess is the retrograde enteric bacterial contamination of the biliary tract from bilioenteric anastomosis or Oddi sphincterectomy. In patients with previous Whipple procedure the incidence of the liver abscess is 40% much more higher than in patients without bilioenteric anastomosis (0.4%) [49]. Considering these, some authors avoid performance of RFA on such patients [2]. In case of performing LRFA for the patients with bilioenteric anastomosis, there should be a close follow-up aiming the early diagnosis and treatment of this complication and a longer antibioprofilaxy. The hepatic abscess can be treated with antibiotics and percutaneous drainage.

Other possible complications are ascitis, liver failure, and respiratory complications.

Thrombocytopenia (excluding patients with preexisting thrombocytemia) and gross mioglobinuria are seldom encountered, being related to the extensive procedure for large or multiple tumors. Acute renal failure due to mioglobinuria is much less encountered as a complication of RFA than cryotherapy and it can be prevented with high hydration of the patient during and after the procedure.

Skin burns are a rare complication with LRFA.

Overall, LRFA is safe and well tolerated, with a per procedure mortality of less than 1%.

3.3. Parietal seeding

Parietal seeding is less a problem in laparoscopic than in percutaneous RFA and can be coped with the aid of a 14 G venous needle or a 2 mm trocar placed through the abdominal wall. The RF electrode is introduced through these large sheaths [53]. For cluster needle such a precaution is not feasible.

3.4. Local recurrence

Local recurrence is defined if the lesion is within 2 cm of the ablated tumor. Remote or distal recurrence is defined when the lesion is at least 2 cm far from the ablated tumor. [53]. Local recurrence is the best measure to assess the technical success of RFA.

Theoretically, the recurrent lesions are due to viable malignant cells that escaped thermal injury during the ablative procedure. This could be the explanation of the recurrences which mainly occur at the periphery of the lesions [50].

The wide range of local recurrence after RFA between 1.8% and 60% reflects difference in tumor type, size, number, liver segmental location, approach, ablation margin, blood vessel proximity, operator experience, and - last but not least - type of RF probe and generator used [54, 55].

The higher rates of recurrence seen within certain tumor histology types are likely a reflection of tumor biology (e.g. density, vascularity, heat conduction) but also of parenchymal milieu (e.g. cirrhosis) [55]. Patients with metastases from colorectal cancer, hepatocellular carcinoma, and melanoma have higher rates of local recurrence comparing with other malignant liver tumors [56].

LRFA results In a tumoral recurrence of 5.8% which is similar with 4.4% obtained in open approach but significant lesser comparing with 16.4% reported with the percutaneous approach [55].

In case of limited hepatic recurrences after other ablative procedures or in selected cases after liver resection, it is our believe that LRFA deserves to be the first-choice treatment. In case of multiple hepatic recurrences, transarterial chemoembolization (TACE) is needed in association with LRFA performed for the larger lesions [57].

3.5. Association of LRFA with other therapeutic methods

In patients with multiple liver masses, LRFA can be performed in association with laparoscopic liver resections [58]. LRFA is indicated for deep-situated (<3 cm) tumors while resection is feasible and safety for exophitic/subcapsular tumors. The association of resection with RFA was found to be a safe procedure with long term outcomes better than the ablation but poorer than resection alone [59].

Due to the progression of the malignant disease most of the patients will develop recurrences after LRFA [53, 60]. Because better survival rates have been obtained with the association of regional chemotherapy, some authors recommend the placement of hepatic arterial infusion pump (HAIP) in all patients who undergo RFA [61]. Concomitant LRFA and HAIP are safe and feasible [62].

LRFA is a therapeutic option for the patients with primary digestive cancer and synchronic liver metastases. A rule of thumb is to perform surgery for the primary indication that brings the patient to the operation (i.e. colorectal, pancreas resection, ileostomy reversal). The surgery for digestive tract can be performed either by laparoscopy or laparotomy and is followed by LRFA. A laparotomy should be converted for LRFA because laparoscopic approach facilitates accurate needle placement [63]. Moreover, LRFA avoids the need of large incision for liver access. For selected cases with colorectal tumors and liver dissemination in which liver resection might increase the operative risk, the ablation of the hepatic lesions is recommended to be performed laparoscopically in the same operative session. The tumor ablation combined with other operative procedures was shown to be safe and not to increase the risk of morbidity and hospital stay [63].

4. Conclusion

Laparoscopic exploration and intraoperative ultrasound permit an accurate staging of malignant disease. In unresectable malignant liver tumors, LRFA represents a safe and effective treatment especially when percutaneus approach to the lesions is deemed difficult. LRFA can also be a substitute for hepatic resection in patients with small malignant tumors or benign liver tumors. LRFA proved to be safe for the treatment of subcapsular tumors due to the possibility of direct visualization, active protection of the surrounding structures, and control of the potential bleeding from these lesions. Deep-situated lesions difficult or impossible to be visualized by percutaneous US and/or punctured percutaneously can be successfully ablated by laparoscopy. Laparoscopic approach is the first choice for ablation of large or multiple liver tumors with possible association of surgical resection or portal vein ligation. LRFA represents a good bridge therapy for prevention of tumor progression and downstaging of multiple lesions for patients with HCC and cirrhosis on the waiting list for liver transplantation. LRFA is associated with less intraoperative blood loss and fewer postoperative complications when compared with open procedure. Due to its minimal surgical trauma, this procedure determines a fast recovery time and short hospital stay. Tumoral recurrence after LRFA is similar to the open approach but significant lesser comparing with percutaneous one. In case of incomplete thermal ablation or tumor recurrence, LRFA can be repeated or followed by transarterial chemoembolization.

Acknowledgements

This chapter was supported by the Sectorial Operational Program Human Resources Development 2007-2013 through the project "Molecular and cellular biotechnologies with medical applications", FSE POSDRU/89/1.5/S/60746.

Author details

Mirela Patricia Sîrb Boeti[1,2*], Răzvan Grigorie[2] and Irinel Popescu[1,2]

*Address all correspondence to: paboet@yahoo.com

1 University of Medicine and Pharmacy "Carol Davila", Bucharest, Romania

2 Fundeni Clinical Institute, Department of General Surgery and Liver Transplantation, Buchares, Romania

References

[1] Mc Gahan, J. P., Browning, P. D., Brock, J. M., & Tesluk, H. (1990). Hepatic ablation using radiofrequency electrocautery. *Invest Radiol*, 25(3), 267-70.

[2] Poon, R. T., Ng, K. K., Lam, C. M., Ai, V., Yuen, J., Fan, S. T., et al. (2004). Learning curve for radiofrequency ablation of liver tumors: prospective analysis of initial 100 patients in a tertiary institution. *Ann Surg*, Apr, 239(4), 441-9.

[3] Hildebrand, P., Leibecke, T., Kleemann, M., Mirow, L., Birth, M., Bruch, H. P., et al. (2006). Influence of operator experience in radiofrequency ablation of malignant liver tumours on treatment outcome. *Eur J Surg Oncol*, May, 32(4), 430-4.

[4] Garcea, G., & Berry, D. P. (2007). Focal liver ablation techniques in primary and secondary liver tumors. *In: P.M.Schlag USS, editor. Regional Cancer Therapy (Cancer Drug Discovery and Development). Humana Press Inc., Totowa, NJ.*

[5] Giovannini, M., Moutardier, V., Danisi, C., Bories, E., Pesenti, C., & Delpero, J. R. (2003). Treatment of hepatocellular carcinoma using percutaneous radiofrequency thermoablation: results and outcomes in 56 patients. *J Gastrointest Surg*, Sep, 7(6), 791-6.

[6] Curley, S. A. (2001). Radiofrequency ablation of malignant liver tumors. *Oncologist*, 6(1), 14-23.

[7] Fan, R. F., Chai, F. L., He, G. X., Wei, L. X., Li, R. Z., Wan, W. X., et al. (2006). Laparoscopic radiofrequency ablation of hepatic cavernous hemangioma. *A preliminary experience with 27 patients. Surg Endosc*, Feb, 20(2), 281-5.

[8] Buscarini, L., Rossi, S., Fornari, F., Di Stasi, M., & Buscarini, E. (1995). Laparoscopic ablation of liver adenoma by radiofrequency electrocauthery. *Gastrointest Endosc*, Jan, 41(1), 68-70.

[9] Rahusen, F. D., Cuesta, Borgstein. P. J., Bleichrodt, R. P., Barkhof, F., Doesburg, T., et al. (1999). Selection of patients for resection of colorectal metastases of the liver using diagnostic laparoscopy and laparoscopic ultrasonography. *Ann Surg*, 230(1), 31-7.

[10] Kim, R. D., Nazarey, P., Katz, E., & Chari, R. S. (2004). Laparoscopic staging and tumor ablation for hepatocellular carcinoma in Child C cirrhotics evaluated for orthotopic liver transplantation. *Surg Endosc*, Jan, 18(1), 39-44.

[11] Lefor, A. T., Hughes, K. S., Shiloni, E., Steinberg, S. M., Vetto, J. P., Papa, M. Z., et al. (1998). Intra-abdominal extrahepatic disease in patients with colorectal hepatic metastases. *Dis Colon Rectum*, 31(2), 100-3.

[12] Bilchik, A. J., Wood, T. F., & Allegra, D. P. (2001). Radiofrequency ablation of unresectable hepatic malignancies: lessons learned. *Oncologist*, 6(1), 24-33.

[13] Kang, C. M., Ko, H. K., Song, S. Y., Kim, K. S., Choi, J. S., Lee, W. J., et al. (2007). Dual-scope guided (simultaneous thoraco-laparoscopic) transthoracic transdiaphragmatic intraoperative radiofrequency ablation for hepatocellular carcinoma located beneath the diaphragm. *Surg Endosc*, Jun 26.

[14] Ishikawa, T., Kohno, T., Shibayama, T., Fukushima, Y., Obi, S., Teratani, T., et al. (2001). Thoracoscopic thermal ablation therapy for hepatocellular carcinoma located beneath the diaphragm. *Endoscopy*, Aug, 33(8), 697-702.

[15] Ishikawa, T., Kohno, T., Teratani, T., & Omata, M. (2002). Thoracoscopic radiofrequency ablation therapy for hepatocellular carcinoma above the diaphragm associated with intractable hemothorax. *Endoscopy*, Oct, 34(10), 843.

[16] Topal, B., Aerts, R., & Penninckx, F. (2003). Laparoscopic radiofrequency ablation of unresectable liver malignancies: feasibility and clinical outcome. *Surg Laparosc Endosc Percutan Tech*, Feb, 13(1), 11-5.

[17] Smith, M. K., Mutter, D., Forbes, L. E., Mulier, S., & Marescaux, J. (2004). The physiologic effect of the pneumoperitoneum on radiofrequency ablation. *Surg Endosc*, Jan, 18(1), 35-8.

[18] Shimata, M., Takenaka, K., Fujiwara, Y., Giot, T., Shirabe, K., Yanaga, K., et al. (1998). Risk factors linked to postoperative morbidity in patients with hepatocellular carcinoma. *Br J Surg*, 85(2), 195-8.

[19] Kew, M. C. (2002). Epidemiology of hepatocellular carcinoma. *Toxicology*, 181-182, 35-8.

[20] Johnson, E. W., Holck, P. S., Levy, A. E., Yeh, M. M., & Yeung, R. S. (2004). The role of tumor ablation in bridging patients to liver transplantation. *Arch Surg*, Aug, 139(8), 825-9.

[21] Montorsi, M., Santambrogio, R., Bianchi, P., Dapri, G., Spinelli, A., & Podda, M. (2002). Perspectives and drawbacks of minimally invasive surgery for hepatocellular carcinoma. *Hepatogastroenterology*, Jan, 49(43), 56-61.

[22] Liu, L. X., Zhang, W. H., & Jiang, H. C. (2003). Current treatment for liver metastases from colorectal cancer. *World J Gastroenterol*, Feb, 9(2), 193-200.

[23] Abdalla, E. K., Vauthey, J. N., Ellis, L. M., Ellis, V., Pollock, R., Broglio, K. R., et al. (2004). Recurrence and outcomes following hepatic resection, radiofrequency ablation, and combined resection/ablation for colorectal liver metastases. *Ann Surg*, Jun, 239(6), 818-25.

[24] Fahy, B. N., & Jarnagin, W. R. (2006). Evolving techniques in the treatment of liver colorectal metastases: role of laparoscopy, radiofrequency ablation, microwave coagulation, hepatic arterial chemotherapy, indications and contraindications for resection, role of transplantation, and timing of chemotherapy. *Surg Clin North Am*, Aug, 86(4), 1005-22.

[25] Curley, S. A., Izzo, F., Delrio, P., Ellis, L. M., Granchi, J., Vallone, P., et al. (1999). Radiofrequency ablation of unresectable primary and metastatic hepatic malignancies: results in 123 patients. *Ann Surg*, Jul, 230(1), 1-8.

[26] Bentrem, D. J., Dematteo, R. P., & Blumgart, L. H. (2005). Surgical therapy for metastatic disease to the liver. *Annu Rev Med*, 56, 139-56.

[27] Touzios, J. G., Kiely, J. M., Pitt, S. C., Rilling, W. S., Quebbeman, E. J., Wilson, S. D., et al. (2005). Neuroendocrine hepatic metastases: does aggressive management improve survival? *Ann Surg*, 241, 776-85.

[28] Mazzaglia, P. J., Berber, E., Milas, M., & Siperstein, A. E. (2007). Laparoscopic radiofrequency ablation of neuroendocrine liver metastases: a 10-year experience evaluating predictors of survival. *Surgery*, Jul, 142(1), 10-9.

[29] Berber, E., Flesher, N., & Siperstein, A. E. (2002). Laparoscopic radiofrequency ablation of neuroendocrine liver metastases. *World J Surg*, Aug, 26(8), 985-90.

[30] Berber, E., Ari, E., Herceg, N., & Siperstein, A. (2005). Laparoscopic radiofrequency thermal ablation for unusual hepatic tumors: operative indications and outcomes. *Surg Endosc*, Dec, 19(12), 1613-7.

[31] Siperstein, A., Garland, A., Engle, K., Rogers, S., Berber, E., String, A., et al. (2000). Laparoscopic radiofrequency ablation of primary and metastatic liver tumors. Technical considerations. *Surg Endosc*, Apr, 14(4), 400-5.

[32] Salmi, A., & Metelli, F. (2003). Laparoscopic ultrasound-guided radiofrequency thermal ablation of hepatic tumors: a new coaxial approach. *Endoscopy*, Sep, 35(9), 802.

[33] Bao, P., Sinha, T. K., Chen, C. C., Warmath, J. R., Galloway, R. L., & Herline, A. J. (2007). A prototype ultrasound-guided laparoscopic radiofrequency ablation system. *Surg Endosc*, Jan, 21(1), 74-9.

[34] String, A., Berber, E., Foroutani, A., Matcho, J. R., Pearl, J. M., & Siperstein, A. (2001). Use of the optical access trocar for safe and rapid entry in various laparoscopic procedures. *Surg Endosc*, 15, 570-3.

[35] Hozumi, M., Ido, K., Hiki, S., Isoda, N., Nagamine, N., Ono, K., et al. (2003). Easy and accurate targeting of deep-seated hepatic tumors under laparoscopy with a forward-viewing convex-array transducer. *Surg Endosc*, Aug, 17(8), 1256-60.

[36] Inamori, H., Ido, K., Isoda, N., Hozumi, M., Onobuchi, Y., Nagae, G., et al. (2004). Laparoscopic radiofrequency ablation of hepatocellular carcinoma in the caudate

lobe by using a new laparoscopic US probe with a forward-viewing convex-array transducer. *Gastrointest Endosc*, Oct, 60(4), 628-31.

[37] Berber, E., Herceg, N. L., Casto, K. J., & Siperstein, A. E. (2004). Laparoscopic radio-frequency ablation of hepatic tumors: prospective clinical evaluation of ablation size comparing two treatment algorithms. *Surg Endosc*, Mar, 18(3), 390-6.

[38] Zhou, X., Strobel, D., Haensler, J., & Bernatik, T. (2005). Hepatic transit time: indicator of the therapeutic response to radiofrequency ablation of liver tumours. *Br J Radiol*, May, 78(929), 433-6.

[39] Rossi, S., Garbagnati, F., De Accocella, F. I., Leonardi, F., Quaretti, L., et, P., et al. (1999). Relationship between the shape and size of radiofrequency induced thermal lesions and hepatic vascularization. *Tumori*, Mar, 85(2), 128-32.

[40] Scott, D. J., Fleming, J. B., Watumull, L. M., Lindberg, G., Tesfay, S. T., & Jones, D. B. (2002). The effect of hepatic inflow occlusion on laparoscopic radiofrequency ablation using simulated tumors. *Surg Endosc*, Sep, 16(9), 1286-91.

[41] Patterson, E. J., Scudamore, C. H., Owen, D. A., Nagy, A. G., & Buczkowski, A. K. (1998). Radiofrequency ablation of porcine liver in vivo: Effects of blood flow and treatment on lesion size. *Surg Oncol*, 227(4), 559-65.

[42] Chang, C. K., Hendy, M. P., Smith, J. M., Recht, M. H., & Welling, R. E. (2002). Radio-frequency ablation of the porcine liver with complete hepatic vascular occlusion. *Ann Surg Oncol*, Jul, 9(6), 594-8.

[43] Goldberg, S. N., Gazelle, G. S., Compton, C. C., Mueller, P. R., & Tanabe, K. K. (2000). Treatment of intrahepatic malignancy with radiofrequency ablation: radiologic-pathologic correlation. *Cancer*, Jun 1, 88(11), 2452-63.

[44] Shen, P., Fleming, S., Westcott, C., & Challa, V. (2003). Laparoscopic radiofrequency ablation of the liver in proximity to major vasculature: effect of the Pringle maneuver. *J Surg Oncol*, May, 83(1), 36-41.

[45] Denys, A., Doenz, F., Qanadli, S. D., & Chevallier, P. (2005). Radiofrequency tumor ablation: from the liver to the lung passing by the kidney]. *Rev Med Suisse*, Jul 13, 1(27), 1774-8.

[46] Jakimowicz, J., Stultines, G., & Smulders, F. (1998). Laparoscopic insufflation in the abdomen reduces portal venous flow. *Surg Endosc*, 12, 129-32.

[47] Elias, D., Sideris, L., Pocard, M., Dromain, C., & de Baere, T. (2004). Intraductal cooling of the main bile ducts during radiofrequency ablation prevents biliary stenosis. *J Am Coll Surg*, May, 198(5), 717-21.

[48] Chapman, W. C., Debelak, J. P., Wright, P. C., Washington, M. K., Atkinson, J. B., Venkatakrishnan, A., et al. (2000). Hepatic cryoablation, but not radiofrequency ablation, results in lung inflammation. *Ann Surg*, May, 231(5), 752-61.

[49] Berber, E., & Siperstein, A. E. (2007). Perioperative outcome after laparoscopic radio-frequency ablation of liver tumors: an analysis of 521 cases. *Surg Endosc*, Apr, 21(4), 613-8.

[50] Berber, E., Foroutani, A., Garland, A. M., Rogers, S. J., Engle, K. L., Ryan, T. L., et al. (2000). Use of CT Hounsfield unit density to identify ablated tumor after laparoscopic radiofrequency ablation of hepatic tumors. *Surg Endosc*, Sep, 14(9), 799-804.

[51] Dromain, C., de Baere, T., Elias, D., Kuoch, V., Ducreux, M., Boige, V., et al. (2002). Hepatic tumors treated with percutaneous radio-frequency ablation: CT and MR imaging follow up. *Radiology*, 223(1), 255-62.

[52] Mason, T., Berber, E., Graybill, J. C., & Siperstein, A. (2007). Histological, CT, and Intraoperative Ultrasound Appearance of Hepatic Tumors Previously Treated by Laparoscopic Radiofrequency Ablation. *J Gastrointest Surg*, Oct, 11(10), 1333-8.

[53] Santambrogio, R., Opocher, E., Costa, M., Cappellani, A., & Montorsi, M. (2005). Survival and intra-hepatic recurrences after laparoscopic radiofrequency of hepatocellular carcinoma in patients with liver cirrhosis. *J Surg Oncol*, Mar 15, 89(4), 218-25.

[54] Ahmad, A., Chen, S. L., Kavanagh, M. A., Allegra, D. P., & Bilchik, A. J. (2006). Radiofrequency ablation of hepatic metastases from colorectal cancer: are newer generation probes better? *Am Surg*, Oct, 72(10), 875-9.

[55] Mulier, S., Ni, Y., Jamart, J., Ruers, T., Marchal, G., & Michel, L. (2005). Local recurrence after hepatic radiofrequency coagulation: multivariate meta-analysis and review of contributing factors. *Ann Surg*, Aug, 242(2), 158-71.

[56] Amersi, F. F., Mc Elrath-Garza, A., Ahmad, A., Zogakis, T., Allegra, D. P., Krasne, R., et al. (2006). Long-term survival after radiofrequency ablation of complex unresectable liver tumors. *Arch Surg*, Jun, 141(6), 581-7.

[57] Nicoli, N., Casaril, A., Marchiori, L., Mangiante, G., & Hasheminia, A. R. (2001). Treatment of recurrent hepatocellular carcinoma by radiofrequency thermal ablation. *J Hepatobiliary Pancreat Surg*, 8(5), 417-21.

[58] Belli, G., D'Agostino, A., Fantini, C., Cioffi, L., Belli, A., Russolillo, N., et al. (2007). Laparoscopic radiofrequency ablation combined with laparoscopic liver resection for more than one HCC on cirrhosis. *Surg Laparosc Endosc Percutan Tech*, Aug, 17(4), 331-4.

[59] Elias, D., Goharin, A., El Otmany, A., Taieb, J., Duvillard, P., Lasser, P., et al. (2000). Usefulness of intraoperative radiofrequency thermoablation of liver tumours associated or not with hepatectomy. *Eur J Surg Oncol*, Dec, 26(8), 763-9.

[60] Santambrogio, R., Podda, M., Zuin, M., Bertolini, E., Bruno, S., Cornalba, G. P., et al. (2003). Safety and efficacy of laparoscopic radiofrequency ablation of hepatocellular carcinoma in patients with liver cirrhosis. *Surg Endosc*, Nov, 17(11), 1826-32.

[61] Bilchik, A. J., Rose, D. M., Allegra, D. P., Bostick, P. J., Hsueh, E., & Morton, D. L. (1999). Radiofrequency ablation: a minimally invasive technique with multiple applications. *Cancer J Sci Am*, Nov, 5(6), 356-61.

[62] Cheng, J., Glasgow, R. E., O'Rourke, R. W., Swanstrom, L. L., & Hansen, P. D. (2003). Laparoscopic radiofrequency ablation and hepatic artery infusion pump placement in the evolving treatment of colorectal hepatic metastases. *Surg Endosc*, Jan, 17(1), 61-7.

[63] Berber, E., Senagore, A., Remzi, F., Rogers, S., Herceg, N., Casto, K., et al. (2004). Laparoscopic radiofrequency ablation of liver tumors combined with colorectal procedures. *Surg Laparosc Endosc Percutan Tech*, Aug, 14(4), 186-90.

Chapter 9

Egyptian Hepatic Veno-Occlusive Disease: Surgical Point of View

Elsayed Ibrahim Salama

Additional information is available at the end of the chapter

1. Introduction

Hepatic veno-occlusive disease (HVOD): was described as a non portal cirrhosis occurring frequently in children and occasionally in adults. Now it is considered an important cause of non cirrhotic portal hypertension particularly in children [1].

Rollins 1989 [2], stated that HVOD is a non-thrombotic obliteration of small intrahepatic veins by loose connective tissues. The venous occlusion may be progressive and lead to massive hepatocellular necrosis. However the precise pathogenesis is still obscure but also most likely relates to venous endothelial injury.

Originally the syndrome was described in South Africa at 1920, but at present it is endemic in Jamaica, encountered in Afghanistan and India. The syndrome was described under different names, from Jamaica the disease was described under the term Jamaican veno-occlusive disease, in India the disease was given the term Indian childhood Cirrhosis (ICC), in Europe HVOD has been called endophlebitis obliterans of which sporadic cases were described, as in Germany. Hepatic veno- occlusive disease was examined by scanning electron microscopy (SEM). SEM correlated its histology and postmortem examination and disclosed microscopic occlusion of the centrilobular and sublobular veins in the liver, these veins were occluded partially or completely by intimal and medial thickening of their walls due to proliferation of collagen and reticulin fibers. In addition to venous obliteration, which had not been demonstrated by other techniques, frequent occlusion of the sinusoidal opening into the central veins was observed by SEM. [4], [5], [6].

Causes of non cirrhotic portal hypertension	
Intrahepatic	**Extrahepatic**
Schistosomiasis	Extrahepatic portal vein thrombosis
Extrahepatic portal vein thrombosis	Splenic vein thrombosis
Biliary cirrhosis, primary and secondary	
Chronic veno-occlusive disease	
Chronic active hepatitis	
Congenital hepatic fibrosis	
Haemochromatosis	
Alcoholic fibrosis	
Sarcoidosis	
Nodular regenerative hyperplasia	
Idiopathic portal hypertension	
Non-cirrhotic portal fibrosis	

Hepatic veno-occlusive disease has been recognized as being due to the toxic effects of some remedies, recently pyrrolizidine alkaloids mostly involved, as in senecio (bush teas) and crotalaria (comfrey trees). It is also now seen as complication of high dose of anti-neoplastic chemotherapy, especially in the setting of bone marrow transplantation. HVOD may be familial, so the term *"veno occlusive familial hepatic disease"* [7], [8], [9].

2. Hepatic veno-occlusive disease (HVOD) in Egypt: Overview

In Egypt Hashem 1939 [7], gave the first reference to this syndrome, in his study of portal cirrhosis among Egyptian children. Since 1939 several reports pointed out the occurrence of a specific syndrome among Egyptian children who rapidly developed abdominal distention with ascites and hepatomegaly. In 1965, Safouh et al [11]; reported that 54 Egyptian children were studied and the term "Hepatic vein occlusion disease in Egyptian children" was applied. At the same year, El Gholmy 1956 [10], studied a group of patients and introduced the term "Infantile cirrhosis of Egypt"

The different reports from Egypt, thereafter, describing the syndrome, the clinical picture, the pathology and the etiology revealed that HVOD is not uncommon among Egyptian infants and young children. They also have shown clearly for the first time that hepatic vein occlusion should be considered in the diagnosis of Egyptian children presenting with hepatosplenomegaly [11].

Safouh 1965 [11], reported that the Egyptian hepatic vein occlusion is the result of enhanced thrombotic activity of the blood with the formation of fibrinous thrombi followed by organization and thickening or closure of the vessels, a finding which seems peculiar to the Egyptian cases and thus differs from the classical HVOD.

3. Clinical Picture of HVOD

Clinical diagnosis is based on; hepatomegaly and/or right upper quadrant pain, ascites or unexplained weight gain and also jaundice may or may not present [7].

The acute stage starts abruptly with abdominal discomfort or pain accompanied by hepatomegaly and ascites, nausea and vomiting are common. Histologically the liver shows an edematous endophlebitis of the central veins associated with centrilobular congestion, hemorrhage and necrosis. Mclean 1969 [12], has shown experimentally that the block occurs first at the outlets of the sinusoids. Patients surviving the acute stage may progress to the subacute stage with persistent hepatomegaly and ascites which then diminish if an adequate collateral circulation becomes established. The chronic stage is a centrilobular type of septal cirrhosis [7].

Clinical picture:
Non febrile onset
Mild continuous dragging pain in right hypochondrium
Anorexia, nausea and vomiting
Rapidly filling ascites
Distended veins over the abdomin
Oliguria and pedal edema
Hepatomegaly
Splenomegaly in some cases

Tandon 1977

4. Diagnosis of HVOD

In the acute phase the diagnosis is usually readily made from the history and the characteristic clinical picture. In the sub-acute and chronic stages the diagnosis may be more difficult. In all stages the diagnosis is confirmed by the characteristic histopathological findings of liver biopsy in the absence of extrahepatic venous obstruction.

4.1. Laboratory Studies:

1. Safouh et al; 1965 [11] reported the following results:

Most of the cases showed some degree of anemia.

Total and differential leukocytic counts did not show any constant deviation from normal.

Liver function tests showed that : * Serum bilirubin was always below 3 mg/dl, * Serum AST varied between 20 and 60 units, * Serum ALT and alkaline phosphatase were found to be normal.

Erythrocyte sedimentation rate (ESR) was low in spite of advanced state of the disease.

The pattern of serum total proteins showed a state of hypoproteinemia ranging from 4-5 gm/dl and the albumen fraction is usually is decreased but globulin fraction may be increased.

2. Millis and Bale 1976 [13], stated that a feature of their cases is the partial immune deficiency. However, such a state of hypogammaglobulinemia reported by them goes parallel with findings in the acute cases only, that their cases were quite a different group of patients suffering from genetic immunodeficiency as observed from the very early appearance of the syndrome in some of them being as early as days.

3. Serum procollagen type III is an early and sensitive marker in VOD after BM transplantation, usually above 100 ng /ml.

4. Serum protein S,C, liedin factor

4.2. Ultrasonographic scaning of the liver:

It is of *definite help* in the diagnosis of this syndrome, it showed that the liver is enlarged especially the caudate lobe, splenic enlargement is usually of mild degree and ascites is always found in acute cases. Narrowing of inferior vena cava could be detected in 40% of cases. Examination of the terminal parts of the hepatic veins demonstrated their occlusion or attenuation, a finding which is considered a new and significant contribution to the early diagnosis of this syndrome [14].

4.3. Inferior vena cava angiogram:

Presented as narrow or closed intra-hepatic portion of the inferior vena cava with marked collaterals [14].

4.4. Liver biopsy:

In the acute stage it shows centrilobular hemorrhage, necrosis and sinusoidal dilatation. In the chronic stage it presents picture of micronodular cirrhosis with normal portal tracts [7].

4.5. Other tools of investigations [14]

- The ascitic fluid is a main laboratory field of investigations. It usually shows protein values ranging between 1-3.5 gms/dl with occasional lymphocytes.

- Other sophisticated modules of investigations might be carried out : liver isotopic scanning, splenoportal venogram and arterio-venography of the portal system.

5. Management of Hepatic veno-occlusive disease:

No effective therapy until now especially in this type of Egyptian children. The target of available line is, may be, to reduce the complications, to reduce the stress of the patients and keep the patients in nearly comfortable life, but the following measures could be used safely [14].

5.1. Preventive measures:

- More investigation for the etiology of the disease especially pyrrolizidine alkaloids.

- Encouraging the breast feeding for two years as Glorious Qura'n says. (Sorra El bakara), regulation and careful inspection of diet after weaning [11].

- Good nutrition of the mother

- What about copper utensils ?? it suspected to play a role in indian cirrhosis !

5.2. Conservative measures :

- Follow up, because a grossly abnormal scan of liver and spleen in a patient with HVOD has been normalized completely without any interference.

- Colonic lavage to wash out the toxic metabolites.

5.3. Medical treatment:

- Low doses of *heparin or anticoagulants*, adapted dose of *prostacyclin*.

- *Anti inflammatory* or *steroids*.

- Use of *Vit C*, use of *Vit. E* and Glutamine (source of glutathione) as antioxidants [15].

- Use of *recombinant tissue plasminogen activator* (rtPA), especially in patients after BM transplantation, *Urokinase* especially in cases with bleeding diathesis leading to thrombotic HVOD [15], [16], [17].

- *Diuretics* for ascites.

- *Large doses of glucose* together with *insulin* to aid glycogen deposition in the liver and so help its nutrition.

- Cupper chelation treatment (Di-penecillamine)

5.4. Surgical treatment [18].

5.4.1. Treatment of ascites :

- Frequent aspiration (partial or full)
- TIPS (transjagular intrahepatic portosystemic shunt)
- Hepatic and portal decompression for interactable ascites.
- LeVeen, peritoneojagular shunt.

5.4.2. Treatment of portal hypertension:

- Porto-systemic shunt as porto-caval, spleno-renal or meso-atrial.
- Acute venous obstruction could be treated by hepatofugal portal flow via veno-venous bypass to drain arterial blood flow.

5.4.3. Liver transplantation:

- It is now a part of the therapeutic armamentarium for this condition.

6. Therapeutic paracentesis [21].

The first study re-evaluating paracentesis as a treatment of cirrhotic patients with ascites consisted of a randomized controlled trial comparing repeated large-volume paracentesis (4-6 l/day until the disappearance of ascites) plus intravenous albumin infusion (40g after each tap) with standard diuretic therapy (frusemide plus spironolactone) in I17 patients with tense ascites and avid sodium retention who were admitted to several hospitals in the Barcelona area. This study, later confirmed by two more trials performed in Milan and Barcelona, showed the following results:

1. paracentesis was more effective than diuretics in eliminating ascites (96.5 versus 72.8%);

2. paracentesis plus albumin infusion did not induce significant changes in hepatic and renal function, serum electrolytes, cardiac output, plasma volume, plasma renin activity and plasma concentration of noradrenaline and antidiuretic hormone.

3. the incidence of hyponatremia, hepatic encephalopathy and renal impairment was much lower in patients treated with paracentesis.

4. the duration of hospital stay was lower in patients treated with paracentesis.

5. there were no significant probability of re-admission, probability of survival and causes of death between the two groups of patients.

Tito et al., later investigated whether ascites can be safely mobilized by total paracentesis (complete removal of ascites by a single paracentesis) plus intravenous albumin infusion

(6-8 g/l removed) in a one day hospitalization regime. The incidence of complications and the clinical course of the disease, as estimated by the probability of readmission to hospital, causes of re-admission, probability of survival and causes of death, were comparable to those reported by the same group of investigators in patients treated with repeated large-volume paracentesis.

In conclusion, these studies demonstrate that mobilization of ascites by paracentesis associated with intravenous albumin infusion does not impair systemic haemodynamics and renal function in patients with cirrhosis and tense ascites. Therapeutic paracentesis should be the treatment of choice for cirrhotic patients admitted to hospital with tense ascites, because it is more effective in mobilizing associated with a lower incidence of complications and reduce the duration of hospitalization. To avoid re-accumulation of ascites, patients treated with paracentesis require dietary sodium restriction and administration of diuretics after the procedures.

Subsequently, a trial was performed to establish whether intravenous albumin infusion is necessary in cirrhotic patients with tense ascites treated with repeated large-volume paracentesis. It was observed that paracentesis plus intravenous albumin does not induce significant changes in standard renal function testes, plasma renin activity and plasma aldosterone concentration. In contrast, paracentesis without albumin was associated with a significant increase in blood urea nitrogen, a marked elevation in plasma renin activity and plasma aldosterone concentration, and a significant reduction in serum sodium concentration. The number of patients developing hyponatremia and renal impairment was remarkably higher in patients treated with repeated large-volume paracentesis without intravenous albumin infusion. There are two detailed investigations assessing the effects of large-volume paracentesis without albumin infusion on systemic haemodynamics vasoactive hormones and renal function. A significant increase in cardiac output was observed 1 hour after treatment in both studies. Some hours later, however, a significant drop below baseline values was observed in cardiac output, pulmonary wedge capillary pressure and central venous pressure. Plasma renin activity increased and plasma atrial natriuretic peptide concentration decreased. The adverse effects observed after complete mobilization of ascites by paracentesis without albumin expansion did not occur in patients in whom ascites was only partially mobilized by paracentesis without colloid replacement. In conclusion, these studies demonstrate that complete mobilization of ascites by paracentesis without plasma volume expansion is followed by a reduction in effective intravascular volume, which leads to activation of the renin-aldosterone system and may impair renal function. The infusion of intravenous albumin is an important measure to prevent these abnormalities in cirrhotic patients with tense ascites treated with large-volume or total paracentesis.

Five randomized controlled trials and one prospective study aimed at investigating whether albumin can be substituted by less expensive plasma expanders (dextran-70, dextran-40, Haemaccel 5% and isotonic saline) have recently been reported. It has been observed that total or repeated large-volume paracentesis associated with intravenous administration of dextran-70 or Haemaccel is not associated with significant changes in renal and hepatic function. The incidence of hyponatremia, renal impairment and hepatic encephalopathy in patients receiving dextran-70 or Haemaccel was comparable with that in patients receiving albumin.

In one study, patients treated with dextran-70 showed a significant increase in plasma renin activity and aldosterone concentration. In a more recent study, however, therapeutic paracentesis plus intravenous dextran-70 administration was not associated with significant changes in plasma renin activity, which was measured 24 and 96 hours after the treatment. Cabrera et al., in one study including 14 patients, have suggested that intravenous isotonic saline infusion can also be a safe and cost effective alternative plasma expander in cirrhotics with tense ascites treated with paracentesis. Further studies are obviously needed to confirm their findings. It seems that dextran-40 is not as effective as albumin in preventing renal and electrolyte complications after therapeutic paracentesis, as renal impairment and/or hyponatremia developed after treatment in a relatively high proportion of patients.

Recently, a multicenter randomized trial comparing therapeutic paracentesis with PVS in cirrhotic patients with refractory or recurrent ascites has been published. More than 40 patients were included in each group. Both treatments were equally effective in mobilizing the ascites during the first hospital stay, although the duration of hospitalization was significantly longer in the shunt group. There were also no significant differences between both groups in the number of patients who developed complications or died. The number of readmissions for any reason or for ascites, was significantly higher, and the time to first readmission for any reason and for ascites significantly shorter in the paracentesis group than in the shunt group. The total time in hospital during follow-up, however, was similar in the two groups. The probability of shunt obstruction was 40 % at 1 -year follow-up. The probability of survival was similar in both groups. In conclusion, this trial shows that, although the LeVeen shunt was better than paracentesis in the long-term control of ascites, it did not reduce the total time in hospital nor prolong survival. On the other hand, patients treated with PVS required frequent re-operations due to obstruction of the prosthesis. Therapeutic paracentesis is therefore an alternative treatment to LeVeen shunt in cirrhotic patients with refractory ascites.

7. Peritoneovenous Shunting

In 1974 LeVeen [19], and colleagues developed a pressure-activated one-way valve for use in a peritoneovenous shunt (PVS). This device consists of a perforated intra-abdominal tube connected through a one-way pressure sensitive valve to a silicone tube that traverses the subcutaneous tissue up to the neck, where it enters one of the jugular veins (usually the internal jugular vein). The tip of the intravenous tube is located in the superior vena cava, near the right atrium or in the right atrium itself. The shunt produces a sustained circulating blood volume expansion by continuous passage of ascitic fluid to the general circulation. Flow in the shunt is maintained if there is a 3-5 cm H2O pressure gradient between the abdominal cavity and the superior vena cava. A loss of this gradient causes the valve to close, preventing blood from flowing back into the tubing. Two additional shunts have been introduced Denver and Cordis-Hakim. These latter shunts include a pumping mechanism that allows flow to be increased or a partially occluded shunt to be cleared.

The intravenous infusion of ascitic fluid through the shunt is associated with an increase in circulating blood volume and cardiac output. Since arterial pressure does not rise, there is a concomitant reduction in peripheral vascular resistance. These hemodynamic changes are associated with an increase in the plasma concentration of atrial natriuretic factor and a suppression of plasma levels of renin, aldosterone, noradrenaline and antidiuretic hormone. Urine volume and free water clearance increase in most patients. However, there is significant natriuresis in less than half of the patients, demonstrating that the PVS does not completely correct the abnormal sodium-retaining state associated with cirrhosis. Finally, in cirrhotic patients with moderate FRF, the PVS may improve renal blood flow and glomerular filtration rate. These hemodynamic and hormonal changes persist in most cases and a significant proportion of patients remains with minimal or no ascites despite a moderate sodium restriction and low diuretic dosage. There are also two studies that suggest that PVS has a positive effect on the nutritional status of patients in whom the shunt functions for a prolonged period of time. Despite these positive effects of PVS, there are a large number of complications, which may occur early in the postoperative period or at any time during follow-up [19], [20].

The role of PVS in the management of cirrhotic patients with ascitcs is still not well established. Only one prospective study showed that PVS is superior to conventional medical therapy in the management of ascites and in improving survival. By contrast, four randomized studies have failed to demonstrate a longer survival time in cirrhotic patients with ascites treated with PVS compared with medical therapy. Of these studies, that which was performed by Stanley et al., 1989 [22], is worth mentioning. They compared PVS with medical treatment (diuretics and occasional paracentesis) in 299 patients with cirrhosis and refractory or recurrent ascites. Although early mortality and probability of survival after randomization were similar in both therapeutic groups, PVS was more effective in the management of ascites than was conventional medical therapy, as indicated by shorter duration of first hospitalization, longer time to recurrence of ascites, and lower diuretic requirements during follow-up. However, these results are not surprising, because PVS was compared with a treatment that by definition was known to be ineffective.

The effect of PVS on survival in patients with FRF has also been studied in a randomized controlled trial. The treated patients had some improvement in renal function, but their survival was unaffected. Several studies have shown that morbidity and survival of cirrhotic patients treated with PVS correlate with the degree of impairment of liver and renal function. Therefore, the best results with this procedure should be expected to occur in those few patients with diuretic-resistant ascites and preserved hepatic function [23].

7.1. Early complications of peritoneovenous shunting

Acute bacterial infection is the most serious early complication. Staphylococcus aureus is a frequent isolate and represents the operative contamination of the shunt in some cases. The prosthesis is usually colonized and the infection cannot be eradicated in most cases unless the shunt is removed a high mortality can be expected. The prophylactic administration of anti-staphylococcal antibiotics 24 hours before and 48 hours after surgery reduces the incidence of early postoperative infection. Biochemical disseminated intravascular coagulation (DIC) is seen in practically every cirrhotic patient treated with PVS in the early postoperative period. Bleeding caused by DIC develops most commonly in those patients with severe liver disease, but is now very uncommon, because many surgeons remove the ascitic fluid before inserting the shunt and replace it with normal saline. DIC is thought to develop because of infusion of factors present in ascitic fluid that activate coagulation (thromboplastin, activated clotting factors, endotoxin, collagen, plasminogen activator and fibrin split products). Postoperative fever, probably related to the passage of endotoxin contained in the ascitic fluid to the general circulation, is almost a constant and disappears spontaneously within the second postoperative week. Rapid expansion of the plasma volume is associated with a rise in portal pressure and may increase the risk of variceal haemorrhage. This complication can also be prevented by removing most ascitic fluid before the insertion of the shunt [24].

7.2. Long-term complications of peritoneovenous shunting

Obstruction of the shunt is the most common complication during follow-up. It occurs in more than 30% of patients and is usually due to deposition of fibrin within the valve or the intravenous catheter, thrombotic obstruction of the venous limb of the prosthesis, or thrombosis of the superior vena cava or right atrium initiated at the venous end of the shunt or damaged endothelium. Shunt obstruction is generally associated with ascites re-accumulation. Shunt patency can be assessed by Doppler ultrasound or by technetium 99m scintigraphy using intraperitoneal radioisotope injection. If the obstruction is confirmed, a shuntogram after the injection of contrast into the proximal limb of the shunt may identify the site of obstruction. Venography or digital angiography is necessary in the case of obstruction of the venous tip of the shunt. Superior vena cava syndrome secondary to total obstruction of the vein and pulmonary embolism are much less common. It is not clear that the insertion of a titanium tip into the venous end of the LeVeen shunt prevents thrombotic obstruction and the development of superior vena cava thrombosis. Finally, another long-term complication of PVS is small-bowel obstruction, which occurs in approximately 10% of patients and is due to intraperitoneal fibrosis [25].

8. Transjugular intrahepatic portosystemic shunt (TIPS)

The feasibility of intrahepatic portosystemic shunting was first demonstrated by Rosch and colleagues 1969 in pigs. Colapinto et al; 1982 [27] reported the first application of this technique to humans. This was attempted following transhepatic obliteration of varices in 20 severely ill patients with variceal hemorrhage. The authors inflated a balloon catheter in the intrahepatic track and left it there for 12 hours. In an initial report all six shunts studied were patent 12 hours after the procedure and one was still patent at autopsy 6 weeks late.

Many demonstrated prolonged patency of the shunt for up to 10 months and ease of recanalizing the radiopaque shunt when occlusion occurred. This expandable stent was then used successfully in patients with portal hypertension. Similar good results were soon reported with the self-expanding Wall stent. Percutaneous portography was used in the early cases to facilitate transjugular portal vein puncture. With increasing experience this has been replaced by ultrasound guidance in most centers [28].

There is now an increasing array of equipment available for transjugular intrahepatic portosytemic shunt (TIPS) insertion. The most widely used needles are a standard transjugular biopsy needle with a straight or reversed bevel (Cook Ltd) or the Richter needle which has a tapered tip and a blunt obturator (Angiomed, Karlsruhe, Germany). Another set with a blunt cannula, through which is passed a sharp style is also available (Cook). There is also a wider choice with regard to the type and dimensions of metal stent. In addition to the original Palmaz and Wall stents, there is the Strecker stent and the Memotherm stent (Angiomed, Karlsruhe, Germany). Claimed advantages for these new stents are increased radioopacity (Strecker stent) and improved delivery systems (Memo stent) [29].

A recent randomized controlled study compared the Palmaz and Wall stent in 90 patients and found little difference in outcome. Early shunt thrombosis was more likely with the Wall stent (9%), whereas stenosis of the hepatic vein was more likely with the Palmaz stent (I3%). Experience with the other stents is limited.

As yet the long-term expectations of TIPS have not been fulfilled in those clinical situations in which long-term efficacy is needed as prevention of variceal rebleeding, ascites, cirrhotic hydrothorax, Budd-Chiari syndrome, and long-term amelioration of clinical status before liver transplantation. All these indications need controlled trials against current best optimal management before TIPS is used routinely even for an individual patient. The high stent obstruction rate is the most important limiting factor, but change in stent shape, coating material or other technical aspects may overcome this [30].

The complications of TIPS are significant if elective and long-term use is considered, thus the need for trials before new therapies are introduced. In an emergency situation the complications due to TIPS are an acceptable risk, but again information from controlled trials is needed. This is particularly true when TIPS is used as a short-term bridge to liver transplantation. TIPS will have a place in the treatment of cirrhotic patients. At present short-term rather than long-term indications appear to be where TIPS will have more beneficial effects [28].

9. Liver transplantation: and hepatic venous obstruction

Liver transplantation for Budd–Chiari syndrome: A European study on 248 patients from 51 centers) [31]: The results of liver transplantation for Budd–Chiari syndrome (BCS) are poorly known and the role and timing of the procedure are still controversial. The aim of this study was to investigate the results of transplantation for BCS, focusing on overall outcome, on prognostic factors and on the impact of the underlying disease. Methods: An enquiry on 248 patients representing 84% of the patients transplanted for BCS in the European Liver Transplantation Registry between 1988 and 1999. Results: Of the 248 patients, 70.4% were female and 29.6% male. The mean age was 35.7 years. The overall actuarial survival was 76% at 1 year, 71% at 5 years and 68% at 10 years. 77% of deaths occurred in the first 3 months: 47% were due to infection and multiple organ failure, and 18% to graft failure or hepatic artery thrombosis. Late mortality (>1 year) occurred in nine patients, due to BCS recurrence in four of them. The only pre-transplant predictors of mortality on multivariate analysis (Cox) were impaired renal function and a history of a shunt.

10. Conclusions

Liver transplantation for BCS is an effective treatment, irrespective of the underlying cause, and should be considered before renal failure occurs [31].

Acknowledgements

We would like to thank all the staff of pediatric department, at National Liver Institute, Menoufya University for supporting our work.

Author details

Elsayed Ibrahim Salama*

Address all correspondence to: elsayedsalama5@yahoo.com

Pediatric Department, National, Menoufia University, Egypt

References

[1] Al, Hasany. M., & Mohamed, A. (1970). Veno occlusive disease of Liver in Iraq. *Archives of disease in childhood*, 45(243), 722-724.

[2] Rollins, B. J. (1989). Hepatic Veno-occlusive Disease. *Am J of Med*, 8, 297.

[3] Bras, G., Jeliffe, D. B., & Stuart, K. L. (1954). *Arch Path, Chicago*, 57, 285.

[4] Stein, H. (1957). Veno-occlusive disease of the liver in African children. *Br Med J*, 1, 1496.

[5] Tandon, B. N., Tandon, R., Tandon, H. D., Narndrunat, L., & Joghi, Y. K. (1976). An epidemic of veno-occlusive disease of liver in central India. *Lancet*, 271-272.

[6]   Shirai, M., Nagashima, K., Iwasaki, S., & Mori, W. (1987). A light and scanning elec-
      tron microscopic study of hepatic veno-occlusive disease. *Acta Path Jpn*, 37(12),
      1961-711.

[7]   Hashem, M. (1939). Etiology and Pathology of types of liver cirrhosis in Egyptian
      children. *J Egypt Med Association*, 22, 1-36.

[8]   Mohabbat, O., Srivastava, R. N., Younos, M. S., Sedio, G. G., Merzad, A. A., & Aram,
      G. N. (1967). An outbreak of Hepatic Veno-occlusive Disease due to toxic Alkaloid in
      herbal tea in north western Afghanistan. *Lancet*, 7950, 269.

[9]   Wilmot, F. C., & Robertson, G. W. (1920). Senecio disease and cirrhosis of liver due to
      senecio boisoning. *Lancet*, 11, 848-849.

[10] El Gholmy, A., El Nabaway, M., Khatab, M., Shukry, Gabr. M., El Sibie, B., Aidaro, S.,
      & Soliman, L. (1956). Infantile liver cirrhosis of Egypt. *Gaz Egypt Ped Assoc*, 4, 320.

[11] Safouh, M. A., Shehata, A., & Elwi, A. (1965). Veno occlusive disease in Egyptian
      Children. *Arch Path*, 79, 505.

[12] Mc Lean, E. K. (1969). The early sinusoidal lesion in experimental veno occlusive dis-
      ease of the liver. *British Journal of Experimental Pathology*, 223 -22.

[13] Mellis, C., & Bale, P. M. (1976). Famelial hepatic Veno occlusive disease with proba-
      ble immune deficiency. *J Pediatrics*, 88, 236-242.

[14] Mc Dermott, W. V., & Ridker, P. M. (1990). The Budd-Chiari syndrome and hepatic
      veno occlusive. Recognition and treatment. *Archives of surgery*, 125(4), 525-527.

[15] Nattakom, T. V., Charlton, A., & Wilmore, D. W. (1995). Use of Vitamine E. and glu-
      tamine in the successful treatment of severe VOD following bone marrow transplan-
      tation. *Nutritionin Clinical Practice*, 10(1), 16-18.

[16] Fogteloo, A. J., Smid, W. M., Kok, T., Van Der Meer, J., Van Imhoff, G. W., & Daenen,
      S. (1993). Successful treatment of veno occlusive disease of the liver with urokinase in
      a patient with non-hodgkin's lymphoma. *Leukemia*, 7(5), 760-763.

[17] Simpson, D. R., Browett, P. J., Doak, P. B., & Palmer, S. J. (1994). Successful treatment
      of veno occlusive disease with recombinant tissue plasminogen activator in a patient
      requiring peritoneal dialysis. *Bone Marrow Transplantation*, 14(4), 635-636.

[18] Cuenoud, P. F., & Mosiman, F. (1992). Surgical treatment of Budd-Chiari syndrome
      and VOD. *Helvetica Chirurgica Acta*, 58(6), 805-808.

[19] Le Veen, H. H., Christoudias, G., Moon, J. P., et al. (1974). Peritoneovenous shunting
      for ascites. *Ann Surg*, 180, 580-591.

[20] Le Veen, H. H., Vujic, ., D'Ovidio, N. J., & Hutto, R. B. (1984). Peritoneovenous shunt
      occlusion: Etiology. diagnosis, therapy. *Ann Surg*, 212-223.

[21] Salemo, F., Badalamenti, S., Incerti, P., et al. (1987). Repeated paracentesis and IV albumin infusion to treat "tense " ascites in cirrhotic patients a safe alternative therapy. *J Hepatol*, 5, 102-108.

[22] Stanley, A. M., Ochi, S., Lee, K. K., et al. (1989). Peritoneovenous shunting as compared with medical treatment in patients with alcoholic cirrhosis and massive ascites. *N Engl J Med*, 321, 1632-1638.

[23] Stanley, M. M. (1985). PVS in patients with cirrhotic ascites and end-stage renal failure. *Am Kidney Dis*, 6, 185-187.

[24] Smajda, C., Tridart, D., & Franco, D. (1986). Recurrent ascites due to central venous thrombosis after peritoneojugular (LeVeen) shunt. *Surgery*, 100, 535-540.

[25] Sale, H. H., Dudley, F. J., Merret, A., et al. (1983). Coagulopathy of peritoneovenous shunt studies on the pathogenic role of ascitic fluid collagen and value of antiplatelet therapy. *Gut*, 24, 412-417.

[26] Rosch, J., Hanafee, W. N., & Snow, H. (1969). Transjugular portal venography and radiological portocaval shunt: an experimental study. *Radiology*, 92, 1112-1114.

[27] Colapinto, R. F., Stonell, R. D., Birch, S. J., et al. (1982). Creation of an intrahepatic portosystemic shunt with a Gruntzig balloon catheter. *Can Med Assoc*, 126, 267-268.

[28] Haag, K., Noldge, G., Sellinger, M., Ochs, A., Gerok, W., & Rossle, M. (1992). Transjugular intrahepatic portosystemic stent shunt (TIPS). Monitoring of function by color duplex sonography. *Gastroenterology*, 102, 817.

[29] Palmaz, I. C., Sibbit, R. R., Reuter, S. R., Garcia, F., & Tio, F. O. (1985). Expandable intraheptic portacaval shunt stents. Early experience in the dog. *Am J Roentgenol*, 145, 821-825.

[30] Conn, H. (1993). Transjugular intrahepatic portal systemic shunts: the state of the art. *Hepatology*, 17, 148-158.

[31] Gilles, Mentha., Giostra, Emiliano, Majno, Pietro E., Bechstein, Wolf. O., Neuhaus, Peter., O'Grady, John., Praseedom, Raaj. K., Burroughs, Andrew. K., Treut, Yves. P., Kirkegaard, Preben., Rogiers, Xavier., Ericzon, Goran -Bo., Hockersted, Krister., Adam, René., & Juergen, Klempnaue. (2005). Liver transplantation for Budd-Chiari syndrome: A European study on 248 patients from 51 centres. *Sciences*, 50(3), 540-546.

Chapter 10

Management of Hepatobiliary Trauma

Rajan Jagad, Ashok Thorat and Wei-Chen Lee

Additional information is available at the end of the chapter

1. Introduction:

The liver is the most commonly injured solid abdominal organ, despite its relative protected location [1, 2]. Treatment of traumatic liver injuries is based on patient physiology, mechanism and degree of injury, associated abdominal and extra-abdominal injuries and local expertise. Non-operative management has evolved into the treatment of choice for most patients with blunt liver injuries who are hemodynamically stable and success rates for non-operative management commonly are greater than 95%. With the sweeping shift towards the non-operative management, most hepatic injuries can be treated conservatively [3, 4, 5].

More recently several authors have highlighted an excessive use of non-operative management (NOM), which for some high grade liver injuries is pushed far beyond the reasonable limits, carrying increased morbidity at short and long term, such as bilomas, biliary fistula, early or late haemorrhage, false aneurysm, arterio-venous fistulae, haemobilia, liver abscess, and liver necrosis [5]. Incidence of complications attributed to NOM increases in concert with the grade of injury. In a series of 337 patients with liver injury grades III-V treated non-operatively, those with grade III had a complication rate of 1%, grade IV 21%, and grade V 63% [6].

2. Mechanism of injury and anatomic consideration:

Road traffic accident, antisocial violent behaviours, industrial and farming accidents are the commonest mode of injury to the liver. Though the liver is protected by the rib cage, as the largest solid organ in the abdomen, the liver is particularly vulnerable to the ability of compressive abdominal blows to rupture its relatively thin capsule. The vasculature consists of wide-bore, thin-walled vessels with a high blood flow, and injury is usually associated with significant blood loss. Blunt trauma in a road traffic accident, or fall from a height, may result in a deceleration injury as the liver continues to move on impact. This leads to tears at sites of fixation to the diaphragm and abdominal wall. A well-recognised deceleration injury involves a fracture between the posterior sector (segments VI and VII) and the anterior sector (segments V and VIII) of the right lobe. This type of injury can lead to rupture of right hepatic vein and significant bleeding. In contrast, direct blow on right upper abdomen during vehicular accident or direct blow by a weapon or fist can lead to stellate type of injury to the central liver (segment IV, V and VIII). This type of injury can lead to massive bleeding from portal vein or hepatic vein and can also lead to bile duct injury.

Penetrating injuries may be associated with a significant vascular injury. For example, a stab injury may cause major bleeding from one of the three hepatic veins or the vena cava and also from the portal vein or hepatic artery if it involves the hilum. Gunshots may similarly disrupt these major vessels; this disruption may be much more marked than with stab wounds due to the cavitation effect, particularly with bullets from high-velocity weapons.

The connection between the thin-walled hepatic veins and the inferior vena cava (IVC), at the site where the ligamentous mechanism anchors the liver to the diaphragm and posterior abdominal wall, represents a vulnerable area, particularly to shearing forces during blunt injury. Disruption here leads to the "juxtahepatic" venous injuries, which are usually associated with major blood loss and present a particularly challenging management problem.

3. Grade of liver injury:

The severity of liver injuries ranges from the relatively inconsequential minor capsular tear to extensive disruption of both lobes with associated hepatic vein, portal vein, or vena caval injury. Several classifications have been advised to grade the liver injury and management accordingly. Following table shows the grade of liver injury. Grade I & II are successfully managed non-operatively in most cases. Grade IV and onward injuries will eventually require emergency exploration. Grade III injuries require observation and if such patients are hemodynamically stable will recover with conservative treatment. Such patients should be closely followed in ICU with serial monitoring of hemoglobin and hematocrit level along with cardio-respiratory monitoring. Any fall in hematocrit or hemodynamic instability not responding to fluid resuscitation warrants urgent exploration.

Liver organ injuriy scale		
Grade		description
I	Hematoma	Subcapsular, <10% surface area
	Laceration	Capsular tear, < 1 cm parenchymal depth
II	Hematoma	Subcapsular, <10%-50% surface area; intraparenchymal, <10 cm in diameter
	Laceration	1-3 cm parenchymal depth, <10 in Length

Liver organ injuriy scale		
III	Hematoma	Subcapsular,>50% surface area or expanding; ruptured subcapsular or parenchymal hematoma
	Laceration	>3cm parenchymal depth
IV	Hematoma	Parenchymal disruption involving 25%-75% of hepatic lobe or 1-3 Couinaud segments within a single lobe
V	Laceration	Parenchymal disruption involving >75% of hepatic lobe >3 Couinaud segments within a single lobe
	Vascular	Juxtahepatic venous injuries; ie, retrohepatic vena cava/central major hepatic vein
VI	Hepatic avulsion	

Table 1. Liver Organ Injury Scale.

4. Early Measures:

4.1. Resuscitation and treatment of Hemodynamic instability:

It is generally accepted that initial resuscitation and management is the same as for any patient with major trauma and should follow the Advanced Trauma Life Support (ATLS) principles of aggressive fluid resuscitation, guided by monitoring of central venous pressure and urinary output [7]. Management should also be directed toward avoidance of any of the sinister triad of hypothermia, coagulopathy, and acidosis, which are associated with significantly increased mortality. Mechanisms to avoid hypothermia are standard now in major centres and include the use of rewarming blankets and heat exchanger pumps for rapid infusion of resuscitation fluids and blood [8].

The next management phase depends largely on the response to resuscitation and the stability of the patient. Liver injury should be suspected in all patients with blunt or penetrating thoracoabdominal trauma but particularly in shocked patients with blunt or penetrating trauma to the right side. There are two major determinants to consider when making decisions in suspected liver trauma: hemodynamic stability and mechanism of injury. In general, hemodynamic instability or peritonism makes decision-making in trauma more straightforward, although ultimately, the surgical procedure required may be complex. Management decisions are more challenging when patients are hemodynamically stable as the array of potential therapeutic modalities are substantial and the patient's future clinical course is unknown [9].

4.2. Advanced Trauma Life Support:

The appropriate evaluation and management of liver injuries results from an organized approach to abdominal trauma. Experience and technical developments over the past several decades make the current approach both logical and effective. It is generally accepted that initial resuscitation and management is the same as for any patient with major trauma and should follow the Advanced Trauma Life Support (ATLS) principles of aggressive fluid resuscitation, guided by monitoring of central venous pressure and urinary output [7]. Management should also be directed toward avoidance of any of the sinister triad of hypothermia, coagulopathy, and acidosis, which are associated with significantly increased mortality.

4.3. Focused assessment by ultrasound for trauma (FAST):

Ultrasonography (USG) is the most important and readily available investigation for any patient with blunt or sharp abdominal injury. It is particularly useful for detecting injury to parenchymal organs and the presence of free intraperitoneal fluid or blood. USG is a quick, non-invasive, inexpensive, and transportable tool, used with increasing frequency in the initial workup of patients with abdominal trauma [10].

The particular relevance to major liver injury is the focused assessment by ultrasound for trauma (FAST), often performed in the emergency department, which involves a rapid examination of several areas, namely, the pericardial region, right upper quadrant (including Morrison's pouch), left upper quadrant, and the pelvis, specifically looking for free fluid. One of the main limitations of USG is that parenchymal injuries, sometimes relevant and requiring surgical or embolization therapy, may be present without combined peritoneal fluid [11,12].

On the basis of detection of free fluid or parenchymal injury, the sensitivity of USG has been found to be 72% to 95% for abdominal organ injuries, 51% to 92% for liver lesions, and 98% for grade III or higher liver injuries [13]. Richards et al reported 56% and 68% sensitivity of FAST and complete USG, respectively, in detecting childhood abdominal trauma [11].

Detection of peritoneal fluid is the first step in FAST. Fluid in the right upper quadrant or in the right upper quadrant and pelvic recess suggests hepatic injury, as opposed to splenic, renal, or enteric injury [14]. Fluid limited to the left upper quadrant or to both upper quadrants is not seen in patients with isolated liver trauma [14]. Hemoperitoneum recognition must prompt further imaging, but its absence does not definitely exclude parenchymal injury. Clinical assessment and observation are also relevant in combination with USG. With special reference to liver trauma, it has been noted that patients with negative USG results but with an aspartate aminotransferase level of greater than 360 IU/L should undergo CT imaging because of potentially overlooked hepatic injury, whereas patients with normal levels can be effectively discharged [15].

Although FAST provides a rapid assessment of liver disruption and intraperitoneal bleeding, it is a limited scan that is highly operator dependent. It is very important to note that a negative FAST scan does not safely rule out injury [12, 16]. Due to the operator dependence of the modality, different end points, and inconsistent comparative gold standards in the studies, the reported specificities, sensitivities, and overall accuracies are variable [17]. It has been demonstrated that up to a quarter of hepatic and splenic injuries, as well as renal, bladder, pancreatic, mesenteric, and gut injuries, can be missed if ultrasound is used as the primary investigative modality in the stable patient. However, while the possibility of false negatives is ever present, the combination of a negative ultrasound scan and normal clinical examination and observations almost excludes liver injury in the event of significant blunt trauma [12, 18].

4.4. Computed Tomography:

The wide availability of high-resolution CT has changed the manner in which blunt abdominal trauma is diagnosed and managed (figure 1). Currently, multi-detector computed tomography (MDCT) scanning with intravenous contrast is the gold standard diagnostic modality in hemodynamically stable patients with intra-abdominal fluid detected with FAST.

CT has a sensitivity of 92% to 97% and a specificity of 98.7% for detection of liver injury. The type and grade of liver injury, the volume of hemoperitoneum, and differentiation between clotted blood and active bleeding can be identified. In addition to increasing the rate of detection of liver lesions following trauma, CT has also helped to improve the understanding of the course of liver injuries [19]. CT scan also allows diagnosis of associated intraperitoneal and retroperitoneal injuries, including splenic, renal, bowel, and chest trauma, and pelvic fractures.

Even though NOM has proven to be of tremendous benefit, a couple of controversies regarding the current management of trauma patients should be discussed. Advances in CT technology have improved the practitioner's ability to determine the degree of injury and to identify patients who are more likely to fail NOM. However, until now, MDCT scanning has not been able to differentiate, in a precise manner, among which patients should be treated conservatively, which would benefit from angio-embolization and which would respond best to a surgical response.

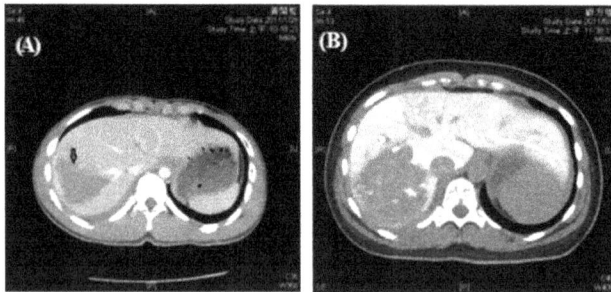

Figure 1. CT scan images of blunt abdominal trauma patients. (A) CT scan of liver showing intraparenchymal hematoma in segment VI. (B) CT scan of liver showing intraparenchymal hematoma in segment VI and extending to segment VII and V.

Although CT is the investigative gold standard, it is important to remember that it involves exposure to high levels of ionising radiation and the use of intravenous contrast may compromise renal function. In the majority of hospitals the use of CT requires movement of the patient away from adequate resuscitation facilities to the X-ray department, highlighting the importance of hemodynamic stability in patients with abdominal trauma being considered for CT examination [16].

4.5. Diagnostic laparoscopy:

The use of laparoscopy for trauma patients has been slower to evolve partly due to factors inherent in the trauma population and some limitations of the laparoscopic technique. Initially, the evaluation of peritoneal violation in hemodynamically stable patients was seen as the greatest benefit of laparoscopy for trauma [20]. Improvements in laparoscopic training and technology have enabled an increase in the use of diagnostic and therapeutic procedures in trauma patients.

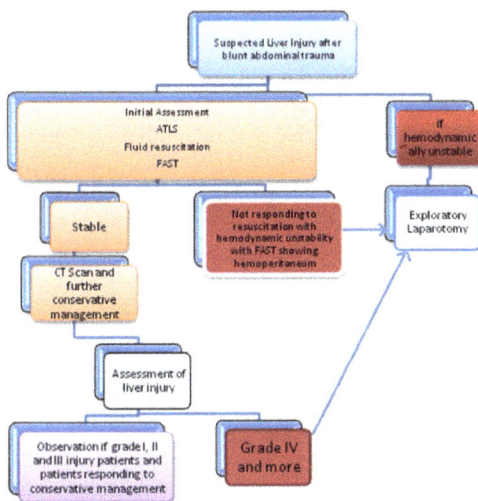

Figure 2. Algorithm - Advanced trauma life support, FAST- focused assessment by ultrasound for trauma. ATLS for managing liver trauma patients.

There are a number of series describing the successful haemostasis of minor liver injuries, in both the civilian [21] and military setting [22], although it is likely that these were self-limiting injuries anyway.

5. Management of hepatic Trauma:

There are two major determinants to consider when making decisions in suspected liver trauma: hemodynamic stability and mechanism of injury. In general, hemodynamic instability or peritonism makes decision-making in trauma more straightforward, although ultimately, the surgical procedure required may be complex (figure 2). Management decisions are more challenging when patients are hemodynamically stable as the array of potential therapeutic modalities are substantial and the patient's future clinical course is unknown [9].

5.1. Non operative management:

Hogarth Pringle, in 1908, provided the first description of operative management of liver trauma. Unfortunately, all eight patients died and Pringle recommended conservative non-operative management of these patients. In the modern surgical literature, non-operative management was first reported in 1972 and has been one of the most significant changes in the treatment of liver injuries over the last two decades [23, 24].

Initiated in pediatric trauma patients [25], nonsurgical management of blunt liver trauma has become recognized as an appropriate treatment option for hemodynamically stable adult patients with blunt hepatic injury [26, 27].

With the wide availability and improved quality of CT scanning, and the more modern, less invasive intervention options, such as angio-embolization, NOM has evolved into the treatment of choice for hemodynamically stable patients. Although angio-embolization has been defined the logical augmentation of damage control techniques for controlling hemorrhage, the overall liver-related complication rate can be as high as 60.6% with 42.2% incidence of major hepatic necrosis [28]. Non-operative management (NOM) consists of close observation of the patient completed with angio-embolization, if necessary. Observational management involves admission to a unit and the monitoring of vital signs, with strict bed rest, frequent monitoring of hemoglobin concentration and serial abdominal examinations [29].

Following factors contribute to conservative management of liver trauma:

i.   Realization that more than 50% of liver injuries stop bleeding spontaneously at the time of exploration

ii.   Availability of CT scan imaging for better assessment of grade of liver injury and associated injuries

iii.   The success of non-operative management in paediatric patients

iv.   Knowledge that the liver has tremendous capacity of healing after injury,

v.   Improved critical care management in specialized unit

vi.   The introduction of angio-embolization which allows patients with specific CT findings to potentially be treated in a minimally invasive manner.

Given the availability of angio-embolization, trauma surgeons are more likely to initiate non-operative treatment, even in higher grade injuries, because, in the event of failure, intervention in the form of angio-embolization is possible and, in the event of angio-embolization failure, surgical intervention is possible. Criteria for non-operative management include foremost, hemodynamic stability, absence of other abdominal injuries that require laparotomy, immediate availability of resources including a fully staffed operating room, and a vigilant surgeon. While non-operative management was initially introduced for minor injuries, it was soon in vogue for more severe injuries (grades III–V) [6, 30]. Close observation and repeated scans are usually recommended to document non-expansion of hematoma and healing of the injuries over time. The shift towards non-operative management of liver injuries has resulted in a lower mortality rate, but still a significant percentage of complications [31]. The current reported success rate of non-operative management of hepatic trauma ranges from 82% to 100%. Twenty-five percent of patients with blunt hepatic injury managed non-operatively, 92% of whom have grade IV or V injury will require an intervention for complications [5].

Despite the reduction of mortality that has been achieved using angio-embolization, some studies describe a rise in severe but treatable complications such as hepatic necrosis, abscesses or bile leakage [6, 28]. Gallbladder ischemia, hepatic parenchymal necrosis and biloma may also occur, and in patients with a high grade liver injury (grade 4 and 5) the incidence of complications can be high [32].

A determinant of the success of NOM is the level of cooperation between different specialists in the hospital. Good teamwork among the trauma surgeon, the anaesthesiologist and the interventional radiologist leads to a quicker understanding of the underlying injuries and thus shortens the time between entering the hospital and the initiation of therapeutic interventions. This seems obvious in level 1 trauma centers, but can be a matter of concern, especially in level II or III trauma centers.

While there has been considerable debate about the grade of liver injury and the acceptable volume of hemoperitoneum, it is now generally accepted that the ultimate decisive factor in favour of non-operative management is the hemodynamic stability of the patient, irrespective of the grade of injury or the volume of hemoperitoneum. It is also essential that appropriate clinical and radiological follow-up is arranged [33].

The rate of liver-related complications is low, and generally ranges from 0% to 7% [31]. Liver-related complication rates in high-grade liver injury patients are 11-13% and can be predicted by the grade of liver injury and the volume of packed red blood cells transfused at 24 hours post-injury [6, 34]. Incidence of complications attributed to NOM increases in concert with the grade of injury. In a series of 337 patients with liver injury grades III-V treated non-operatively, those with grade III had a complication rate of 1%, grade IV 21%, and grade V 63% [6]. Patients with grades IV and V injuries are more likely to require operation, and to have complications of non-operative treatment. Therefore, although it is not essential to perform liver resection at the first laparotomy, if bleeding has been effectively controlled, increasing evidence suggests that liver resection should be considered as a surgical option in patients with complex liver injury, as an initial or delayed strategy, which can be accomplished with low mortality and liver related morbidity in experienced hands [3].

Some of the complications related to conservative management of liver injuries are bile leaks, liver abscess, delayed haemorrhage, false aneurysm, arterio-venous fistulae, haemobilia, liver and gall bladder necrosis. Carrillo described complications in up to 85% of patients with a high (≥4) Abbreviated Injury Score (AIS) in a series of 32 patients who were treated non-operatively [27].

High grade liver injury (>3) treated with NOM and angio-embolization may be associated with severe complications like liver necrosis, bile leaks and severe sepsis. Mortality has been noted in up to 11% of patients in high grade liver injury treated conservatively [35]. Although angio-embolization has been defined the logical augmentation of damage control techniques for controlling hemorrhage, the overall liver-related complication rate can be as high as 60.6% with 42.2% incidence of major hepatic necrosis [28]. Early liver lobectomy in such cases required lesser number of procedures and achieved lower complication rate and lower mortality compared to less aggressive approaches such as serial operative debridements and/or percutaneous drainage [36].

5.2. Transarterial Embolization (TAE):

TAE of blunt hepatic injury was first recognized as a safe and effective treatment for the control of recurrent postoperative hemorrhage, hemobilia and hepatic artery-portal vein fistulas in the late 1970s [37]. Hashimoto et al. [38] also showed the efficacy of emergency TAE in four patients with severe complex hepatic injury and suggested that this method may be useful in nonsurgical management of unstable patients with severe hepatic injury. This multidisciplinary approach to the management of complex hepatic injuries is becoming much more important as the role of interventional radiology expands. Denton et al. [39] reported successful use of a combination of arterial embolization and transhepatic venous stenting in the management of a grade V injury involving the retrohepatic vena cava in a patient whose injury had been temporarily controlled by perihepatic packing. Recent more extensive series of angiography for control of hepatic haemorrhage have reported increasing success, with identification and control of bleeding rates ranging from 68 to 87%. [40] Angiography and embolization or stenting is a very useful adjunctive technique in the stable patient who is being managed non-operatively or in the patient who either has been stabilised by perihepatic packing or has re-bled after a period of initial stability.

The recent literature reveals that the increased use of angio-embolization and decreased mortality rates result in increased frequencies of severe complications, such as liver necrosis, bile leakage and intra-abdominal abscesses [28, 32, 41]. Indications of angiography in hemodynamically stable patients are high grade liver injury in CT scan, evidence of arterial vascular injury, and the presence of hepatic venous injury [41]. Angio-embolization can be used immediately after a damage control laparotomy as part of the primary haemorrhage control strategy [42]. Alternatively, angio-embolization can be used in post-operative patients to manage ongoing bleeding not associated with hemodynamic compromise [32]. This can involve not only angio-embolization, but also the placement of stents to reconstruct vasculature [39].

5.3. Complications of non-operative management:

5.3.1. Biliary complications:

Bile leaks are a frequent complication in the non-operative management of liver injuries, occurring in 6% to 20% of cases. Bile leaks present either as trauma, drainage of bile through surgically placed drain, or percutaneously placed catheter to drain biloma. The time of presentation of biliary leaks is variable. Ultrasound and CT scan are used to diagnose a biloma, whereas a hepatobiliary iminodiacetic acid scan is used to show an active bile leak.

Majority of bile leaks can be treated by ultrasound or CT-guided percutaneous drainage or ERCP and stenting.

5.3.2. Delayed haemorrhage:

The prevalence of delayed haemorrhage following non-operative management of blunt liver injury ranges from 1.7 to 5.9% [27, 43]. The mechanism of delayed hemorrhage may be related to an expanding injury or to a pseudoaneurysm induced by a biloma which eventually causes an expanding hematoma and free rupture into the peritoneal cavity. Early bleeding episodes are attributed directly to the traumatic insult, while late hemorrhage is probably related to infectious hepatic complications. Angio-embolization may prove an useful technique to deal with such complications.

5.4. Operative management:

Patients with associated liver and spleen injuries are twice as likely to fail non-operative therapy as those with only a single organ injured [44]. Missing associated intra-abdominal injury and delayed treatment, significantly affects the outcome. This occurs more often in conjunction with liver than with splenic injury, especially pancreas and bowel injury are significantly associated with liver injury in blunt trauma.

Patients with high grade liver injury who are hemodynamically unstable require surgical management. Failure of NOM also requires urgent exploration and appropriate surgical management.

Anesthesia must ensure that blood products are already in the room. The massive transfusion protocol should be activated so that the blood bank is always ahead of the patient's needs for packed red blood cells, fresh frozen plasma, platelets, and cryoprecipitate. Adequate vascular access and arterial blood pressure monitoring are essential. It is important to preferentially have venous access above the diaphragm. Resuscitation fluids infused under pressure through femoral access will exacerbate hepatic venous bleeding, at times dramatically so. Massive transfusion protocols should be activated early to prevent any delay in resuscitation with blood products.

The most widely adopted incision for the patient with liver trauma is a long midline laparotomy, which can be extended to the right chest if a posterior right lobe injury, major hepatic venous injury, or vena caval injury is encountered. An effective alternative, which gives good exposure and avoids a thoracotomy, is a right subcostal extension. A bilateral subcostal incision is sometimes favoured by hepatobiliary surgeons if there is an obvious penetrating through-and-through liver injury. This allows excellent exposure of the right lobe of the liver, the hepatic veins, and vena cava without having to open the chest or diaphragm; however, it does compromise access to the lower abdomen.

If a major liver injury is encountered, immediate control of bleeding is an absolute priority because the greatest threat to the patient's life at this juncture is exsanguination. Liver should immediately be manually closed and compressed. Patients with massive hemoperitoneum are at risk of coagulopathy, hypothermia and acidosis. Measures should be taken to prevent and treat all these consequences of massive bleeding. If this still does not control the bleeding, pedicle occlusion (Pringle manoeuvre) should be applied using an atraumatic vascular clamp or non-crushing bowel clamp. If bleeding stops after Pringle manoeuvre, the bleeding is from branches of portal vein or hepatic artery. If bleeding continuous after this manoeuvre, the bleeding is likely to be from hepatic vein or IVC. The time of Pringle manoeuvre is controversial, but it can be applied up to 1 hour without compromising the blood supply to the liver.

5.4.1. Damage control surgery:

The concept of damage control was introduced by Stone et al [45] in the 1980s and promulgated by the group at Ben Taub in 1992 [46]. This came after the report by Denver General in patients sustaining fatal hepatic hemorrhage.

After trauma, hemostasis was not possible as patients were hypothermic, acidotic, and receiving large volumes of packed red cells before blood component or fresh blood [47]. This led to the concept of the "bloody vicious cycle." The term "damage control" was popularized by the group at the University of Pennsylvania in the 1993 [48]. They described initial control of haemorrhage and contamination followed by packing and temporary abdominal closure, ICU restoration of normal physiology, and delayed definitive repair of intra-abdominal injuries. The decision for damage control should be made very early in the operation before the onset of severe coagulopathy, acidosis, and hypothermia. Early institution of packing as a damage control technique has been shown to lessen mortality [49].

The damage control concept is very appropriate for the management of major liver injuries. The three key factors that interact to produce a deteriorating metabolic situation are hypothermia, coagulopathy, and acidosis. Patients in this condition are at the limit of their physiological reserve and persistence with prolonged and complex surgical repair attempts will cause exceptionally high mortality [50]. Early recognition of hypo-thermia, coagulopathy, and acidosis is the key to the damage control approach. It is recommended that definitive surgery should cease and a damage control approach be adopted when hypothermia is deteriorating or a temperature of 34°C is reached, when coagulopathy has developed (nonsurgical oozing or prothrombin time greater than 50% above normal), or when acidosis exists (pH<7.2 despite adequate volume resuscitation).

Once the patient is stabilized, patient is returned to the operation theatre and definitive surgery is undertaken if needed.

5.4.2. Perihepatic packing:

Tamponade which is achieved by manual compression that can then be maintained by packs, which can also be manually compressed if bleeding continues. Packs placed in an anterio-posterior axis will often distract the injured liver further and worsen the bleeding. The lobes of the liver must be compressed back to normal position, essentially back toward midline. Simultaneously, the liver is pushed toward the diaphragm. Maintenance of this anatomic compression by the first or second assistant is critical to reduce bleeding as the surgeon assesses the liver injury or mobilizes the liver. Perihepatic packing can help to maintain this tamponade. Most minor venous bleeding and small lacerations to the parenchyma can be temporized by this manoeuvre. Haemostatic agents such as surgicell, thrombin-soaked gel foam, or fibrin glue are useful adjuncts.

Packing is not as effective for the injuries to the left hemiliver, because with the abdomen open, there is insufficient abdominal and thoracic wall anterior to the left hemiliver to provide adequate compression. Fortunately, haemorrhage from the left hemiliver can be controlled by dividing the left triangular and left coronary ligaments and compressing the left hemiliver between the hands.

Packs must be placed around the liver to reconstitute its anatomical shape. Packs should never be inserted into the hepatic wound, as it will tear the vessels and will increase the bleeding. It is also important to avoid excessive packing, as compression of IVC can lead to resultant decreased venous return, and reduces left ventricular filling. Excessive packing can also lead to compartment syndrome and multi-organ failure [51]. Conversely under-packing is associated with increased transfusion requirements and unplanned re-look laparotomies [52]. To reduce the risk of abdominal compartment syndrome, some advocate closing the upper part of the wound to enhance the tamponade effect but leaving the lower two-thirds open and temporarily covered with a silastic sheet sutured to the skin edges [53, 54].

Perihepatic packing will control profuse haemorrhage in up to 80% of patients undergoing laparotomy and will allow intraoperative resuscitation (resuscitative packing) [50, 55]. In the management of severe injuries of the liver, packing has emerged as the key to effective damage control [56]. However, more definitive "therapeutic" packing is also a very effective technique, particularly when used judiciously to prevent the cascade of hypothermia, coagulopathy, and acidosis [57].

Once the patient is stabilized, temporary closure of the abdomen is done and patient is shifted to the ICU. Packs can be removed after 36-48 hours. Broad spectrum antibiotics should be started to prevent sepsis. The exact timing of the removal of packs is controversial, but they should not be removed before 24 hours as this is related to re-bleeding and leaving them in place for 24 hours or more does improve outcome [58]. Even delayed removal (up to 1 week) has been reported without increasing the morbidity [59]. During removal, the packs should gently be removed after soaking with saline. Liver should be checked for re- bleeding and if adequate hemostasis is achieved, closure of the abdomen can be done after putting a drain.

5.4.3. Hepatorrhaphy:

This is an older technique which involves passing deep parenchymal sutures to bring disrupted tissue together compressing bleeding vessels and reducing dead space. The major drawback of this procedure is ischemic necrosis and infection of the liver parenchyma. However, some advocate hepatorrhaphy for "hard-to-reach" areas such as the dome and posterior portion of the right lobe.

5.4.3.1. Mesh Wrapping:

Mesh-wrapping is a quick and technically feasible method to achieve definitive hemostasis in severe liver trauma. It can be combined ideally with conventional procedures. Mesh-wrapping technique provides a highly selective, tight compression confined to the liver and does not produce an increased intra-abdominal pressure. Emphasis should be given in two important technical aspects while mesh wrapping. First, the traumatized liver has to be slung with the mesh under enough tension to create a tamponade effect. In addition the mesh should be attached into two anchoring stable points. The diaphragmatic crus and the falciform ligament provide the best options to stabilize the mesh. The mesh is resorbable and therefore reoperation for removal is not necessary. Furthermore, the resulting product of mesh hydrolysis has a bacteriostatic effect, minimizing the risk of infection [60].

5.4.4. Hepatotomy and selective vascular ligation:

Combined hepatotomy and selective vascular ligation has emerged as the preferred method of management for major hepatic venous, portal venous, and arterial injuries in many centres [61]. For control of major vascular injuries, Pachter et al. recommend a rapid and extensive finger fracture, often through normal parenchyma, to reach the site of injury. However, it is important to emphasise that with a major hepatic venous injury, significant haemorrhage may occur while attempting to extend a deep liver laceration and that this bleeding will not be controlled by a Pringle clamp and increased morbidity may be incurred. Hepatotomy is done under Pringle manoeuvre and finger fracture method is used to divide the parenchyma to ligate the bleeding vessels. Pringle clamp is released intermittently to identify bleeding vessels.

5.4.5. Non-anatomical resection of liver:

This refers to removal of devitalised parenchyma using the line of injury as the boundary of the resection rather than standard anatomical planes [62]. Resectional debridement is indicated for peripheral portion of nonviable hepatic parenchyma. Debridement is rarely a technique practised in isolation and is frequently used in conjunction with inflow control and hepatotomy. This allows for haemorrhage control prior to resection of all devitalised tissue while usually involves crossing traditional anatomical boundaries hence the term "non-anatomical resection". All devitalized tissues should be removed without making any attempt to resect normal parenchyma. Operative time should be as short as possible.

Except in rare circumstances, the amount of tissue removed should not be more than 25% of the liver. In some cases simple completion of an extensive parenchymal avulsion may suffice, e.g., when there has been an avulsion of the posterior sector of the right lobe (segments VI and VII). This type of injury is often associated with a right hepatic vein laceration and completion of the "resection" will allow control and suture of this. In such situations, vascular stapling devices are extremely useful for rapid and secure division of major veins.

5.4.6. Anatomical resection of liver:

The final alternative for patients with extensive injury to one hemiliver is anatomic hepatic resection. In elective circumstances, anatomic hemi-hepatectomies can be performed with excellent results; however, in the setting of trauma, the mortality associated with this procedure exceeds 50% in most series [63, 64]. This, plus the fact that the time and magnitude of the surgery goes against the later principles of conservative surgery and damage control, has resulted in anatomical resection being practised rarely and it is now performed in only approximately 2–4% major liver trauma cases [51].

Hepatic resection for an injured segment of the liver definitively controls bleeding, potential bile leak, and removes devitalized tissue. However, the role of hepatic resection in the management of liver injury remains controversial. The traditional poor results and lack of enthusiasm for this technique have been contradicted by the results of some recent series particularly that from Strong et al. who achieved excellent results in a series of 37 patients, 11 of whom (33%) had grade V juxtahepatic venous injuries [61]. These results probably reflect the fact that this procedure was performed in a specialist liver resection and transplantation unit, and while the majority of liver injuries continue to be managed initially in trauma centres or district hospitals, it is likely that more conservative and damage control procedures will remain the most widely practised techniques.

5.4.7. Intrahepatic balloon tamponade:

Intrahepatic balloon tamponade is useful for transhepatic penetrating injury. A device can either be fashioned from a Foley catheter and Penrose drain [65] or a Sengstaken-Blakemore tube. The device is gently delivered into the length of the tract and then inflated, often with a radio-opaque contrast fluid so integrity and position can be later confirmed radiologically if required. Once the patient is stabilized and coagulation and acidosis is corrected, the balloon can be deflated and removed during re-laparotomy.

5.4.8. Total vascular exclusion:

Total vascular exclusion of liver is sometimes used for extensive retrohepatic venous injuries. The technique involves clamping of the portal triad and infra- and supra-hepatic IVC and therefore requires experience with mobilisation of the liver as done in liver resection and transplantation. Excellent results were reported for this technique by Khaneja et al. [66] who used it to manage grade V penetrating injuries with 90% of patients surviving the operation and an overall survival rate of 70%.

The major drawback of this technique is decreased venous return due to clamping of IVC. This will lead to further hypotension in patient who is already in hypothermia and hypotension. This procedure can only be feasible in experienced hand in high volume centres.

5.4.9. Liver transplantation:

This remains a therapy of last resort limited to specialist centres with the literature limited to occasional case reports and series [67]. While liver transplantation may be life-saving for major liver trauma, the logistical problems will mean that it remains a limited option, available only in specialist centres.

6. Postoperative complications and mortality:

Overall mortality for patients with hepatic injuries is approximately 10%. The most common cause of death is exsanguination, followed by MODS and intracranial haemorrhage. Liver trauma is a morbid injury with complication rates from recent series ranges from between 8.1% to 30% [68].

6.1. Postoperative haemorrhage:

Primary exsanguinating haemorrhage is a major source of mortality, but most studies report secondary haemorrhage occurring in 3- 6% of survivors with no significant difference between blunt and penetrating mechanisms [69]. Surgical haemorrhage (ie discrete bleeding) and disseminated intravascular coagulation account for the majority of causes in even proportions. In patients managed by peri-hepatic packing, patients who had packs removed at <36hrs had more episodes of haemorrhage requiring re-packing than those with removal between 36 hours and 72 hours.

In most instances of persistent postoperative haemorrhage, the patient is best served by being returned to the operation room. Angiography with embolization may be considered in selected patients. If the reason for haemorrhage is coagulopathy, it should be corrected first and then patients should be reassessed.

6.2. Sepsis and abscess:

Post-operative sepsis occurs in 12-32% of patients. Minor morbidity occurs with urinary tract, surgical wound and respiratory tract sepsis. More serious are intra-abdominal abscesses which occur in up 24% of patients and are associated with concomitant bowel injury, higher grades of liver injury (IV and V) and massive transfusion [70].

An abdominal CT with intravenous and oral contrast should be performed to diagnose the cause of sepsis. Majority of the abscesses can be drained percutaneously under USG or CT-guidance; however, infected hematoma and infected necrotic liver tissue cannot be expected to respond to percutaneous drainage. Operative drainage may be a better option in such type of patients.

6.3. Biloma:

Bilomas are loculated collection of bile, which is with or without infection. CT-guided percutaneous drainage is the best option for infected bilomas. If the biloma is sterile, it will eventually be resorbed. Biliary ascites is caused by disruption of major bile duct. Reoperation after the establishment of appropriate drainage is the prudent course.

Biliary fistulas occur in approximately 3% of the patients with major liver injury [71]. They are usually of little consequences and generally close without specific treatment.

7. Injuries to the Bile ducts and gall bladder:

Extrahepatic bile ducts are rarely injured during blunt or penetrating abdominal injuries [72, 73]. Diagnosis is usually made during surgery or sometimes postoperatively. Management of bile duct injury detected postoperatively has already been described. If laparotomy is performed for patient with trauma, collection of bile in to the right upper quadrant suggest major bile duct injury. Sometimes it is very difficult to detect the site of bile duct injury, as associated disruption of liver parenchyma and haemorrhage makes detection a challenging task.

Management of bile duct injury is further complicated by small calibre and thin wall of the bile duct. Bile duct injury ranges from small laceration to tissue loss or complete disruption. Primary repair may be attempted when there is small laceration and no tissue loss. When there is a tissue loss or the laceration is larger than 25% to 50% of the diameter of the duct, the treatment option is a Roux-en-Y choledocho-jejunostomy [74, 75]. Isolated injury to left or right hepatic duct is even more challenging and should only be managed by experienced hepatobiliary surgeon. If expertise is not available, large bore tube should be kept and patient should be transferred to higher centre. If both the ducts are injured, both the ducts should be intubated by separate tubes and brought out. Elective repair should be undertaken once the patient is stable and after adequate assessment of injury by cholangiogram.

Injury to the gall bladder is treated either by repair or cholecystectomy.

8. Summary:

The management of injuries of the liver has evolved significantly throughout the last two decades. Non-operative techniques for the management of grade IV–V injuries in stable patients have been established, although there is a higher failure rate for these injuries compared with grade I–III injuries. Because of the progress that has been made in the quality and wide availability of the MDCT scan combined with minimally invasive intervention options like angio-embolization, NOM has evolved to be the treatment of choice for hemodynamically stable patients. In terms of surgical management there has been a definite move away from major, time-consuming procedures toward conservative surgery and damage control. The preferred surgical technique for inaccessible bleeding within a laceration is rapid finger fracture hepatotomy, Kelly –crush hepatic transection and direct suture or ligation. Prolonged attempts at surgical control and repair should be avoided, and definitive perihepatic packing should be employed at an early stage in the persistently unstable patient or at the first signs of coagulopathy. Formal anatomical resection carries a high morbidity when used for haemorrhage control, although in an experienced centre this may be appropriate. Hepatorrhaphy has become discouraged due to complications of sepsis and bleeding, but may be a useful technique in penetrating trauma where the liver is difficult to access.

Author details

Rajan Jagad*, Ashok Thorat and Wei-Chen Lee

*Address all correspondence to:

Division of Liver and Transplantation Surgery, Department of General Surgery, Chang-Gung Memorial Hospital at Linkou, Chang-Gung University College of Medicine, Taiwan

References

[1] Miller, P. R., Croce, M. A., Bee, T. K., et al. (2002). Associated injuries in blunt solid organ trauma: the implications for missed injury in non-operative management. *J Trauma*, 53, 238-242.

[2] Shanmuganathan, K., Mirvis, S. E., & Chiu, W. C. (2004). Penetrating torso trauma: triple-contrast helical CT in peritoneal violation and organ injury. *A prospective study in 200 patients. Radiology*, 231, 775-784.

[3] Polanco, P., Leon, S., Pineda, J., et al. (2008). Hepatic resection in the management of complex injury to the liver. *J Trauma*, 65(6), 1264-9, 1269-70.

[4] Badger, S. A., Barclay, R., Diamond, T., et al. (2009). Management of liver trauma. *World J Surg*, 33, 2522-37.

[5] Trunkey, D.D. (2004). Hepatic trauma: contemporary management. *Surg Clin North Am*, 84, 437-50.

[6] Kozar, R. A., Moore, J. B., Niles, S. E., et al. (1999). Complications of non-operative management of high-grade blunt hepatic injuries. *J Trauma 2005* 59:1066-1071.

[7] American College of Surgeons. (1997). Advanced Trauma Life Support manual. *American College of Surgeons*, Chicago, IL.

[8] Peng, R. Y., & Bongard, F. S. (1999). Hypothermia in trauma patients. *J Am Coll Surg*, 188, 688-696.

[9] Mac, Kenzie. S., Kortbeek, J. B., Mulloy, R., & Hameed, S. M. (2004). Recent experiences with a multidisciplinary approach to complex hepatic trauma. *Injury*, 35, 869-77.

[10] Dolich, M. O., Mc Kenney, M. G., Varela, J. E., Compton, R. P., Mc Kenney, K. L., & Cohn, S. M. (2001). ultrasounds for blunt abdominal trauma. *J Trauma*, 50, 108-112.

[11] Richards, J. R., Knopf, N. A., Wang, L., & Mc Gahan, J. P. (2002). Blunt abdominal trauma in children: evaluation with emergency US. *Radiology*, 222, 749-754.

[12] Sirlin, C. B., Brown, M. A., Andrade-Barreto, O. A., et al. (2004). Blunt abdominal trauma: clinical value of negative screening US scans. *Radiology*, 230, 661-668.

[13] Poletti, P. A., Kinkel, K., Vermeulen, B., Irmay, F., Unger, P. F., & Terrier, F. (2003). Blunt abdominal trauma: should US be used to detect both free fluid and organ injuries? *Radiology*, 227, 95-103.

[14] Sirlin, C. B., Casola, G., Brown, M. A., Patel, N., Bendavid, E. J., & Hoyt, D. B. (2001). Patterns of fluid accumulation on screening ultrasonography for blunt abdominal trauma: comparison with site of injury. *J Ultrasound Med*, 20, 351-357.

[15] Stassen, N. A., Lukan, J. K., Carrillo, E. H., et al. (2002). Examination of the role of abdominal computed tomography in the evaluation of victims of trauma with increased aspartate aminotransferase in the era of focused abdominal sonography for trauma. *Surgery*, 132, 642-646.

[16] Jansen, J. O., Yule, S. R., & Loudon, M. A. (2008). Investigation of blunt abdominal trauma. *BMJ*, 336, 938-942.

[17] Rozycki, G. S., Ballard, R. B., Feliciano, D. V., et al. (1998). Surgeonperformed ultrasound for the assessment of truncal injuries: lessons learned from 1540 patients. *Ann Surg*, 228, 557-567.

[18] Stengel, D., Bauwens, K., Sehouli, J., et al. (2005). Emergency ultrasound based algorithms for diagnosing blunt abdominal trauma. *Cochrane Database Syst Rev* (2):CD004446.

[19] Taourel, P., Vernhet, H., Suau, A., et al. (2007). Vascular emergencies in liver trauma. *Eur J Radiol*, 64, 73-82.

[20] Smith, R.S. (2001). Cavitary endoscopy in trauma. *Scand J Surg.*, 91, 67-71.

[21] Kawahara, N. T., Alster, C., Fujimura, I., Poggetti, R. S., & Birolini, D. (2009). Standard examination system for laparoscopy in penetrating abdominal trauma. *J Trauma*, 67:589.

[22] Israelit, S. H., & Krausz, M. M. (2006). Laparoscopic management of a combat military injury during the Lebanon War in August., *J Trauma*, 108-10.

[23] Haan, J. M., Bocchicchio, G. V., Kramer, N., et al. (2005). Nonoperative management of blunt splenic injury: a 5-year experience. *J Trauma*, 58, 492-498.

[24] Stein, D. M., & Scalea, T. M. (2006). Nonoperative management of spleen and liver injuries. *J Intensive Care Med*, 21, 296-304.

[25] Cywes, B. S., Rode, H., & Millar, A. J. (1985). Blunt liver trauma in children: nonoperative management. *J Pediatr Surg*, 20, 14-18.

[26] Sherman, H. F., Savage, B. A., Jones, L. M., et al. (1994). Nonoperative management of blunt hepatic injuries: safe at any grade? *J Trauma*, 37, 616-621.

[27] Carrillo, E. H., Spain, D. A., Wohltmann, C. D., et al. (1999). Interventional techniques are useful adjuncts in nonoperative management of hepatic injuries. *J Trauma*, 46, 619-624.

[28] Dabbs, D. N., Stein, D. M., & Scalea, T. M. (2009). Major hepatic necrosis: a common complication after angioembolization for treatment of high-grade liver injuries. *J Trauma*, 66(3), 621-7.

[29] Pachter, H. L., Guth, A. A., Hofstetter, S. R., & Spencer, F. C. (1998). Changing patterns in the management of splenic trauma: the impact of nonoperative management. *Ann Surg*, 227, 708-717.

[30] Meyer, A. A., Crass, R. A., Lim, R. C., et al. (1985). Selective nonoperative management of blunt liver injury using computed tomography. *Arch Surg*, 120, 550-554.

[31] Velamhaos, G. C., Konstantinos, T., Radan, R., Chan, L., Rhee, P., Tillou, A., & Demetriades, D. (2003). High success with nonoperative management of blunt hepatic trauma. *Arch Surg*, 138, 475-81.

[32] Misselbeck, T. S., Teicher, E. J., Cipolle, M. D., Pasquale, M. D., Shah, K. T., Dangleben, D. A., & Badellino, M. M. (2009). Hepatic angioembolization in trauma patients: indications and complications. *J Trauma*, 67, 769-773.

[33] Yaman, I., Nazli, O., Tugrul, T., et al. (2007). Surgical treatment of hepatic injury: morbidity and mortality analysis of 109 cases. *Hepatogastroenterology*, 54, 1507-1511.

[34] Kozar, R. A., Moore, F. A., Cothren, C. C., Moore, E. E., Sena, M., Bulger, E. M., Miller, C. C., Eastridge, B., Acheson, E., Brundage, S. I., Tataria, M., Mc Carthy, M., & Holcomb, J. B. (2006). Risk factors for hepatic morbidity following nonoperative management: multicenter study. *Arch Surg*, 141, 451-8.

[35] Goldman, R., Zilkoski, M., Mullins, R., Mayberry, J., Deveney, C., & Trunkey, D. (2003). Delayed celiotomy for the treatment of bile leak, compartment syndrome, and other hazards of nonoperative management of blunt liver injury. *Am J Surg*, 185(5), 492-7.

[36] Dabbs, D. N., Stein, D. M., Philosophe, B., & Scalea, T. M. (2010). Treatment of major hepatic necrosis: lobectomy versus serial debridement. *J Trauma*, 69(3), 562-7.

[37] Hashimoto, 5., Hiramatsu, K., Ido, K., Yosii, H., et al. (1990). Expanding role of emergency embolization in the management of severe blunt hepatic trauma. *Cardiovasc Intervent Radiol*, 1, 193-199.

[38] Denton, J. R., Moore, E. E., & Coldwell, D. M. (1997). Multimodality treatment for grade 5 hepatic injuries: 'perihepatic packing', arterial embolisation and venous stenting. *J Trauma*, 42, 964-968.

[39] Asensio, J. A., Demetriades, D., Chahwan, S., et al. (2000). Approach to the management of complex hepatic injuries. *J Trauma*, 48, 66-72.

[40] Gaarder, C., Naess, P. A., Eken, T., Skaga, N. O., Pillgram-Larsen, J., Klow, N. E., et al. (2007). Liver injuries- improved results with a formal protocol including angiography., *Injury*, 38, 1075-1083.

[41] Lin, B. C., Wong, Y. C., Lim, K. E., et al. (2010). Management of ongoing arterial haemorrhage after damage control laparotomy: optimal timing and efficacy of transarterial embolisation. *Injury*, 41, 44-9.

[42] Griffen, M., Ochoa, J., & Boulanger, B. R. (2000). A minimally invasive approach to bile peritonitis after blunt liver injury. *Am Surg*, 66, 309-12.

[43] Malhotra, A. K., Latifi, R., Fabian, T. C., et al. (2003). Multiplicity of solid organ injury: influence on management and outcomes after blunt abdominal trauma. *J Trauma*, 54, 925-9.

[44] Stone, H. H., Strom, P. R., & Mullins, R. J. (1983). Management of the major coagulopathy with onset during laparotomy., *Ann Surg.*, 197, 532-535.

[45] Burch, J. M., Ortiz, V. B., Richardson, R. J., Martin, R. R., Mattox, K. L., & Jordan, G. L. (1992). Abbreviated laparotomy and planned reoperation for critically injured patients., *Ann Surg.*, 215, 476-483.

[46] Elerding, S. C., Arragon, G. E., & Moore, E. E. (1979). Fatal hepatic hemorrhage after trauma., *Am J Surg*, 138, 883-888.

[47] Rotondo, M. F., Schwab, C. W., Mc Gonigal, M. D., et al. (1993). Damage control': an approach for improved survival in exsanguinating penetrating abdominal injury., *J Trauma.*, 35, 375-383.

[48] Asensio, J. A., Roldan, G., Petrone, P., et al. (2003). Operative management and outcomes in 103 AAST-OIS grades IV and V complex hepatic injuries: trauma surgeons still need to operate, but angioembolization helps. J Trauma.; , 54, 647-654.

[49] Hoey, B. A., & Schwab, C. W. (2002). Damage control surgery. *Scand J Surg*, 91, 92-103.

[50] Parks, R. W., Chrysos, E., & Diamond, T. (1999). Management of liver trauma. *Br J Surg*, 86, 1121-35.

[51] Aydin, U., Yazici, P., Zeytunlu, M., & Coker, A. (2008). Is it more dangerous to perform inadequate packing?, *World J Emerg Surg*, 3:1.

[52] Sheridan, R., Driscoll, D., & Felsen, R. (1997). Packing and temporary closure in liver injury. *Injury*, 28, 711-712.

[53] Cue, J. I., Cryer, H. G., Miller, F. B., et al. (1990). Packing and planned re-exploration for hepatic and retroperitoneal haemorrhage: critical refinements of a useful technique. *J Trauma*, 30, 1007-1013.

[54] Nicol, A. J., Hommes, M., Primrose, R., et al. (2007). Packing for control of hemorrhage in major liver trauma. *World J Surg*, 31, 569-574.

[55] Krige, J.E.J. (2000). Liver fracture and bleeding. *Br J Surg*, 87, 1615-1616.

[56] Moore, F. A., Moore, E. E., & Seagraves, A. (1985). Non-resectional management of major hepatic trauma. *Am J Surg*, 150, 725-729.

[57] Walt A.J. (1986). Discussion: packing for control of hepatic haemorrhage. *J Trauma*, 26, 741-756.

[58] Balogh, Z., Mc Kinley, B. A., Cox, C. S., et al. (2003). Abdominal compartment syndrome: the cause or the effect of multiple organ failure? *Shock*, 20, 483-492.

[59] Meldrum, D. R., Moore, F. A., Moore, E. E., et al. (1997). Prospective characterisation and selective management of the abdominal compartment syndrome. *Am J Surg*, 174, 667-673.

[60] Dellaportas, D., Nastos, C., Psychogiou, V., Tympa, A., et al. (2011). Iatrogenic liver trauma managed with mesh-wrapping and ligation of portal vein branch: A case report. *Int J Surg Case Rep.*, 2(8), 261-263.

[61] Fang, J. F., Chen, R. J., Lin, B. C., et al. (2000). Blunt hepatic injury: minimal intervention in the policy of treatment. *J Trauma* 49:722-728.

[62] Duane, T. M., Como, J. J., Bochichio, G. V., et al. (2004). Re-evaluating the management and outcomes of severe blunt liver injury. *J Trauma*, 57, 494-500.

[63] Jacobson, L. E., Kirton, O. C., & Gomez, G. A. (1992). The use of an absorbable mesh wrap in the management of major liver injuries. *Surgery* 111:455.

[64] Poggetti, R. S., & Moore, E. E. (1992). Balloon tamponade for bilobar transfixing hepatic gunshot wounds., *J Trauma*, 33:694.

[65] Khaneja, S. C., Pizzi, W. F., Barie, P. S., et al. (1997). Management of penetrating juxtahepatic inferior vena cava injuries under total vascular exclusion. *J Am Coll Surg*, 184, 469-474.

[66] Angstadt, J., Jarrell, B., Moritz, M., et al. (1989). Surgical management of severe liver trauma: a role for liver transplantation., *J Trauma*, 29, 606-8.

[67] Aldrete, J. S., Halpern, N. B., Ward, S., & Wright, J. O. (1979). Factors determining the mortality and morbidity in hepatic injuries. Analysis of 108 cases., *Ann Surg*, 189, 466-74.

[68] Degiannis, E., Levy, R. D., Sa, F. C. S., Velmahos, G. C., Mokoena, T., & Daponte, A. (1995). Gunshot injuries of the liver : The Baragwanath experience. *Surgery I:*, 359-364.

[69] Caruso, D. M., Battistella, F. D., Owings, J. T., Lee, S. L., & Samaco, R. C. (1999). Perihepatic packing of major liver injuries: complications and mortality. *Arch Surg*, 134:958.

[70] Donovan, A. J., Michaelian, M. J., & Yellin, A. E. (1973). Anatomical hepatic lobectomy in trauma to the liver. *Surgery* 73:833.

[71] Fabian, T. C., Croce, M. A., Stanford, G. G., et al. (1991). Factors affecting morbidity after liver trauma. *Ann Surg* 213:540.

[72] Jurkovich, G. J., Hoyt, D. B., Moore, F. A., et al. (1995). Portal triad inuries: a multi-institutional study: *J trauma* 39:426.

[73] Sheldon, G. F., Lim, R. C., Yee, E. S., et al. (1985). Management of injuries to the porta hepatis. *Ann Surg* 202: 539.

[74] Feliciano, D. V., Bitando, C. V., Burch, J. M., et al. (1985). Management of traumatic injuries to the extrahepatic biliary ducts. *Am J Surg* 150:705.

[75] Bade, P. G., Thomson, S. R., Hirshberg, A., et al. (1989). Surgical options in traumatic injury to the extrahepatic biliary tract. *Br J Surg* 76:256.

Chapter 11

Progressive Familial Intrahepatic Cholestasis

Ahmad Mohamed Sira and Mostafa Mohamed Sira

Additional information is available at the end of the chapter

1. Introduction

Neonatal cholestasis is one of the commonest presentations in the field of pediatric hepatology and gastroenterology and constitutes the major indication for liver transplantation below two years of age. Unfortunately, in spite of being common, fewer categories are amenable to curative or palliative therapy. Moreover, delayed referral to specialized centers is still a problem adding a more difficulty to neonatal cholestasis management. Hepatobiliary surgery is a major line of therapy in some etiologies of neonatal cholestasis. Biliary atresia, choledochal cyst, spontaneous perforation of the bile duct and inspissated bile syndrome are among the commonest known causes for hepatobiliary surgeons. However, there is less orientation about other causes, resulting in progression to cirrhosis and end stage liver disease without being diagnosed. One of these is the progressive familial intrahepatic cholestasis (PFIC) group of diseases [1].

PFIC is an autosomal recessive liver disorder characterized by an intrahepatic cholestasis due to bile canalicular transport defects. It is subdivided into three types with slightly different clinical, biochemical and histological features. PFIC types 1, 2 and 3 are due to mutations in *ATP8B1* (adenosine triphosphatase, type 8B, member 1), *ABCB11* (adenosine triphosphate-binding cassette, subfamily B, member 11) and *ABCB4* (adenosine triphosphate-binding cassette, subfamily B, member 4) genes, respectively. Each of these genes encodes a hepatocanalicular transporter which is essential for the proper secretion and formation of bile [2].

PFIC1 and PFIC2 usually appear in the first months of life, whereas onset of PFIC3 may also occur later in infancy, in childhood or even during young adulthood. The shared main clinical manifestations in all types are cholestasis and pruritus. PFIC represents 10-15 % of causes of cholestasis in children and 10-15% of indications of liver transplantations in children [3].

In this chapter, we want to highlight the etiology, pathophysiology, clinical presentation and the role of surgery in the management of this disease category, especially that medical therapy is of limited value in a magnitude of cases. Moreover, liver transplant is not without significant side effects. So, raising the orientation about this not uncommon condition will help in timely surgical intervention and improving patients' outcome.

2. Historical background

This disorder was first described by Clayton in 1965, and was termed Byler's disease after an American Amish kindred in which it was discovered [4]. Clinical features included severe pruritus, steatorrhea, poor growth and progression to cirrhosis in early childhood. A prominent finding was a low or normal serum gamma glutamyl transpeptidase (GGT), which was discordant with the severe cholestasis. Since its discovery, similar clinical features were described in non-Amish children. Therefore, the more descriptive term, PFIC, is preferred [5].

However, this PFIC nomenclature is not always entirely satisfactory. A preferable term is "bile canalicular transport disorders," especially as it has become apparent that these genetic disorders have numerous clinical phenotypes across all age brackets. For example, benign recurrent intrahepatic cholestasis (BRIC) and intrahepatic cholestasis of pregnancy (ICP) can occur in association with abnormalities in any of the three affected genes [2,6]. However, the PFIC nomenclature is still in use due to its popularity in the literature.

Benign recurrent intrahepatic cholestasis, first described in 1959, is an intermittent form of intrahepatic cholestasis characterized by variable periods of intense pruritus often associated with jaundice [7]. The age of onset is variable, but it typically occurs during childhood or adolescence. The severity and duration of attacks also vary and triggering features are not well known. The benign designation of BRIC refers to the general lack of progressive liver disease, although the pruritus is far from benign during an intense episode [8-10].

As the clinical spectrum between BRIC and PFIC (formerly named Byler's disease) may be a continuum, thus the historical nomenclature of Byler's disease and BRIC may be outdated [11]. So, many clinicians now refer to all these diseases in a general sense as ATP8B1, ABCB11 and ABCB4 deficiency diseases to express the wide continuum of disease severity between the PFIC and BRIC phenotypes [2].

3. Etiology and pathophysiology

3.1. PFIC 1 (ATP8B1 "FIC-1" deficiency)

PFIC1 is an autosomal recessive disease caused by mutations in *ATP8B1* (formerly named *FIC1*) gene on chromosome 18, locus q21-22. This gene encodes a transporter localized on the canalicular membrane of hepatocytes (Figure 1), named FIC1 (ATP8B1), a P-type ATPase [12].

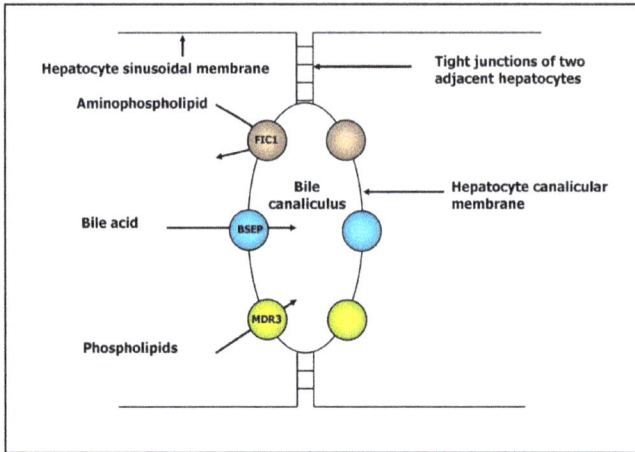

Abbreviations: FIC1: familial intrahepatic cholestasis 1; BSEP: bile salt export pump; MDR3: multidrug resistence protein 3.

Figure 1. A schematic representation of the hepatocyte with its canalicular membrane transporters involved in bile formation. FIC1 is an aminophospholipid flippase, encoded by the *ATP8B1* (*FIC1*) gene. BSEP (bile salt export pump) (formerly sister of P-glycoprotein "SPGP") is a bile acids transporter to the bile canalicular lumen against a high concentration gradient. It is encoded by the *ABCB11* (*BSEP*) gene. The MDR3 is a phospholipid transporter. It is encoded by the *ABCB4* (*MDR3*) gene.

The most widely accepted hypothesis for FIC1 function is that of an aminophospholipid flippase, translocating phospholipids such as phosphatidylserine from the outer to the inner leaflet of the plasma membrane [13]. So, deficiency of FIC1 in the hepatocyte results in the loss of asymmetric distribution of phospholipids in the canalicular membrane, decreasing both membrane stability and function of transmembrane transporters including the bile salt export pump (BSEP) and, as such, causing bile salt retention in hepatocytes with consequent defective bile formation; resulting in cholestasis [14-16].

Different studies have shown that ATP8B1 deficiency is associated with diminished FXR (farnesoid X receptor) activity. The FXR is a nuclear receptor that is highly expressed in the liver and regulates bile acid homeostasis so as to reduce its hepatocyte toxicity. Diminished FXR activity leads to upregulation of bile acid synthesis, reduced expression of the canalicular BSEP, and increased expression of the ileal apical sodium dependent bile acid transporter (ASBT). The net effect of these changes would be increased synthesis of bile acids and diminished its canalicular excretion, coupled with enhanced reabsorption of intestinal bile acids, yielding marked hepatocyte bile acid overload [17,18].

ATP8B1 is abundantly expressed in a wide variety of tissues such as the small intestine, bladder and stomach and to a lesser extent also in the liver and pancreas. This results in the multitude of the extrahepatic manifestations such as the hearing loss, pancreatitis and diarrhea, found in patients with ATP8B1 deficiency [19,20]. Over 50 distinct mutations in

ATP8B1 are described. The mutations G308V found in Amish, D554N found in Inuits and I661T are amongst the most frequently detected [21,22].

In vitro studies showed that ATP8B1 deficiency due to common missense mutations such as G308V, D554N and I661T, can be regarded as a protein folding disease, with different degrees of retention of the mutant protein in the endoplasmic reticulum, resulting in a decreased protein expression at the plasma membrane [23]. The pathophysiologic concept of being a protein folding disease can be used in new therapeutic interventions [24]. Incubation at a reduced temperature could improve proper folding of some of the mutated proteins. Similarly, the pharmacological chaperone 4-phenylbutyrate acid (4-PBA) could stabilize misfolded proteins, partially restoring cell surface expression [25].

Mutations in ATP8B1 are also responsible for:

1. Greenland Eskimo cholestasis (Nielsen syndrome) [26].

2. Benign recurrent intrahepatic cholestasis-1 (BRIC1) [12].

3. Intrahepatic cholestasis of pregnancy-1 (ICP1) [27].

4. Down regulation of CFTR (cystic fibrosis transmembrane regulator): ATP8B1 is highly expressed in biliary epithelial cells, and when it is abnormal in PFIC1, CFTR down regulation in cholangiocytes has been reported which could contribute to impairment of bile secretion [28].

3.2. PFIC 2 (ABCB11 "BSEP" deficiency)

PFIC2 is an autosomal recessive disease caused by mutations in the *ABCB11* (formerly named *BSEP*) gene encoding the BSEP, a liver-specific adenosine triphosphate (ATP)-binding cassette transporter formerly known as sister of P-glycoprotein (SPGP). BSEP is located in the hepatocyte canalicular membrane (Figure 1). *ABCB11* gene is located on chromosome 2, locus q24 [29-31].

The defective canalicular BSEP expression leads to markedly diminished bile salt secretion. This leads to bile secretory failure with secondary retention of bile salts and other biliary constituents in the hepatocytes leading to progressive liver damage and progressive cholestasis. BSEP deficiency represents also a phenotypic continuum between BRIC2 and PFIC2. Different mutations may cause different kinds of BSEP dysfunction, including protein lack, misfolded protein, or protein not delivered from the Golgi to the bile canalicular membrane [31].

Generally missense mutations, e.g. E297G or D482G, lead to a less severe phenotype than mutations that are predicted to result in premature protein truncation or total failure of protein production [31,32]. In vitro, the residual transport function of mutant proteins correlates with the phenotypic differences between BRIC2 and PFIC2, with generally a diminished function in BRIC2 mutants, while complete abolishment is more often seen in PFIC2 mutants [33].

Heterozygous *ABCB11* mutations have also been identified in cases of ICP (ICP2) [34], drug induced cholestasis [35] and transient neonatal cholestasis [36].

3.3. PFIC 3 (ABCB4 "MDR3" deficiency)

PFIC3 is an autosomal recessive disorder due to mutations in the *ABCB4* (formerly named *MDR3*) gene located on chromosome 7, locus q21, which codes for the class III multidrug resistance P-glycoprotein (MDR3). MDR3 is located exclusively on the canalicular membrane of the hepatocyte and serves as a phospholipid translocator (Figure 1) essential for biliary phospholipid (e.g. phosphatidylcholine "PC") secretion [37].

PC in bile normally protects cholangiocytes from bile salt toxicity by forming mixed micelles with it. However, a mutation of the *ABCB4* gene results in decreased biliary PC secretion and high biliary bile salt -to-PC ratio, leading to bile duct injury (cholangitis and ductular proliferation). Also, a decreased biliary PC concentration leads to high biliary cholesterol -to-PC ratio. The high biliary cholesterol saturation promotes crystallization of cholesterol and the lithogenicity of bile [2,38].

Whereas biliary bile salt concentrations are normal in patients with PFIC3, serum bile salt levels are elevated. It is explained by:

1. Downregulation of the bile acid importers to the hepatocyte, NTCP (Na+/taurocholate cotransporting polypeptide) and OATP (organic acid transporting polypeptide) [39].
2. Upregulation of the bile acid exporter from hepatocyte at the sinusoidal membrane, MRP4 (multidrug resistance–related protein 4), mediating bile salt efflux into serum [40].

Over 45 disease-causing mutations in *ABCB4* have been identified [41]. Children with missense mutations seem to have a less severe phenotype, with later onset of disease, slower progression and better response to treatment, as compared to patients with mutations leading to a truncated protein [42]. Possibly this is due to residual transport activity in MDR3 protein affected by missense mutations.

Heterozygous mutations in the *ABCB4* gene can also cause or predispose for a variety of other liver diseases, such as adult biliary cirrhosis, cholelithiasis, transient neonatal cholestasis, drug induced cholestasis and ICP. Mutations can even lead to a cascade of several phenotypes in one patient, indicating the wide phenotypical spectrum of ABCB4 deficiency [43,44].

A small proportion of PFIC phenotypes are not due to mutations in these three genes and therefore additional genes might be involved [2,45].

4. Clinical picture

Mutations in *ATP8B1* and *ABCB11* can result both in progressive cholestatic disease termed PFIC1 and PFIC2, as well as in episodic cholestasis, referred to as BRIC type 1 and 2 respectively. This suggests that PFIC and BRIC are the two ends of a clinical spectrum, with different degrees of severity in between. Therefore, these diseases are preferably referred to as ATP8B1 deficiency and ABCB11 deficiency. While mutations in *ABCB4* can result in progressive cholestatic disease only designated PFIC type 3. Similarly PFIC3 is best designated as *ABCB4* deficiency. Heterozygous mutations in any of these three genes can also be associated with ICP. It is a transient form of cholestasis, characterized by the onset of pruritus during pregnancy, with postnatal resolution [2].

Pruritus is the prominent clinical feature of PFIC; however, until an episode of jaundice intervenes, the diagnosis is often overlooked. Even then, because of the rarity of the condition, children sometimes receive a misdiagnosis of obstructive jaundice caused by the occasionally associated choledocholithiasis in PFIC types 2 and 3 [5].

4.1. PFIC1 "Byler's disease"

- Cholestasis is a major clinical sign in PFIC1 as in all PFIC forms. It usually appears in the first months of life in patients with PFIC1, and is characterized by recurrent episodes of jaundice, which become permanent later in the course of the disease [3]. The variable clinical features are:

1. *Jaundice*: It presents with conjugated hyperbilirubinemia in the first 3–6 months of life. The degree of jaundice may vary [46].

2. *Pruritus*: It is the dominant feature in the majority of patients and is often out of proportion to the level of jaundice [46]. It may initially vary in intensity and may be exacerbated during intercurrent illness. Pruritus may not be noticed until 6 months of age because the neural pathways necessary for concerted scratching are not fully developed. However, affected infants often are irritable and sleep poorly with onset of cholestasis. Scratching is usually evident first as digging at the ears and eyes, which are the first areas to show evidence of excoriation. By one year of age, patients may show generalized mutilation of skin, usually most severe on the extensor surfaces of the arms and legs and on the flanks of the back. The pruritus is very disabling and often responds poorly to medical therapies [12,45].

3. *Hepatomegaly* is present early in life and persists with progression to cirrhosis. The rate of progression to cirrhosis is variable, but usually develops in early childhood without treatment. With progression to cirrhosis splenomegaly develops.

4. *Fat-soluble vitamin deficiencies*, including rickets, may be severe.

5. *Extrahepatic disorders* [19]:

   - Persistent diarrhea with fat malabsorption and protein loss, leading to poor growth and short stature.

   - Bouts of pancreatitis.

   - Recurrent pneumonia may also compromise growth.

   - Sensorineural hearing loss may occur.

- As it has been mentioned before, ATP8B1 deficiency can lead to a continuum of disease severity ranging from the progressive form PFIC1 to the recurrent form, BRIC1. BRIC1 will be discussed briefly in the next paragraphs.

BRIC is an intermittent form of intrahepatic cholestasis characterized by variable periods of intense pruritus often associated with jaundice, separated by symptom-free intervals. The benign designation of BRIC refers to the general lack of progressive liver disease, although the pruritus is far from benign during an intense episode [10]. Two types of BRIC are present according to the gene defect. BRIC1 is due to a mutation of *ATP8B1* gene and BRIC2, due to *ABCB11* gene mutations.

The age of presentation of the first attack of jaundice ranges from 1–50 years, but jaundice usually occurs before the age of twenty years. Attacks usually are preceded by a minor illness and consist of a preicteric phase of 2–4 weeks (characterized by malaise, anorexia, and pruritus) and an icteric phase that may last from 1–18 months. In some patients, hormonal factors such as the use of oral contraceptives and pregnancy have been associated with precipitation of an attack [10,47]. Patients may have severe coughing during episodes, as is seen sometimes in patients with PFIC1 [48].

During the icteric phase, the concentrations of serum bile acid, bilirubin, and alkaline phosphatase (ALP) are increased. Serum GGT concentration, however, remains low. Liver biopsy results are very benign, often showing no pathologic change even during an episode. Some specimens show hepatocellular cholestasis and cholate injury, mostly centrilobular. During the asymptomatic period, all parameters (clinical, laboratory and liver histology) are normal [49].

4.2. PFIC2 "Byler's syndrome"

• PFIC2 affected children differ from those with PFIC1 in some important respects:

The initial presentation and the evolution seem to be more severe than PFIC1, with permanent jaundice from the first months of life and rapid appearance of cirrhosis and liver failure within the first years of life [3].

They do not have extrahepatic involvement such as pancreatitis or diarrhea [45].

Early hepatocellular carcinoma (before one year of age) may complicate the course of PFIC2 [3]. Up to 15% of the patients with ABCB11 deficiency will develop hepatocellular carcinoma (HCC) or cholangiocarcinoma. Close surveillance for hepatobiliary malignancy is therefore warranted in these patients [31,32,45].

At diagnosis, the cholestasis in ABCB11 deficiency results in a more detectable fat-soluble vitamin deficiency manifestations [45].

The development of cholelithiasis in approximately one third of the patients, probably due to the low bile salt concentration in bile, secondary to impaired BSEP function, which might cause supersaturation of cholesterol [32].

• Patients fitting the phenotype of BRIC have been described with mutations in *ABCB11*. They are called BRIC2 and are characterized by:

The age of onset and total number of recurrent episodes were highly variable. Cholelithiasis occurred in many patients with BRIC2. Several patients had a relatively early onset of the disease and developed permanent cholestasis as adults after initial periods of recurrent attacks.

Occasionally BRIC will progress to the more severe and permanent form of PFIC, indicative of a clinical continuum, with intermediate phenotypes between mild and progressive disease [2,11].

4.3. PFIC3 "MDR3 deficiency"

Mutations in the *ABCB4* gene can cause or predispose to a variety of liver diseases with different age of presentation. Moreover, it can even lead to a cascade of several phenotypes in one patient, indicating the wide phenotypical spectrum of ABCB4 deficiency [43].

1. *PFIC3*: it is characterized by:

    - *Cholestasis* developing within the first year of life in about one third of patients and rarely in the neonatal period. It may also manifest later in infancy, in childhood or even in young adulthood [3,45].

    - *Pruritus* occurs less frequently than in the other types of PFIC and is usually mild.

    - *Jaundice* may be less prominent than pruritus.

    - *Height and weight* may be below normal as the disease progresses.

    - *Hepatomegaly*, and at later stages splenomegaly, as a manifestation of portal hypertension is often observed. Liver disease tends to evolve slowly to biliary cirrhosis with or without overt cholestatic jaundice [42,50].

    - *Cholelithiasis* may develop in older children.

    - *No extrahepatic features* or occurrence of malignancies are described in association with PFIC3 [42,50].

2. *Adult biliary cirrhosis*: gastrointestinal bleeding due to portal hypertension and cirrhosis may be the presenting symptom in adolescent or young adult patients [3].

3. *ICP*: some cases of ICP have been associated with heterozygous mutations in *ABCB4* [43].

4. Heterozygous mutations in the *ABCB4* gene can also cause or predispose for transient neonatal cholestasis and drug induced cholestasis [44].

5. Diagnosis

Diagnosis is dependent firstly on suspicion. The most alarming point making PFIC in the scope of diagnosis is the presence of significant pruritus out of proportion to the level of jaundice especially in the setting of low GGT. However, accurate diagnosis is dependent on a constellation of a clinical, biochemical, radiological, histopathological, immunohistochemical studies and finally can be confirmed by genetic testing for mutations (Table 1).

1. *Biochemical parameters*:

- *Serum GGT* is repeatedly normal or low in PFIC1 & PFIC2, while it is elevated in PFIC3 often more than ten times the normal value. In PFIC1 and PFIC2, the serum GGT concentration may increase to greater than 100 IU/L in patients receiving microsomal inducers such as phenobarbital and rifampicin [51].

The mechanism for the low serum concentration of GGT in PFIC1 and 2 is not clear. GGT is normally bound to the canalicular membrane by a glycosyl phosphatidyl inositol (GPI) anchor. In obstructive cholestasis, when excessive amounts of bile salts accumulate in the canalicular lumen under increased pressure, GGT is released from the membrane by detergent action and refluxes back into serum, possibly via leaky intercellular junctions. However, in PFIC and BRIC types 1 and 2, the reduced concentrations of biliary bile acids preserve canalicular GGT localization. This explanation is not entirely satisfactory as serum GGT is elevated in most other forms of intrahepatic cholestasis in which biliary bile acid levels are low. Preliminary studies indicate that some canalicular proteins, including GGT and carcinoembryonic antigen (CEA), are poorly expressed at the canaliculus in PFIC1 and 2. It is possible that low serum GGT levels result from the lack of canalicular GGT available for elution as well as from the inadequate concentrations of intracanalicular bile acids to act as detergents [51,52].

- *Serum transaminases*: In PFIC1 serum transaminases are mildly elevated. While in patients with PFIC2, serum transaminases levels are usually elevated to at least five times normal values. In PFIC3, serum aminotransferases, conjugated bilirubin, and ALP are all significantly elevated [2,45].

- *Serum cholesterol*: it is characteristically low or normal in all the three types [3].

- *Serum bile acid concentration*: it is elevated in all the three types [44,45].

- *Alpha-fetoprotein*: it is elevated at diagnosis in PFIC2 than that in PFIC1 [12,45].

- *Absent serum lipoprotein X (LPX) in PFIC3*: because measurement of biliary phospholipids is impractical in the evaluation of most patients, measurement of serum LPX may serve as a surrogate marker for PFIC3. LPX is the predominant lipoprotein in the plasma of cholestatic patients. LPX is absent from the serum of patients with homozygous *ABCB4* mutations. LPX is probably composed of biliary vesicles that are formed at the subapical compartment of the hepatocyte, transcytosed to sinusoidal membrane, and released into plasma. This process is absolutely dependent on MDR3, but the precise mechanism has not been defined [50,53].

2.   *Biliary bile analysis*:

Biliary bile analysis is performed on gallbladder bile or on bile collected by duodenal aspiration (pure choledochal bile). In case of gallbladder punction, bile contamination by blood may falsify bile analysis. In case of duodenal aspiration, bile dilution or bile contamination by alimentary phospholipids may falsify bile analysis [3].

The biliary bile salt concentration is dramatically decreased (<1 mmol/L) in PFIC2 patients [54] and only mildly decreased in PFIC1 patients (3–8 mmol/L) [19]. The normal concentration of biliary primary bile salts distinguishes PFIC3 patients from those with PFIC1 and PFIC2 [42].

In PFIC3 patients, the cardinal feature is the dramatically decreased biliary phospholipid level (1–15% of total biliary lipids; normal range 19–24%). Biliary bile salt-to-phospholipid is approximately 5-fold higher than in wild type bile, as is also biliary cholesterol-to-phospholipid [3].

3. *Radiological*:

Initial ultrasonography of the liver is performed to exclude biliary tract disease. Typically, ultrasonography is normal but may reveal a huge gallbladder in PFIC3. Sometimes, biliary stones may be identified in both PFIC2 and PFIC3 [3].

Cholangiography performed in a limited number of patients with PFIC3 showed a normal biliary tree, excluding sclerosing cholangitis, and allowed bile to be collected for biliary lipid analysis [42].

4. *Histopathology: Liver biopsy shows*:

- *In PFIC1*

  Light microscopy (LM): on routine hematoxylin and eosin (H & E) staining, liver biopsy shows bland cholestasis with almost no inflammation. It shows canalicular bile plugs of distinctive color. Small-duct paucity may be present. Fibrosis starts early, with approximately 75 % of patients having some fibrosis by 2 years of age. Fibrosis may appear initially either as pericentral sclerosis or portal fibrosis, or sometimes both. Portal to central bridging then develops in association with lacy lobular fibrosis and eventually leads to cirrhosis. Proliferating bile ductules are observed at the edge of the portal tracts in patients with significant fibrosis. The rate of progression of the fibrosis is highly variable but correlates loosely with the severity of the clinical disease [45].

  On electron microscopy (EM), canalicular bile plugs shows characteristic granular appearance "chunky bile".

- *In PFIC2*

  LM: on H & E stains, there is inflammation with giant cell hepatitis, fibrosis and duct reaction [45].

  On EM, bile appears amorphous [45].

- *In PFIC3*

  LM: on H & E stains, bile ductular proliferation and mixed inflammatory infiltrates are observed in the early stages despite patency of intra- and extrahepatic bile ducts. Cholestasis with slight giant cell transformation and isolated eosinophilic necrotic hepatocytes may also be present. Periductal sclerosis affecting the interlobular bile ducts eventually occurs. Extensive portal fibrosis evolves into biliary cirrhosis in older children [42].

  EM of liver has not been reported in proven cases.

5. *Immunohistochemical staining*:

Commercially available MDR3 and BSEP antibodies allow liver immunostaining to be performed. Absence of canalicular or mild immunostaining is in favor of a gene defect. However, normal staining does not exclude a gene defect as a mutation may induce a loss of function but normal synthesis [31,42].

6. *Genetic testing*:

Molecular analysis remains the definitive diagnostic technique for PFIC. Gene analysis is usually performed by DNA sequencing of the 27 coding exons (coding exons 2-28) of the *ATP8B1*, *ABCB11*, and *ABCB4* genes and their splice junctions [3]. The use of a resequensing chip dedicated to genetic cholestasis could facilitate identification of gene mutation [55].

	PFIC-1	PFIC-2	PFIC-3
Synonyms	Byler disease ATP8B1 deficiency FIC1 deficiency	Byler syndrome ABCB11 deficiency BSEP deficiency	ABCB4 deficiency MDR3 deficiency
Gene defect	*ATP8B1 (FIC1)*	*ABCB11 (BSEP)*	*ABCB4 (MDR3)*
Locus	18q21-22	2q24	7q21
Transport defect	Aminophospholipid	Bile acid	Phospholipids
Pathophysiology	Impaired inward translocation of aminophospholipids over cellular membranes	Impaired canalicular bile salt transport secondary to malfunction of BSEP	Impaired canalicular translocation of phosphatidylcholine
Clinical picture:			
Onset of cholestasis	Neonatal	Neonatal	Variable
Pruritus	Severe	Severe	Moderate
Extrahepatic manifestations	Present	Absent	Absent
Cholelithiasis	Absent	Increased incidence	Increased incidence
HCC	No	Risk from the 1st year	No
Clinical spectrum of gene defect	PFIC1, BRIC1, and ICP	PFIC2, BRIC2, and ICP	PFIC3, ICP, adult biliary cirrhosis, cholelithiasis, transient neonatal cholestasis, drug induced cholestasis
Biochemical:			
GGT	Normal or low	Normal or low	Elevated
Transaminases	Mildly elevated	More elevated	Elevated
Bile acids	Elevated	More elevated	Elevated
Cholesterol	Normal	Normal	Normal
Alpha fetoprotein	Not significantly elevated	More elevated	--
Histopathological	Bland cholestasis (LM) Coarse granular bile (EM)	Giant cell hepatitis (LM) Amorphous bile (EM)	Ductular proliferation (LM)
Immunohistochemical	--	Absent or reduced BSEP staining in the majority of patients	Absent or reduced MDR3 staining in about 50 % of patients

Table 1. Summary of the criteria of different PFIC types.

6. Differential diagnosis

Two groups of diseases are in differential diagnosis with PFIC group of disorders. For PFIC1 and PFIC2, it is to be differentiated from other cholestatic disorders with low GGT. While for PFIC3, when it presents early it, is to be differentiated from cholestatic disorders with high GGT and when it presents in an older age, childhood or adolescence, it is to be differentiated from other causes of chronic liver diseases at respective ages.

- *Cholestasis with low GGT*:

    1. Inborn errors of bile acid metabolism [6].

    2. Familial hypercholanemia: familial hypercholanemia represents a PFIC-like disorder due to a bile canalicular tight junction protein defect combined with a defect of primary bile acid conjugation. Cholestasis is due to impaired transport of unconjugated bile acids into bile and to bile leakage into plasma through abnormal canalicular tight junctions increasing paracellular permeability [56].

    3. Arthrogryposis- renal dysfunction cholestasis (ARC) syndrome is a complex disease due to mutation of *VPS33B* involved in intracellular trafficking and targeting of apical proteins. The gene defect results in a loss of apical protein expression in the liver and kidneys [57].

- *Cholestasis with high GGT*:

    1. Biliary atresia [58].

    2. Neonatal sclerosing cholangitis [59].

    3. Congenital cytomegalovirus (CMV) infection.

    4. Alpha1-antitrypsin deficiency disease [60].

    5. North American Indian Childhood Cirrhosis (NAIC) [61].

    6. Aagenaes syndrome (hereditary cholestasis with lymphedema): a very rare familial cholestatic disorder with cholestasis and lower limb edema [62].

- *Causes of chronic liver disease*:

    1. Chronic viral hepatitis.

    2. Autoimmune liver diseases: autoimmune hepatitis and autoimmune sclerosing cholangitis.

    3. Metabolic liver disorders, e.g., Wilson disease and alpha1-antitrypsin deficiency.

7. Treatment

Initial treatment of PFIC includes the use of cholestyramine, ursodeoxycholic acid, rifampicin, and phenobarbital [63-65]. Until the late 1980s, liver transplantation was the only effective therapy for those who did not respond to medical treatment [66,67]. Later on, less invasive non-transplant surgical approaches were proposed and undertaken early in the course of the disease with promising initial results [68]. In this section, a brief overview about the different lines of management for PFIC patients will be given.

7.1. Medical therapy

Unfortunately, most forms of medical therapy for PFIC types 1, 2, and 3 are of limited effectiveness. Nevertheless, several treatment modalities can be used in specific patients to improve quality of life or prevent progression of the disease [2,69].

- *Cholestyramine* is an anion-exchange resin that binds bile salts, preventing their re-absorption in the enterohepatic circulation. In PFIC, relief of pruritus and normalization of biochemical parameters is only described rarely with cholestyramine. However, in patients with BRIC it can be helpful in shortening episodes [2].

- *Rifampicin*, although it accelerates the hepatic detoxification and excretion of compounds, such as bilirubin and bile salts, it has been used with limited efficacy in patients with PFIC [51]. Nevertheless, in patients with BRIC it can completely abort an episode.

- *Ursodeoxycholic acid (UDCA)* is a relatively hydrophilic bile salt, which is less cytotoxic than endogenous bile salts. Upon oral administration (20 mg/kg/day), it will partially replace endogenous bile salts in the bile salt pool, reducing injury of the hepatocytes during cholestasis. In PFIC3 regular administration of UDCA normalizes liver function tests and improves clinical parameters in up to 50% of the patients. The therapeutic effect appears to be dependent on the type of mutation, with premature stop codons leading to a truncated protein being associated with nearly no response to therapy. UDCA should therefore be the first choice in the initial therapeutic management of patients with ABCB4 deficiency, especially when a missense mutation in the corresponding gene is found [42]. In patients with PFIC1 or PFIC2, the results of UDCA treatment are conflicting, ranging from clear improvement to no effect at all.

In this respect, the recommended treatment strategy is to start with UDCA therapy in all types of PFIC, especially PFIC3. If no appropriate response, especially regarding pruritus, add the other medical lines of therapy. Those who will not respond are shifted to surgical treatment [3,45,65,66].

7.2. Surgical treatment

Surgical treatment for PFIC is an important major line of therapy. If no complete clinical or biochemical improvement is obtained with medical therapy, more invasive therapy such as biliary diversion or even liver transplantation is necessary [2,70].

Interruption of the enterohepatic circulation through biliary diversion has yielded excellent clinical, biochemical, and histologic response in a number of children with PFIC, provided the procedure is performed before the development of significant hepatic fibrosis [46]. It reduces the accumulation of toxic bile salts by decreasing their intestinal re-uptake. It is unclear if these approaches are optimal for specific genetic forms of PFIC rather than others. It is possible that these interventions may be best for severe PFIC1 and milder phenotypic variants of PFIC2. Nasobiliary drainage may help to select potential responders to biliary diversion [71].

There are three major non-transplant surgical techniques to permanently interrupt the enterohepatic circulation, namely partial external biliary diversion (PEBD), ileal bypass (IB) and partial internal biliary diversion (PIBD).

• *Partial external biliary diversion (PEBD):*

PEBD interrupts the enterohepatic circulation of bile salts by partially diverting bile from the gallbladder through a loop of jejunum connecting the gallbladder to the abdominal skin [72].

In 1988, Whitington and Whitington [68] introduced cholecystojejunocutaneostomy as a PEBD for the surgical treatment of PFIC, to increase the elimination of bile acids accumulated within the body and thus control the intractable pruritus. In this procedure, one end of a loop of jejunum is anastamosed to the dome of the gallbladder, whereas the other is used to form a cutaneous ostomy (Figure 2A). Bile in the gallbladder then flows either out of the ostomy or into the intestine. Typically 30–50% of bile drains out of the ostomy and is discarded. Two variants on the original PEBD have also been described; one using a laparoscopic technique [73] and the other using an appendiceal conduit [74].

Results of PEBD are promising with respect to pruritus, jaundice and histology, both in patients with PFIC1 and PFIC2, with at least partial improvement in more than 75% of the patients [66,72]. Although this seems promising, at present it is unclear whether in patients responding to PEBD liver transplantation can also be avoided at long-term follow-up [75]. Moreover, some patients do not benefit from biliary surgery at all. Obviously in these patients liver transplantation should be considered [72].

The type of mutation seems to be associated with the outcome of PEBD, with better prognosis in disease caused by milder mutations, especially for the ABCB11 mutations E297G and D482G [32,45]. However, when severe fibrosis is already present at the moment of PEBD, prognosis is worse [72]. One patient with PFIC3 who underwent PEBD was described in literature; this patient showed no improvement [67].

No serious PEBD complications are reported, although problems with the stoma (stenosis, recurrent bleeding) (Figure 2) sometimes make a re-operation necessary. In addition excessive stomal losses can cause dehydration and electrolyte imbalance, while cholangitis can also develop [72,75].

The permanent character of the PEBD makes it less suitable for patients with episodic cholestasis (BRIC). In these patients temporary nasobiliary drainage (NBD) to interrupt the enterohepatic circulation can be endoscopically introduced. This procedure is effective in most of these patients, resolving pruritus and normalising bile salts within short time [10,71].

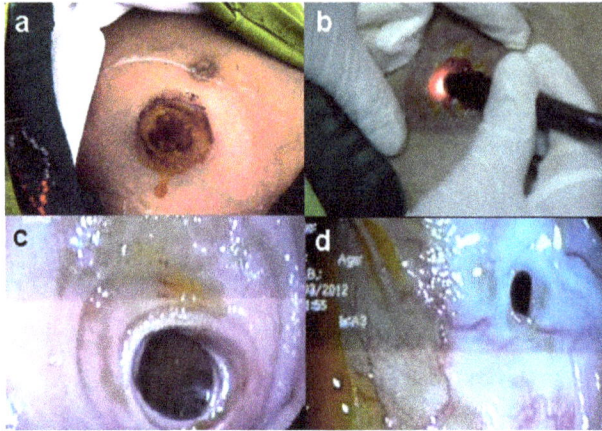

Figure 2. A seven years old child diagnosed as PFIC2 underwent PEBD at the age of 2 years old with good outcome. He had recurrent bleeding from the osteal opening (a). Endoscopy through the osteal opening (b) showed free jejunal loop (c) till its proximal end at the gall bladder (d). The source of bleeding was the stoma itself.

• *Terminal ileal exclusion or ileal bypass (IB)*:

Although most of PFIC patients and their parents tolerate well PEBD with its external biliary fistula and the need for stoma care, sometimes it becomes a real problem, particularly for children of school age and teenagers, who may feel uncomfortable to participate in all activities with their friends. Moreover, there is still a group of patients who cannot undergo PEBD because of a previous cholecystectomy, or who develop postoperative electrolyte inbalance due to the excessive daily amount of bile [5,76].

To deal with these problems, an IB technique was proposed. In IB, the terminal ileum is skipped by an ileocolonic anastomosis. It was developed as an alternative treatment to PEBD, that avoids a long-term stoma complications. In 1994, Whitington et al. described a good initial outcome of IB in two patients after cholecystectomy, but a chronic diarrhea occurred one year later. In 1998, Holland et al. described this procedure in PFIC children after cholecystectomy. All patients were supplemented with vitamin B12 and folic acid. Interestingly, no diarrhea was reported postoperatively. Early results were very promising, with a relief of pruritus and normalization of bilirubin level. Nevertheless, relapse of cholestatsis occurred in half of the patients. The authors underline that IB is not as effective as PEBD and therefore it should not be considered as the primary treatment in children with PFIC [5,51].

The rational of this technique was that the vast majority of intestinal bile salts are reabsorbed in the distal ileum; that is the distal 15% of the small intestine. Therefore, exclusion of this segment of intestine may lead to bile acid wasting. The small intestine is transected at a point that demarcates the distal 15% of the small intestine, and a blind loop is formed with the distal ileal segment. The proximal loop of the intestine is sewn end-to-side to the cecum, completing the internal bypass of the distal ileum. Accurate assessment of the appropriate amount of ileum for bypass is likely to be critical; too little is unlikely to be therapeutic and too much is likely to yield bile acid–induced diarrhea. Mutational analysis may be used eventually to predict which patients are most likely to benefit from surgery. After IB, symptoms may recur within one year requiring conversion to PEBD [5,77].

- *Partial internal biliary diversion (PIBD):*

PIBD interrupts the enterohepatic circulation of bile salts by partially diverting bile from the gallbladder through a loop of jejunum connecting the gallbladder to the colon [46,76].

This operation combines the advantages of partially diverting the biliary flow from the enterohepatic cycle (such as the PEBD does), while at the same time avoiding an external biliary fistula. In addition, this operation lacks the potential for malabsorption that may result from partially excluding the terminal ileum from the intestinal transit. There is, however, a potential for choleretic diarrhea, which may result from large amounts of bile salts entering the colon. Because of this, it was strongly emphasized that the conduit should be made at least 15 cm long to create a certain resistance to the bile flow; it is believed that this stimulates a certain amount of bile to flow through the normal biliary tract to the duodenum. This problem occurred in a transient way in a few of the patients and it can be controlled with the use of cholestyramine for a limited span of time [46].

Through an upper midline abdominal incision, the gallbladder and the liver are evaluated. An intestinal conduit is constructed using a 15- to 20-cm segment of midjejunum, which is sutured initially to the gallbladder wall and then terminolaterally to the midportion of the ascending colon. The distal end of the jejunum is slightly tapered in a way that the jejunum could reach the colon in an isoperistaltic direction to prevent colonic contents from entering the conduit. The clinical and laboratory results described for PIBD make it a very attractive surgical option for the treatment of PFICs in children with a normal gallbladder. However, long-term follow-up is necessary to evaluate late results and eventual complications associated with this technique [46].

If all previously described therapies fails in controlling pruritus, when there is an end-stage PFIC liver disease, or when the disease is progressive despite treatment; orthotopic liver transplantation (OLT) remains the only alternative [78-80]. Before the development of liver transplantation, therapy for these patients was generally ineffective. With the advent of liver transplantation, many PFIC patients were treated with this life-saving procedure [70,78]. At one time, PFIC was among the 5 most common indications for liver transplantation in children [81,82].

Although OLT is associated with serious surgical risks and lifetime immunosuppressive therapy is necessary, it usually gives complete correction of phenotype in patients with PFIC2 and PFIC3 deficiency in which the disease is hepatocyte specific. However, phenotypic recurrence of severe PFIC2 deficiency post-transplantation can occur as a result of the formation of autoantibodies against BSEP [83,84]. Intensifying immunosuppressive therapy may resolve this problem.

In contrast, in PFIC1, liver transplantation is potentially fraught with a number of potential complications related to the extrahepatic expression of the *ATP8B1* gene. The most prominent posttransplantation problems include intractable diarrhea, hepatic steatosis, poor growth, and recurrent pancreatitis. Worsening diarrhea post liver transplant might be due to an imbalance between bile salt excretion and re-absorption, since the hepatic graft excretes a normal amount of bile salts, whereas the intestine remains functionally impaired. The resulting increased amount of bile salts in the ileum and colon induces or worsens diarrhea, which might respond to cholestyramine treatment [19,85]. Therefore, in PFIC1, non-transplant surgical approaches should be considered the preferred first-line of therapy.

In summary, children with PFIC do better with non-transplant surgical interventions than they do with the natural history of disease, which is uniformly fatal. Successful outcomes have been demonstrated, with marked improvements in clinical symptoms, laboratory values, growth and histology. It appears that the success rate is high enough that many patients may do better with a non-transplant procedure than transplant given the posttransplant morbidities associated with immunotherapy. Those with more advanced disease are most likely to have a poor outcome with non-transplant surgical procedures. This may encourage clinicians to consider a surgical intervention early in the course of disease before significant hepatic scarring develops [76].

Some authors proposed that the treatment strategy is to perform PEBD rapidly after diagnosis in patients with PFIC1 & PFIC2 and to consider OLT when treatment fails. In patients with PFIC3, UDCA treatment is the first-line therapy; if not successful it is followed by liver transplantation. In patients with episodic cholestasis (BRIC) medical treatment with rifampicin with or without cholestyramine can be attempted at the start of an attack. If medication is not successful in aborting the cholestatic episode NBD can be performed [2,69]. In BRIC patients who progress to a more permanent form of cholestasis, or in patients with very frequent or debilitating attacks, a biliary diversion can be considered [69].

7.3. New and future therapies

New and future therapies for PFIC patients include hepatocyte transplantation, the use of nuclear receptor ligands, enhancing the expression of the mutated transporter protein by employing chaperones and mutation specific therapy [2,69].

Hepatocyte transplantation has been successful in partially repopulating the liver, diminishing pathology in a mouse model of ABCB4 deficiency, but unfortunately not yet in patients [86]. In ABCB11 deficiency it is doubtful whether hepatocyte transplantation is a good therapeutic option since possible premalignant cells are left in place.

Certain nuclear receptors regulate bile formation. The key nuclear receptor in bile formation is the bile salt sensor FXR. Activated FXR transactivates a number of genes, resulting in improved bile salt excretion and detoxification. Targeting FXR with synthetic ligands is explored as a possible therapeutic option for cholestasis syndromes [87].

A pharmacological chaperone is defined as a small molecule that specifically binds to its target protein and induces or promotes proper folding and trafficking of the protein [88]. Some researchers have investigated the usefulness of pharmacological chaperones for treatment of diseases caused by folding-defective membrane proteins [24,89,90]. Pharmacological chaperones such as 4-phenylbutyrate acid (4-PBA) have been shown to stabilize proteins misfolded due to missense mutations, thereby preventing degradation in the endoplasmic reticulum. In vitro, 4-PBA enhances cell surface protein expression for some of the missense mutations found in ATP8B1 deficiency and ABCB11 deficiency [25,91]. Misawa et al [24], showed that bile acids do act as pharmacological chaperones of E297G BSEP. They also described the discovery and structural development of non-steroidal compounds with potent pharmacological chaperone activity for E297G BSEP.

Author details

Ahmad Mohamed Sira* and Mostafa Mohamed Sira

*Address all correspondence to: asira@liver-eg.org

Department of Pediatric Hepatology, National Liver Institute, Menofiya University, Egypt

References

[1] De Bruyne, R., Van Biervliet, S., Vande, Velde S., & Van Winckel, M. (2011). Clinical practice: neonatal cholestasis. *Eur J Pediatr*, 170(3), 279-284.

[2] Van der Woerd, W. L., van Mil, S. W., Stapelbroek, J. M., Klomp, L. W., van de Graaf, S. F., & Houwen, R. H. (2010). Familial cholestasis: progressive familial intrahepatic cholestasis, benign recurrent intrahepatic cholestasis and intrahepatic cholestasis of pregnancy. *Best Pract Res Clin Gastroenterol*, 24(5), 541-553.

[3] Davit-Spraul, A., Gonzales, E., Baussan, C., & Jacquemin, E. (2009). Progressive familial intrahepatic cholestasis. *Orphanet J Rare Dis*, 4(1).

[4] Clayton, R. J., Iber, F. L., Ruebner, B. H., & McKusick, V. A. (1969). Byler disease. Fatal familial intrahepatic cholestasis in an Amish kindred. *Am J Dis Child*, 117(1), 112-124.

[5] Hollands, C. M., Rivera-Pedrogo, F. J., Gonzalez-Vallina, R., Loret-de-Mola, O., Nahmad, M., & Burnweit, C. A. (1998). Ileal exclusion for Byler's disease: an alternative surgical approach with promising early results for pruritus. *J Pediatr Surg;*, 33(2), 220-224.

[6] Jankowska, I., & Socha, P. (2012). Progressive familial intrahepatic cholestasis and inborn errors of bile acid synthesis. *Clin Res Hepatol Gastroenterol*, 36(3), 271-274.

[7] Summerskill, W. H., & Walshe, J. M. (1959). Benign recurrent intrahepatic "obstructive" jaundice. *Lancet*, 2(7105), 686-690.

[8] Luketic, V. A., & Shiffman, M. L. (2004). Benign recurrent intrahepatic cholestasis. *Clin Liver Dis*, 8(1), 133-149, vii.

[9] Folvik, G., Hilde, O., & Helge, G. O. (2012). Benign recurrent intrahepatic cholestasis: review and long-term follow-up of five cases. *Scand J Gastroenterol*, 47(4), 482-488.

[10] Toros, A. B., Ozerdenen, F., Bektas, H., & Sari, N. D. (2012). A case report: nasobiliary drainage inducing remission in benign recurrent intrahepatic cholestasis. *Turk J Gastroenterol*, 23(1), 75-78.

[11] Van Ooteghem, N. A., Klomp, L. W., van Berge-Henegouwen, G. P., & Houwen, R. H. (2002). Benign recurrent intrahepatic cholestasis progressing to progressive familial intrahepatic cholestasis: low GGT cholestasis is a clinical continuum. *J Hepatol*, 36(3), 439-443.

[12] Van Mil, S. W., Klomp, L. W., Bull, L. N., & Houwen, R. H. (2001). FIC1 disease: a spectrum of intrahepatic cholestatic disorders. *Semin Liver Dis*, 21(4), 535-544.

[13] Verhulst, P. M., van der Velden, L. M., Oorschot, V., van Faassen, E. E., Klumperman, J., Houwen, R. H., Pomorski, T. G., Holthuis, J. C., & Klomp, L. W. (2010). A flippase-independent function of ATP8B1, the protein affected in familial intrahepatic cholestasis type 1, is required for apical protein expression and microvillus formation in polarized epithelial cells. *Hepatology*, 51(6), 2049-2060.

[14] Cai, S. Y., Gautam, S., Nguyen, T., Soroka, C. J., Rahner, C., & Boyer, J. L. (2009). ATP8B1 deficiency disrupts the bile canalicular membrane bilayer structure in hepatocytes, but FXR expression and activity are maintained. *Gastroenterology*, 1060-1069.

[15] Paulusma, C. C., Groen, A., Kunne, C., Ho-Mok, K. S., Spijkerboer, A. L., Rudi de, Waart. D., Hoek, F. J., Vreeling, H., Hoeben, K. A., van Marle, J., Pawlikowska, L., Bull, L. N., Hofmann, A. F., Knisely, A. S., & Oude, Elferink. R. P. (2006). Atp8b1 deficiency in mice reduces resistance of the canalicular membrane to hydrophobic bile salts and impairs bile salt transport. *Hepatology*, 44(1), 195-204.

[16] Paulusma, C. C., de Waart, D. R., Kunne, C., Mok, K. S., & Elferink, R. P. (2009). Activity of the bile salt export pump (ABCB11) is critically dependent on canalicular membrane cholesterol content. *J Biol Chem*, 284(15), 9947-9954.

[17] Alvarez, L., Jara, P., Sanchez-Sabate, E., Hierro, L., Larrauri, J., Diaz, M. C., Camarena, C., De la Vega, A., Frauca, E., Lopez-Collazo, E., & Lapunzina, P. (2004). Reduced hepatic expression of farnesoid X receptor in hereditary cholestasis associated to mutation in ATP8B1. *Hum Mol Genet*, 13(20), 2451-2460.

[18] Chen, F., Ananthanarayanan, M., Emre, S., Neimark, E., Bull, L. N., Knisely, A. S., Strautnieks, S. S., Thompson, R. J., Magid, M. S., Gordon, R., Balasubramanian, N., Suchy, F. J., & Shneider, B. L. (2004). Progressive familial intrahepatic cholestasis, type 1, is associated with decreased farnesoid X receptor activity. *Gastroenterology*, 126(3), 756-764.

[19] Lykavieris, P., van Mil, S., Cresteil, D., Fabre, M., Hadchouel, M., Klomp, L., Bernard, O., & Jacquemin, E. (2003). Progressive familial intrahepatic cholestasis type 1 and extrahepatic features: no catch-up of stature growth, exacerbation of diarrhea, and appearance of liver steatosis after liver transplantation. *J Hepatol*, 39(3), 447-452.

[20] Stapelbroek, J. M., Peters, T. A., van Beurden, D. H., Curfs, J. H., Joosten, A., Beynon, A. J., van Leeuwen, B. M., van der Velden, L. M., Bull, L., Oude, Elferink R. P., van Zanten, B. A., Klomp, L. W., & Houwen, R. H. (2009). ATP8B1 is essential for maintaining normal hearing. *Proc Natl Acad Sci, U S A*, 106(24), 9709-9714.

[21] Klomp, L. W., Vargas, J. C., van Mil, S. W., Pawlikowska, L., Strautnieks, S. S., van Eijk, M. J., Juijn, J. A., Pabon-Pena, C., Smith, L. B., De Young, J. A., Byrne, J. A., Gombert, J., van der Brugge, G., Berger, R., Jankowska, I., Pawlowska, J., Villa, E., Knisely, A. S., Thompson, R. J., Freimer, N. B., Houwen, R. H., & Bull, L. N. (2004). Characterization of mutations in ATP8B1 associated with hereditary cholestasis. *Hepatology*, 40(1), 27-38.

[22] Liu, L. Y., Wang, X. H., Wang, Z. L., Zhu, Q. R., & Wang, J. S. (2010). Characterization of ATP8B1 gene mutations and a hot-linked mutation found in Chinese children with progressive intrahepatic cholestasis and low GGT. *J Pediatr Gastroenterol Nutr*, 50(2), 179-183.

[23] Folmer, D. E., van der Mark, V. A., Ho-Mok, K. S., Oude Elferink, R. P., & Paulusma, C. C. (2009). Differential effects of progressive familial intrahepatic cholestasis type 1 and benign recurrent intrahepatic cholestasis type 1 mutations on canalicular localization of ATP8B1. *Hepatology*, 50(5), 1597-1605.

[24] Misawa, T., Hayashi, H., Sugiyama, Y., & Hashimoto, Y. (2012). Discovery and structural development of small molecules that enhance transport activity of bile salt export pump mutant associated with progressive familial intrahepatic cholestasis type 2. *Bioorg Med Chem.*

[25] Van der Velden, L. M., Stapelbroek, J. M., Krieger, E., van den Berghe, P. V., Berger, R., Verhulst, P. M., Holthuis, J. C., Houwen, R. H., Klomp, L. W., & van de Graaf, S. F. (2010). Folding defects in P-type ATP 8B1 associated with hereditary cholestasis are ameliorated by 4-phenylbutyrate. *Hepatology*, 51(1), 286-296.

[26] Klomp, L. W., Bull, L. N., Knisely, A. S., van Der Doelen, M. A., Juijn, J. A., Berger, R., Forget, S., Nielsen, I. M., Eiberg, H., & Houwen, R. H. (2000). A missense mutation in FIC1 is associated with greenland familial cholestasis. *Hepatology*, 32(6), 1337-1341.

[27] Mullenbach, R., Bennett, A., Tetlow, N., Patel, N., Hamilton, G., Cheng, F., Chambers, J., Howard, R., Taylor-Robinson, S. D., & Williamson, C. (2005). ATP8B1 mutations in British cases with intrahepatic cholestasis of pregnancy. *Gut*, 54(6), 829-834.

[28] Demeilliers, C., Jacquemin, E., Barbu, V., Mergey, M., Paye, F., Fouassier, L., Chignard, N., Housset, C., & Lomri, N. E. (2006). Altered hepatobiliary gene expressions in PFIC1: ATP8B1 gene defect is associated with CFTR downregulation. *Hepatology*, 43(5), 1125-1134.

[29] Gerloff, T., Stieger, B., Hagenbuch, B., Madon, J., Landmann, L., Roth, J., Hofmann, A. F., & Meier, P. J. (1998). The sister of P-glycoprotein represents the canalicular bile salt export pump of mammalian liver. *J Biol Chem*, 273(16), 10046-10050.

[30] Strautnieks, S. S., Bull, L. N., Knisely, A. S., Kocoshis, S. A., Dahl, N., Arnell, H., Sokal, E., Dahan, K., Childs, S., Ling, V., Tanner, M. S., Kagalwalla, A. F., Nemeth, A., Pawlowska, J., Baker, A., Mieli-Vergani, G., Freimer, N. B., Gardiner, R. M., & Thompson, R. J. (1998). A gene encoding a liver-specific ABC transporter is mutated in progressive familial intrahepatic cholestasis. *Nat Genet*, 20(3), 233-238.

[31] Strautnieks, S. S., Byrne, J. A., Pawlikowska, L., Cebecauerova, D., Rayner, A., Dutton, L., Meier, Y., Antoniou, A., Stieger, B., Arnell, H., Ozcay, F., Al-Hussaini, H. F., Bassas, A. F., Verkade, H. J., Fischler, B., Nemeth, A., Kotalova, R., Shneider, B. L., Cielecka-Kuszyk, J., Mc Clean, P., Whitington, P. F., Sokal, E., Jirsa, M., Wali, S. H., Jankowska, I., Pawlowska, J., Mieli-Vergani, G., Knisely, A. S., Bull, L. N., & Thompson, R. J. (2008). Severe bile salt export pump deficiency: 82 different ABCB11 mutations in 109 families. *Gastroenterology*, 134(4), 1203-1214.

[32] Pawlikowska, L., Strautnieks, S., Jankowska, I., Czubkowski, P., Emerick, K., Antoniou, A., Wanty, C., Fischler, B., Jacquemin, E., Wali, S., Blanchard, S., Nielsen, I. M., Bourke, B., Mc Quaid, S., Lacaille, F., Byrne, J. A., van Eerde, A. M., Kolho, K. L., Klomp, L., Houwen, R., Bacchetti, P., Lobritto, S., Hupertz, V., Mc Clean, P., Mieli-Vergani, G., Shneider, B., Nemeth, A., Sokal, E., Freimer, N. B., Knisely, A. S., Rosenthal, P., Whitington, P. F., Pawlowska, J., Thompson, R. J., & Bull, L. N. (2010). Differences in presentation and progression between severe FIC1 and BSEP deficiencies. *J Hepatol*, 53(1), 170-178.

[33] Kagawa, T., Watanabe, N., Mochizuki, K., Numari, A., Ikeno, Y., Itoh, J., Tanaka, H., Arias, I. M., & Mine, T. (2008). Phenotypic differences in PFIC2 and BRIC2 correlate with protein stability of mutant Bsep and impaired taurocholate secretion in MDCK II cells. *Am J Physiol Gastrointest Liver Physiol*, 294(1), G 58-67.

[34] Pauli-Magnus, C., Lang, T., Meier, Y., Zodan-Marin, T., Jung, D., Breymann, C., Zimmermann, R., Kenngott, S., Beuers, U., Reichel, C., Kerb, R., Penger, A., Meier, P. J., & Kullak-Ublick, G. A. (2004). Sequence analysis of bile salt export pump (ABCB11) and multidrug resistance p-glycoprotein 3 (ABCB4, MDR3) in patients with intrahepatic cholestasis of pregnancy. *Pharmacogenetics*, 14(2), 91-102.

[35] Pauli-Magnus, C., & Meier, P. J. (2006). Hepatobiliary transporters and drug-induced cholestasis. *Hepatology*, 44(4), 778-787.

[36] Hermeziu, B., Sanlaville, D., Girard, M., Leonard, C., Lyonnet, S., & Jacquemin, E. (2006). Heterozygous bile salt export pump deficiency: a possible genetic predisposition to transient neonatal cholestasis. *J Pediatr Gastroenterol Nutr*, 42(1), 114-116.

[37] De Vree, J. M., Jacquemin, E., Sturm, E., Cresteil, D., Bosma, P. J., Aten, J., Deleuze, J. F., Desrochers, M., Burdelski, M., Bernard, O., Oude Elferink, R. P., & Hadchouel, M.

(1998). Mutations in the MDR3 gene cause progressive familial intrahepatic cholestasis. *Proc Natl Acad Sci*, U S A, 95(1), 282-287.

[38] Oude Elferink, R. P., & Paulusma, C. C. (2007). Function and pathophysiological importance of ABCB4 (MDR3 P-glycoprotein). *Pflugers Arch*, 453(5), 601-610.

[39] Noe, J., Kullak-Ublick, G. A., Jochum, W., Stieger, B., Kerb, R., Haberl, M., Mullhaupt, B., Meier, P. J., & Pauli-Magnus, C. (2005). Impaired expression and function of the bile salt export pump due to three novel ABCB11 mutations in intrahepatic cholestasis. *J Hepatol*, 43(3), 536-543.

[40] Keitel, V., Burdelski, M., Warskulat, U., Kuhlkamp, T., Keppler, D., Haussinger, D., & Kubitz, R. (2005). Expression and localization of hepatobiliary transport proteins in progressive familial intrahepatic cholestasis. *Hepatology*, 41(5), 1160-1172.

[41] Degiorgio, D., Colombo, C., Seia, M., Porcaro, L., Costantino, L., Zazzeron, L., Bordo, D., & Coviello, D. A. (2007). Molecular characterization and structural implications of 25 new ABCB4 mutations in progressive familial intrahepatic cholestasis type 3 (PFIC3). *Eur J Hum Genet*, 15(12), 1230-1238.

[42] Jacquemin, E., De Vree, J. M., Cresteil, D., Sokal, E. M., Sturm, E., Dumont, M., Scheffer, G. L., Paul, M., Burdelski, M., Bosma, P. J., Bernard, O., Hadchouel, M., & Elferink, R. P. (2001). The wide spectrum of multidrug resistance 3 deficiency: from neonatal cholestasis to cirrhosis of adulthood. *Gastroenterology*, 120(6), 1448-1458.

[43] Lucena, J. F., Herrero, J. I., Quiroga, J., Sangro, B., Garcia-Foncillas, J., Zabalegui, N., Sola, J., Herraiz, M., Medina, J. F., & Prieto, J. (2003). A multidrug resistance 3 gene mutation causing cholelithiasis, cholestasis of pregnancy, and adulthood biliary cirrhosis. *Gastroenterology*, 124(4), 1037-1042.

[44] Gonzales, E., Davit-Spraul, A., Baussan, C., Buffet, C., Maurice, M., & Jacquemin, E. (2009). Liver diseases related to MDR3 (ABCB4) gene deficiency. *Front Biosci*, 14, 4242-4256.

[45] Davit-Spraul, A., Fabre, M., Branchereau, S., Baussan, C., Gonzales, E., Stieger, B., Bernard, O., & Jacquemin, E. (2010). ATP8B1 and ABCB11 analysis in 62 children with normal gamma-glutamyl transferase progressive familial intrahepatic cholestasis (PFIC): phenotypic differences between PFIC1 and PFIC2 and natural history. *Hepatology*, 51(5), 1645-1655.

[46] Bustorff-Silva, J., Sbraggia Neto, L., Olimpio, H., de Alcantara, R. V., Matsushima, E., De Tommaso, A. M., Brandao, M. A., & Hessel, G. (2007). Partial internal biliary diversion through a cholecystojejunocolonic anastomosis--a novel surgical approach for patients with progressive familial intrahepatic cholestasis: a preliminary report. *J Pediatr Surg*, 42(8), 1337-1340.

[47] Jansen, P. L., & Sturm, E. (2003). Genetic cholestasis, causes and consequences for hepatobiliary transport. *Liver Int*, 23(5), 315-322.

[48] Chatila, R., Bergasa, N. V., Lagarde, S., & West, A. B. (1996). Intractable cough and abnormal pulmonary function in benign recurrent intrahepatic cholestasis. *Am J Gastroenterol*, 91(10), 2215-2219.

[49] Mizuochi, T., Kimura, A., Tanaka, A., Muto, A., Nittono, H., Seki, Y., Takahashi, T., Kurosawa, T., Kage, M., Takikawa, H., & Matsuishi, T. (2012). Characterization of urinary bile acids in a pediatric BRIC-1 patient: Effect of rifampicin treatment. *Clin Chim Acta*, 413(15-16), 1301-1304.

[50] Jacquemin, E. (2001). Role of multidrug resistance 3 deficiency in pediatric and adult liver disease: one gene for three diseases. *Semin Liver Dis*, 21(4), 551-562.

[51] Whitington, P. F., Freese, D. K., Alonso, E. M., Schwarzenberg, S. J., & Sharp, H. L. (1994). Clinical and biochemical findings in progressive familial intrahepatic cholestasis. *J Pediatr Gastroenterol Nutr*, 18(2), 134-141.

[52] Cabrera-Abreu, J. C., & Green, A. (2002). Gamma-glutamyltransferase: value of its measurement in paediatrics. *Ann Clin Biochem*, 39(pt1), 22-5.

[53] Elferink, R. P., Ottenhoff, R., van Marle, J., Frijters, C. M., Smith, A. J., & Groen, A. K. (1998). Class III P-glycoproteins mediate the formation of lipoprotein X in the mouse. *J Clin Invest*, 102(9), 1749-1757.

[54] Jansen, P. L., Strautnieks, S. S., Jacquemin, E., Hadchouel, M., Sokal, E. M., Hooiveld, G. J., Koning, J. H., De Jager-Krikken, A., Kuipers, F., Stellaard, F., Bijleveld, C. M., Gouw, A., Van Goor, H., Thompson, R. J., & Muller, M. (1999). Hepatocanalicular bile salt export pump deficiency in patients with progressive familial intrahepatic cholestasis. *Gastroenterology*, 117(6), 1370-1379.

[55] Liu, C., Aronow, B. J., Jegga, A. G., Wang, N., Miethke, A., Mourya, R., & Bezerra, J. A. (2007). Novel resequencing chip customized to diagnose mutations in patients with inherited syndromes of intrahepatic cholestasis. *Gastroenterology*, 132(1), 119-126.

[56] Carlton, V. E., Harris, B. Z., Puffenberger, E. G., Batta, A. K., Knisely, A. S., Robinson, D. L., Strauss, K. A., Shneider, B. L., Lim, W. A., Salen, G., Morton, D. H., & Bull, L. N. (2003). Complex inheritance of familial hypercholanemia with associated mutations in TJP2 and BAAT. *Nat Genet*, 34(1), 91-96.

[57] Gissen, P., Johnson, C. A., Morgan, N. V., Stapelbroek, J. M., Forshew, T., Cooper, W. N., Mc Kiernan, P. J., Klomp, L. W., Morris, A. A., Wraith, J. E., Mc Clean, P., Lynch, S. A., Thompson, R. J., Lo, B., Quarrell, O. W., Di Rocco, M., Trembath, R. C., Mandel, H., Wali, S., Karet, F. E., Knisely, A. S., Houwen, R. H., Kelly, D. A., & Maher, E. R. (2004). Mutations in VPS33B, encoding a regulator of SNARE-dependent membrane fusion, cause arthrogryposis-renal dysfunction-cholestasis (ARC) syndrome. *Nat Genet*, 36(4), 400-404.

[58] Moreira, R. K., Cabral, R., Cowles, R. A., & Lobritto, S. J. (2012). Biliary atresia: a multidisciplinary approach to diagnosis and management. *Arch Pathol Lab Med*, 136(7), 746-760.

[59] Hadj-Rabia, S., Baala, L., Vabres, P., Hamel-Teillac, D., Jacquemin, E., Fabre, M., Lyonnet, S., De Prost, Y., Munnich, A., Hadchouel, M., & Smahi, A. (2004). Claudin-1 gene mutations in neonatal sclerosing cholangitis associated with ichthyosis: a tight junction disease. *Gastroenterology*, 127(5), 1386-1390.

[60] Stoller, J. K., & Aboussouan, L. S. (2012). A review of alpha1-antitrypsin deficiency. *Am J Respir Crit Care Med*, 185(3), 246-259.

[61] Chagnon, P., Michaud, J., Mitchell, G., Mercier, J., Marion, J. F., Drouin, E., Rasquin-Weber, A., Hudson, T. J., & Richter, A. (2002). A missense mutation (R565W) in cirhin (FLJ14728) in North American Indian childhood cirrhosis. *Am J Hum Genet*, 71(6), 1443-1449.

[62] Bull, L. N., Roche, E., Song, E. J., Pedersen, J., Knisely, A. S., van Der Hagen, C. B., Eiklid, K., Aagenaes, O., & Freimer, N. B. (2000). Mapping of the locus for cholestasis-lymphedema syndrome (Aagenaes syndrome) to a 6.6-cM interval on chromosome 15q. *Am J Hum Genet*, 67(4), 994-999.

[63] Lazaridis, K. N., Gores, G. J., & Lindor, K. D. (2001). Ursodeoxycholic acid 'mechanisms of action and clinical use in hepatobiliary disorders'. *J Hepatol*, 35(1), 134-146.

[64] Cohran, V. C., & Heubi, J. E. (2003). Treatment of Pediatric Cholestatic Liver Disease. *Curr Treat Options Gastroenterol*, 6(5), 403-415.

[65] Jacquemin, E., Hermans, D., Myara, A., Habes, D., Debray, D., Hadchouel, M., Sokal, E. M., & Bernard, O. (1997). Ursodeoxycholic acid therapy in pediatric patients with progressive familial intrahepatic cholestasis. *Hepatology*, 25(3), 519-523.

[66] Ismail, H., Kalicinski, P., Markiewicz, M., Jankowska, I., Pawlowska, J., Kluge, P., Eliadou, E., Kaminski, A., Szymczak, M., Drewniak, T., & Revillon, Y. (1999). Treatment of progressive familial intrahepatic cholestasis: liver transplantation or partial external biliary diversion. *Pediatr Transplant*, 3(3), 219-224.

[67] Wanty, C., Joomye, R., Van Hoorebeek, N., Paul, K., Otte, J. B., Reding, R., & Sokal, E. M. (2004). Fifteen years single center experience in the management of progressive familial intrahepatic cholestasis of infancy. *Acta Gastroenterol Belg*, 67(4), 313-319.

[68] Whitington, P. F., & Whitington, G. L. (1988). Partial external diversion of bile for the treatment of intractable pruritus associated with intrahepatic cholestasis. *Gastroenterology*, 95(1), 130-136.

[69] Stapelbroek, J. M., van Erpecum, K. J., Klomp, L. W., & Houwen, R. H. (2010). Liver disease associated with canalicular transport defects: current and future therapies. *J Hepatol*, 52(2), 258-271.

[70] Kaur, S., Sharma, D., Wadhwa, N., Gupta, S., Chowdhary, S. K., & Sibal, A. (2012). Therapeutic interventions in progressive familial intrahepatic cholestasis: experience from a tertiary care centre in north India. *Indian J Pediatr*, 79(2), 270-273.

[71] Stapelbroek, J. M., van Erpecum, K. J., Klomp, L. W., Venneman, N. G., Schwartz, T. P., van Berge Henegouwen, G. P., Devlin, J., van Nieuwkerk, C. M., Knisely, A. S-, & Houwen, R. H. (2006). Nasobiliary drainage induces long-lasting remission in benign recurrent intrahepatic cholestasis. *Hepatology*, 43(1), 51-53.

[72] Schukfeh, N., Metzelder, M. L., Petersen, C., Reismann, M., Pfister, E. D., Ure, B. M., & Kuebler, J. F. (2012). Normalization of serum bile acids after partial external biliary diversion indicates an excellent long-term outcome in children with progressive familial intrahepatic cholestasis. *J Pediatr Surg*, 47(3), 501-505.

[73] Metzelder, M. L., Bottlander, M., Melter, M., Petersen, C., & Ure, B. M. (2005). Laparoscopic partial external biliary diversion procedure in progressive familial intrahepatic cholestasis: a new approach. *Surg Endosc*, 19(12), 1641-1643.

[74] Rebhandl, W., Felberbauer, F. X., Turnbull, J., Paya, K., Barcik, U., Huber, W. D., Whitington, P. F., & Horcher, E. (1999). Biliary diversion by use of the appendix (cholecystoappendicostomy) in progressive familial intrahepatic cholestasis. *J Pediatr Gastroenterol Nutr*, 28(2), 217-219.

[75] Arnell, H., Bergdahl, S., Papadogiannakis, N., Nemeth, A., & Fischler, B. (2008). Preoperative observations and short-term outcome after partial external biliary diversion in 13 patients with progressive familial intrahepatic cholestasis. *J Pediatr Surg*, 43(7), 1312-1320.

[76] Davis, A. R., Rosenthal, P., & Newman, T. B. (2009). Nontransplant surgical interventions in progressive familial intrahepatic cholestasis. *J Pediatr Surg*, 44(4), 821-827.

[77] Kalicinski, P. J., Ismail, H., Jankowska, I., Kaminski, A., Pawlowska, J., Drewniak, T., Markiewicz, M., & Szymczak, M. (2003). Surgical treatment of progressive familial intrahepatic cholestasis: comparison of partial external biliary diversion and ileal bypass. *Eur J Pediatr Surg*, 13(5), 307-311.

[78] Bassas, A., Chehab, M., Hebby, H., Al, Shahed. M., Al Husseini, H., Al Zahrani, A., & Wali, S. (2003). Living related liver transplantation in 13 cases of progressive familial intrahepatic cholestasis. *Transplant Proc*, 35(8), 3003-3005.

[79] Englert, C., Grabhorn, E., Richter, A., Rogiers, X., Burdelski, M., & Ganschow, R. (2007). Liver transplantation in children with progressive familial intrahepatic cholestasis. *Transplantation*, 84(10), 1361-1363.

[80] Torri, E., Lucianetti, A., Pinelli, D., Corno, V., Guizzetti, M., Maldini, G., Zambelli, M., Bertani, A., Melzi, M. L., Alberti, D., Doffria, E., Giovanelli, M., Torre, G., Spada, M., Gridelli, B., & Colledan, M. (2005). Orthotopic liver transplantation for Byler's disease. *Transplant Proc*, 37(2), 1149-1150.

[81] Esquivel, C. O., Iwatsuki, S., Gordon, R. D., Marsh, W. W., Jr., Koneru, B., Makowka, L., Tzakis, A. G., Todo, S., & Starzl, T. E. (1987). Indications for pediatric liver transplantation. *J Pediatr*, 111(6), Pt 2, 1039-1045.

[82] Whitington, P. F, & Balistreri, W. F. (1991). Liver transplantation in pediatrics: indications, contraindications, and pretransplant management. *J Pediatr*, 118(2), 169-177.

[83] Keitel, V., Burdelski, M., Vojnisek, Z., Schmitt, L., Haussinger, D., & Kubitz, R. (2009). De novo bile salt transporter antibodies as a possible cause of recurrent graft failure after liver transplantation: a novel mechanism of cholestasis. *Hepatology*, 50(2), 510-517.

[84] Jara, P., Hierro, L., Martinez-Fernandez, P., Alvarez-Doforno, R., Yanez, F., Diaz, M. C., Camarena, C., De la Vega, A., Frauca, E., Munoz-Bartolo, G., Lopez-Santamaria, M., Larrauri, J., & Alvarez, L. (2009). Recurrence of bile salt export pump deficiency after liver transplantation. *N Engl J Med*, 361(14), 1359-1367.

[85] Egawa, H., Yorifuji, T., Sumazaki, R., Kimura, A., Hasegawa, M., & Tanaka, K. (2002). Intractable diarrhea after liver transplantation for Byler's disease: successful treatment with bile adsorptive resin. *Liver Transpl*, 8(8), 714-716.

[86] De Vree, J. M., Ottenhoff, R., Bosma, P. J., Smith, A. J., Aten, J., & Oude Elferink, R. P. (2000). Correction of liver disease by hepatocyte transplantation in a mouse model of progressive familial intrahepatic cholestasis. *Gastroenterology*, 119(6), 1720-1730.

[87] Zollner, G., & Trauner, M. (2009). Nuclear receptors as therapeutic targets in cholestatic liver diseases. *Br J Pharmacol*, 156(1), 7-27.

[88] Morello, J. P., Petaja-Repo, U. E., Bichet, D. G., & Bouvier, M. (2000). Pharmacological chaperones: a new twist on receptor folding. *Trends Pharmacol Sci*, 21(12), 466-469.

[89] Chen, Y., & Liu-Chen, L. Y. (2009). Chaperone-like effects of cell-permeant ligands on opioid receptors. *Front Biosci*, 14, 634-643.

[90] Ohgane, K., Dodo, K., & Hashimoto, Y. (2010). Retinobenzaldehydes as proper-trafficking inducers of folding-defective P23H rhodopsin mutant responsible for retinitis pigmentosa. *Bioorg Med Chem*, 18(19), 7022-7028.

[91] Hayashi, H., & Sugiyama, Y. (2007). 4-phenylbutyrate enhances the cell surface expression and the transport capacity of wild-type and mutated bile salt export pumps. *Hepatology*, 45(6), 1506-1516.

[92] Hacein-Bey-Abina, S., von Kalle, C., Schmidt, M., Le Deist, F., Wulffraat, N., Mc Intyre, E., Radford, I., Villeval, J. L., Fraser, C. C., Cavazzana-Calvo, M., & Fischer, A. (2003). A serious adverse event after successful gene therapy for X-linked severe combined immunodeficiency. *N Engl J Med*, 348(3), 255-256.

Chapter 12

Hepatic Trauma

Bilal O. Al-Jiffry and Owaid AlMalki

Additional information is available at the end of the chapter

1. Introduction

The word liver was derived from the old English word "life" [1]. Survival without the liver is impossible for more than a few hours except in very unusual circumstances. The liver is the largest intra-abdominal solid organ; with its friable parenchyma, its thin capsule, and its relatively fixed position in relation to the spine, makes it particularly prone to injury. As a result of its larger size and proximity to the ribs, the right hemi-liver is injured more commonly than the left. It's the second most commonly injured organ in abdominal trauma, but damage to the liver is the most common cause of death after abdominal injury [2], [3]. Management of Liver Trauma may vary widely from non operative management (NOM) with or without angioembolization to Damage Control Surgery (DCS) [4]. DCS is mainly centered on stopping the bleeding by packing, Pringles, and vascular exclusion to totally replacing the liver by a liver transplant [5].

Although blunt liver trauma accounts for 15-20% of abdominal injuries, it is responsible for more than 50% of deaths resulting from blunt abdominal trauma. The mortality rate is higher with blunt abdominal trauma than with penetrating injuries[6]. In Europe, blunt trauma predominates (80-90 per cent of all liver injuries)[6]-[8], while penetrating injuries account for 66 per cent of liver trauma in South Africa [9] and up to 88 per cent in North America [10]-[13]. Unfortunately, we don't have enough data for the Arab countries though we are one of the highest countries in motor vehicle accidents with more than 9000 deaths per year.

As a result of this high mortality rate, emergency surgery was frequently indicated in patients with hepatic injury in the past. However, advances in diagnostic imaging, better monitoring facilities and the introduction of damage control strategy in trauma has influenced our approach in the management of liver trauma [14].

2. Anatomy

In this part we will describe the anatomy of the liver and its attachments in relation to what is needed in liver trauma, to achieve good mobilization with haemorrhage control to reach the first stage of damage control.

2.1. Surface anatomy

It's important to know the location of the liver and its surface anatomy to be able to choose the best incision, to determine if it is involved in a penetrating trauma, and to think of it when you have a chest trauma especially on the right lower chest. When viewed from the front (fig. 1), the normal liver surface markings are [15]:

Upper margin: at the xiphisternal joint arching upwords on both sides. On the left it runs for 7-8cm from the mid-line. On the right, it reaches the fifth rib.

Right boarder: it curves downword from the seventh to the eleventh rib in the mid axillary line.

Inferior boarder: along a line that joins both right lower and upper left points.

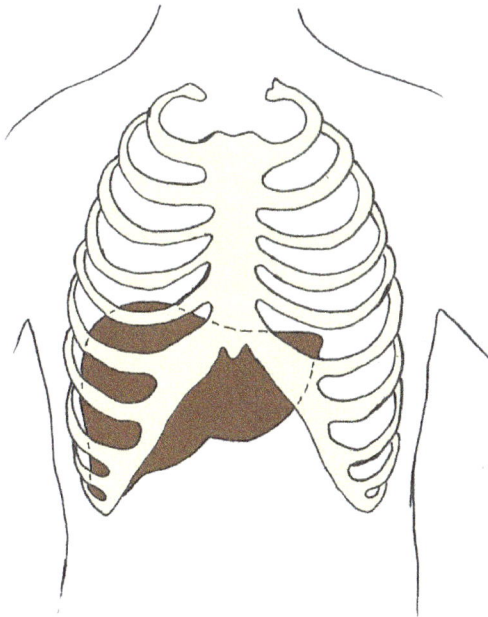

Figure 1. Surface anatomy of the liver

2.2. Gross anatomy

The liver has three surfaces [16]

• Diaphragmatic Surface:

This is covered with peritoneum to act as a sheath around the liver. In the midline the falciform ligament is attached and divides the liver into the right and left anatomical liver, or better descried it runs between the left lateral section (segment 2 and 3) and the left medial section (segment 4).

• Visceral Surface:

The sharp inferior border of the liver joins the diaphragmatic surface with the visceral surface of the liver. The main structures are lined in an H shaped. The cross part is made of the porta hepatis (hilum of the liver). The right limb is made of the inferior vena cava. The left limb is made of the contiuity of the fissures for the ligamentum teres anteriorly and the ligamentum venosum posteriorly. On the left side lies the caudate lobe and on the right lies the bare area of the liver.

• Posterior Surface (fig 2):

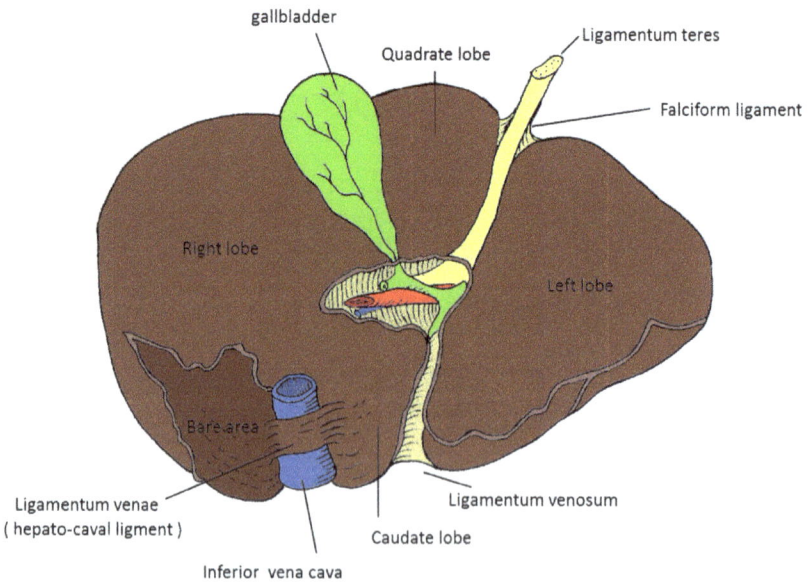

Figure 2. Visceral surface of the Liver

The IVC runs in the centre of the posterior surface. A firous band called the ligamentum venae cavae (hepato-caval ligament) covers part of the IVC posteriorly. The rest of the posterior surface is made of by the ligaments (the left and right triangular ligaments, and the coronary ligament) which attach the liver to the diaphragm.

2.3. Ligaments of the liver

The falciform ligament consists of two closely layers of peritoneum. The ligamentum teres runs on its free edge with a small paraumbilical vein. On the right it forms the upper layer of the coronary ligament, witch continues inferiorly to form the right triangular ligament, then to the lower coronary ligament. On the left, the falciform ligament forms the anterior layer of the left triangular ligament. (fig 3 &4)

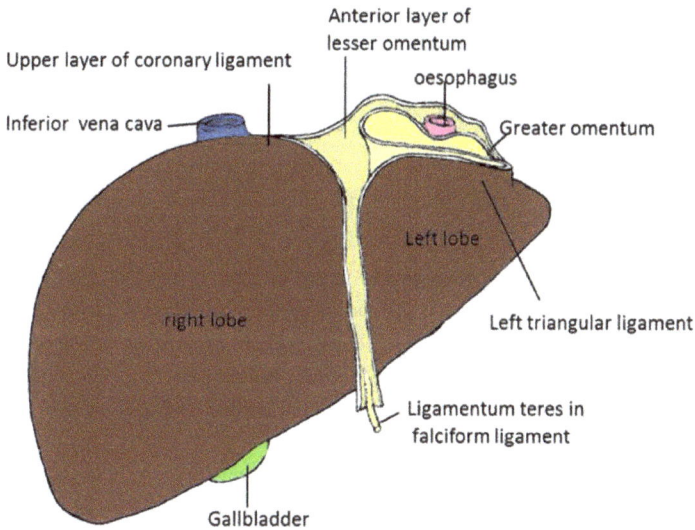

Figure 3. Diaphragmatic surface of the liver and its ligaments

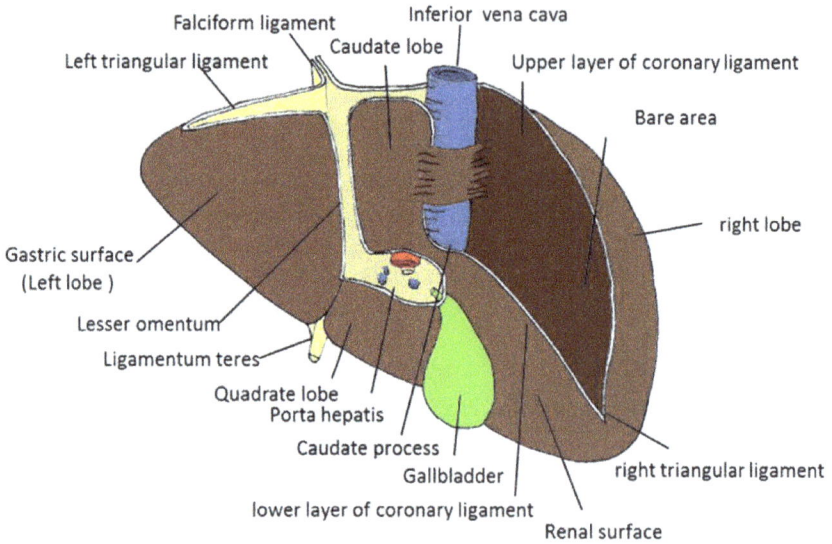

Figure 4. Posterior surface of the liver and its ligaments

2.4. Caudate lobe

The caudate lobe is the dorsal portion of the liver lying posteriorly and embracing the retro-hepatic IVC in a semi circumferential fashion. It lies between the IVC posteriorly, the portal triad inferiorly and the hepatic veins superiorly. There is a series of short hepatic veins which drains directly from the caudate lobe to the retrohepatic IVC. Thus it is surrounded by important structures that can be involved in liver trauma 17 (Fig 5).

2.5. The glissonian sheath

Glisson's capsule which covers the liver extends into the liver at the hilus and covers the portal triad were it is called the Glisson's sheath. With relation to liver trauma it is impor-tant to know only the extrahepatic portion of the Glissonian pedicle which is called the hep-atodudenal ligament. This is very important when a Pringle manoeuvre is needed. It usually composed of connective tissue and peritoneum up to the hepatic hilum. They surround the portal vein posteriorly, the hepatic artery anteriorly and to the left, and the common bile duct anteriorly and to the right (fig 6) 18.

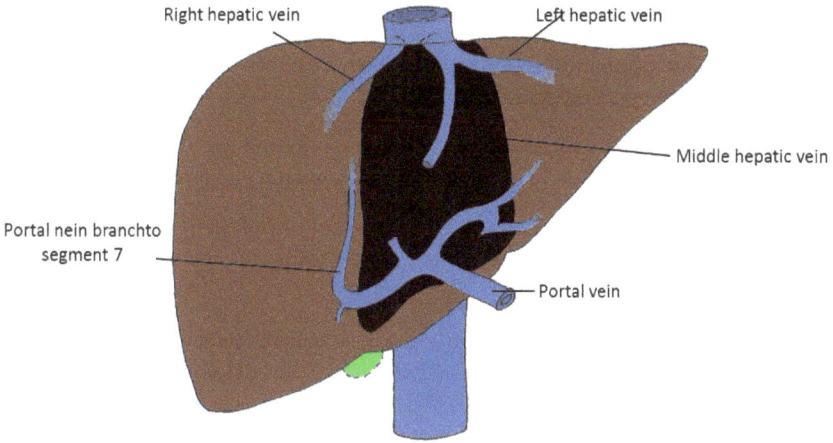

Figure 5. The caudate lobe: front view

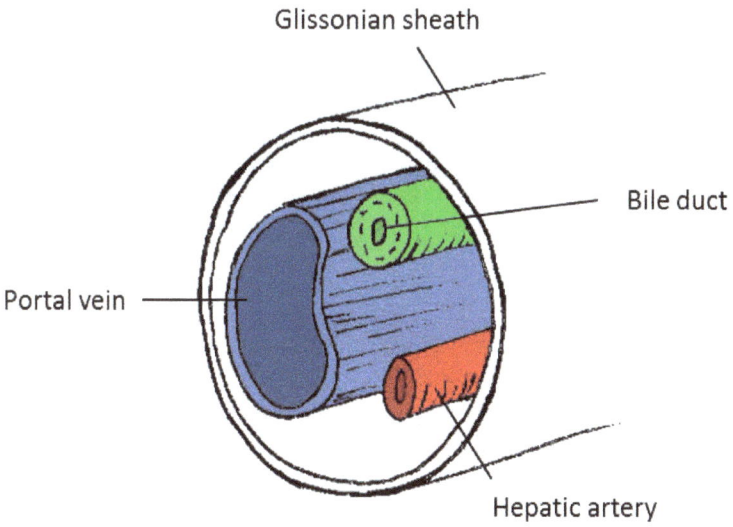

Figure 6. Structures within the glissonian sheath

2.6. Retrohepatic IVC and its branches (fig 7)

In relation to liver trauma we can divide the retrohepatic IVC into four parts:

The suprahepatic group; which is composed of both right and left inferior phrenic veins which drain the right and left diaphragm.

The hepatic veins; which are composed of the right, middle and left hepatic vein. There are multiple variations that can exist and its knowledge is important in liver surgery.

The retrohepatic group; which is composed of short veins that drain part of the right hemi-liver and the caudate lobe directly into the IVC. These veins are short and very fragile and are prone to injury.

Lastly, the infrahepatic group; which consists mainly of both the right and left adrenal veins. These veins are frequently injured in trauma and if not considered during mobilizing the right liver [19].

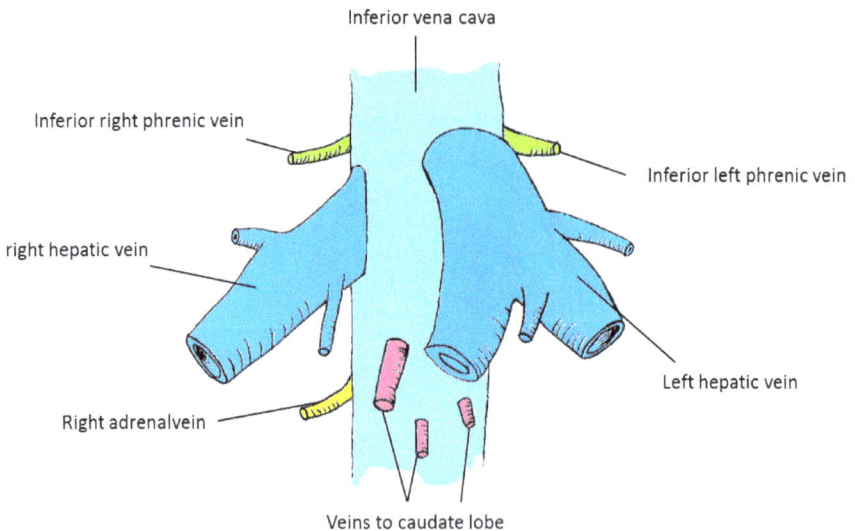

Figure 7. The abdominal inferior vena cava and its suprarenal branches

3. Mechanism

Penetrating and blunt trauma are the two principal mechanisms for liver trauma. Motor vehicle accidents account for the majority of blunt trauma, whereas knife and gunshot wounds constitute the major cause of penetrating injuries

Two types of blunt liver trauma have been described: deceleration (shearing) injuries occur in motor vehicle accidents and in falls from a height where there is movement of the liver in its relatively fixed position, thereby producing a laceration of its relatively thin capsule and parenchyma at the sites of attachment to the diaphragm[13].

The other type of liver injuries is crush injury. Crush injuries follow direct trauma to the abdomen over the liver area. Decelerating injuries typically create lacerations between the right posterior section (segments 6 and 7) and the right anterior section (segments 5 and 8), which can extend to involve major vessels. Crush injuries can lead to damage to the central portion of the liver (segment 4, 5 and 8) and also may cause bleeding from the caudate lobe (segment 1)[12]-[13]. Blunt trauma can cause parenchymal hepatic injury with intact Glisson's capsule, leading to an intraparenchymal or subcapsular haematoma[12]-[13].

Penetrating injuries are usually associated with gunshot or stab wounds, with the former usually resulting in more tissue damage due to the cavitation effect as the bullet traverses the liver substance [13]-[20]. These injuries usually require surgery more often than blunt injuries when the liver is involved.

4. Diagnosis

Signs and symptoms of hepatic injuries are related to the amount of blood loss, peritoneal irritation, right upper quadrant tenderness, and guarding. Rebound abdominal tenderness is common but nonspecific. Occasionally, patients with blunt abdominal trauma do well initially, but they subsequently develop a liver abscess, presumably due to unrecognized liver damage. These patients present with signs and symptoms of deep-seated infection [21]. Patients may present with severe peritonism due to bile peritonitis resulting from bile leaks. Signs of blood loss, such as shock, hypotension, and a falling hematocrit level, may dominate the picture [21] As resuscitation proceeds, a detailed physical examination is carried out. Most conventional texts emphasis the need for a careful history and physical examination of the abdomen. While this is undoubted importance, it is extremely difficult to assess the abdomen in the trauma situation as the history may not be available and all the existing physical signs are misleading. Fresh blood is not a peritoneal irritant [22]. The mechanism of injury is critically important in assessing the potential for abdominal injury. This information may be obtained from the patient, relatives, police or emergency care personnel [22]

Following initial assessment, a conscious patient, who is haemodynamically unstable following blunt trauma and has generalized peritonism, should undergo immediate laparotomy without further investigation [13]. Urgent laparotomy is also indicated in patients who have sustained a stab wound to the abdomen and are haemodynamically unstable. If the patient is stable and a liver injury is suspected, imaging studies should be performed [21]-[23] However, haemodynamically stable patients with suspected liver injury can be investigated at this stage to define the nature of the injury.

Ultrasonography (FAST) has gained increased acceptance, particularly in the emergency department, for the rapid evaluation of patients with blunt or penetrating abdominal trauma [24]-[29]. It is cheap, portable and noninvasive, compare to peritoneal lavage and it does not use radiation or iodinated contrast media [30]-[32]. Its sensitivity for the presence of intra-abdominal fluid in patients with trauma ranges from 75 to 93.8% and the specificity from 97 to 100% [24]-[25]. However, some pitfalls remain in abdominal ultrasonography. Injuries at the dome or lateral segments of the liver can easily by missed with ultrasound, especially in the presence of ileus or if the patient cannot cooperate because of pain. Hepatic laceration or hematomas are usually difficult to distinguish, especially in the acute phase, because they are isoechoic to the normal liver [33]-[34].

Kalogeropoulu and colleagues (2006) demonstrated the usefulness of contrast enhanced ul-trasonography in penetrating liver trauma [35]. It increases the sensitivity and the specificity of ultrasound in evaluation of abdominal trauma not only in detection of free peritoneal flu-id but also in the visualization of the parenchymal lacerations. The use of contrast in addition to the conventional ultrasound scanning does not significantly prolong the examination time, compared with a contrast enhanced CT scan. Furthermore repeated doses of the contrast can be injected to scan the rest of the solid abdominal organs such spleen and kidneys if a more complex trauma is suspected [35]. However, US is operator dependent, were you may not find an expert ultrasonographer in the middle of the night. In addition, US contrast is not wildly available in every casualty.

Computed tomography (CT) is the gold standard investigation for the evaluation of a stable patient with suspected liver trauma [36]-[39]. CT has high sensitivity and specificity for detecting liver injuries which increase as the time between injury and scanning increases, evidently because haematomas and lacerations become better defined [40]. Contrast-enhanced CT, is accurate in localizing the site and extent of liver and associated injuries, providing vital information for treatment in patients. CT without intravenous contrast enhancement is of limited value in hepatic trauma, but it can be useful in identifying or following up a hemo-peritoneum [41]-[43].

CT scanning allows reasonably accurate grading of liver injuries and provides crude quantitation of the degree of hemoperitoneum. CT scanning is mandatory for patients with blunt trauma whose liver injury is to be managed nonoperatively. CT has also been useful for detecting missile tracts in penetrating trauma patients. Such information is imperative for surgeons who want to attempt nonoperative management of penetrating wounds [44]-[47]

Although CT is very useful in the evaluation of stable patients with abdominal trauma, most authors agree that unstable patients, with either blunt or penetrating trauma, are unlikely to benefit from this investigation because of the valuable time that it requires [44] (Fig 8)

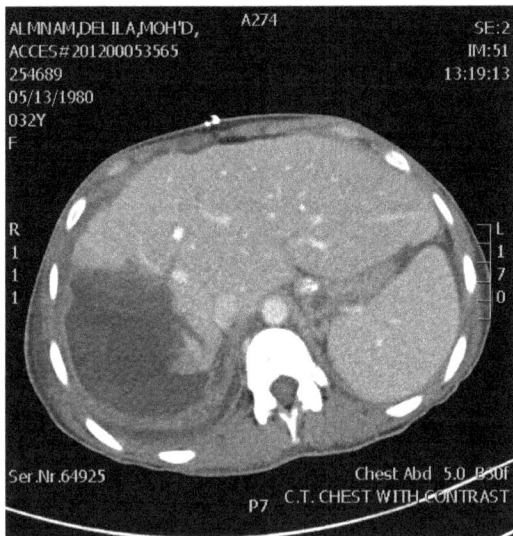

Figure 8. A CT demonstrating a grade 4 liver injury that was treated surgically

False-positive errors in the diagnosis of liver injury with CT scans may occur as a result of beam-hardening artifacts from adjacent ribs, which can mimic contusion or hematoma. An air-contrast level within the stomach in a patient with a nasogastric tube can produce streak artifacts throughout the left lateral section of the liver; these may mimic intrahepatic lacerations and/or hemorrhage. The nature of these artifacts can be confirmed if the patient is scanned in a decubitus position [48].

False-negative findings may occur in the setting of a fatty liver only when contrast-enhanced CT scan are obtained. On these images, the enhanced fatty liver may become isoattenuating relative to the laceration or hematoma. In this situation, a nonenhanced CT scan may provide useful information regarding hepatic injury. Focal fatty infiltration may also mimic hepatic hematoma, laceration, or infarction. Hepatic lacerations with a branching pattern can mimic unopacified portal or hepatic veins or dilated intrahepatic bile ducts. Careful evaluation of all branching intrahepatic structures is important and the diagnosis is made with serial images to differentiate the various structures [48]-[49]

MRI has a limited role in the evaluation of blunt abdominal trauma, and it has no advantage over CT scanning. Theoretically, MRI can be used in follow-up monitoring of patients with blunt abdominal trauma, and MRI may be useful in young and pregnant women with abdominal trauma in whom the radiation dose is a concern [6], [50].

MRCP has been used in the assessment of pancreatic duct trauma and its sequelae, and it can be used to image biliary trauma. Another potential use of MRI is in patients with renal failure and in patients who are allergic to radiographic contrast medium. MRI offers no sig nificant advantage over CT scanning for routine evaluation of acute abdominal trauma. Experience is insufficient for assessing the value of the special circumstances mentioned above. Sufficient experience has not been gained in the use of MRI to establish false-positive and false-negative findings [6]

Angiography has no role in the evaluation of unstable patients. However, if the patient is stable, cross-sectional imaging may provide sufficient detail to treat the patient conservatively. A dynamic angiographic study may demonstrate the site of active bleeding. This when combined with angiographic embolization, especially in high-grade liver injury is of significant value and may be the only treatment required [51]-[52]. Although angiography is useful in selected patients, both false-positive and false-negative results occur in patients with hepatic trauma [6]

Endoscopic retrograde cholangiopancreatography (ERCP) may help in the delineation of the biliary tree in patient with liver trauma, and stents may be used to treat biliary Leaks [53]-[54] (Fig 9).

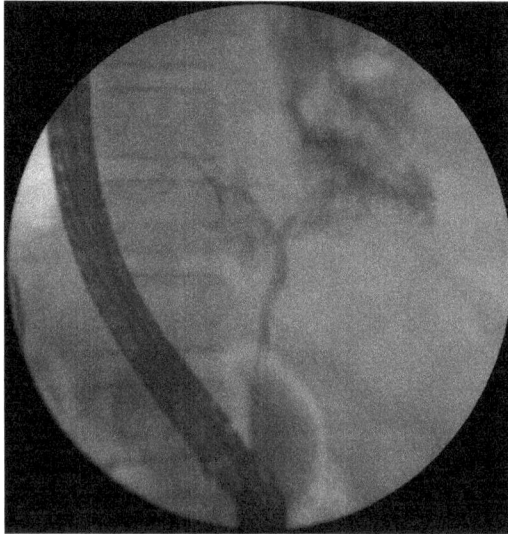

Figure 9. ERCP demonstrating a bile leak from the main right duct

Diagnostic laparoscopy has been used successfully in patients with abdominal trauma [55]-[58], and laparoscopic fibrin glue in managing liver injuries has also been reported [60].The benefits of laparoscopic assessment include reducing negative and non-therapeutic laparotomy rates, patient morbidity rates, hospital stay and treatment costs [56]-[57]. Raphael and colleagues(1999) reviewed 37 studies with more than 1,900 trauma patients (including those with liver trauma), and laparoscopy was analyzed as a screening, diagnostic, or therapeutic tool. They came out with the conclusion that "Laparoscopy has been applied safely and effectively as a screening tool in stable patients with acute trauma. Because of the large number of missed injuries when used as a diagnostic tool, its value in this context is limited. Laparoscopy has been reported infrequently as a therapeutic tool in selected patients, and its use in this context requires further study.[61].

5. Classification of liver injury

Liver trauma ranges from a minor capsular tear, with or without parenchymal injury, to extensive disruption involving both hemi liver with associated hepatic vein or vena caval injury. In 1989, the Organ Injury Scaling Committee of the American Association for the Surgery of Trauma produced a Hepatic Injury Scale [62] by which hepatic injuries are described in most major trauma centers (Table 1). Grade I or II injuries are considered minor; they represent 80-90 per cent of all cases and usually require minimal or no operative treatment [1], [63]. Grade III-V injuries are generally considered severe and often require surgical intervention, while grade VI injuries are regarded as incompatible with survival.

Grade	Type of Injury	Description of injury
I (fig 10)	Hematoma	Subcapsular, < 10% surface area
	Laceration	Capsular tear, < 1cm parenchymal depth
II (Fig 11)	Hematoma	Subcapsular, 10% to 50% surface area
	Laceration	Capsular tear, 1-3cm parenchymal depth and < 10cm in length
III (Fig 12)	Hematoma	Subcapsular, > 50% surface area or expanding
	Laceration	Intraparenchymal hematoma > 2cm or expanding
		Capsular tear, >3cm parenchymal depth
IV (Fig 13)	Hematoma	Ruptured intraparenchymal hematoma with active bleeding
	Laceration	Parenchymal disruption involving 25-50% of hepatic lobe
V	Laceration	Parenchymal disruption involving >50% of hepatic lobe
	Vascular	Juxtahepatic venous injuries
VI	Vascular	Hepatic avulsion

Table 1. Classification of liver injury

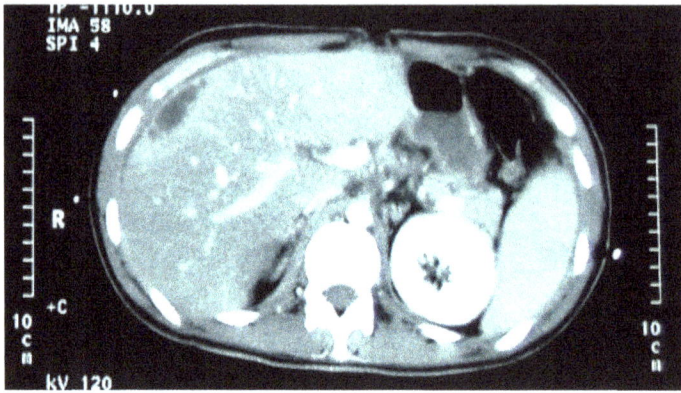

Figure 10. Grade 1 liver injury treated non surgically

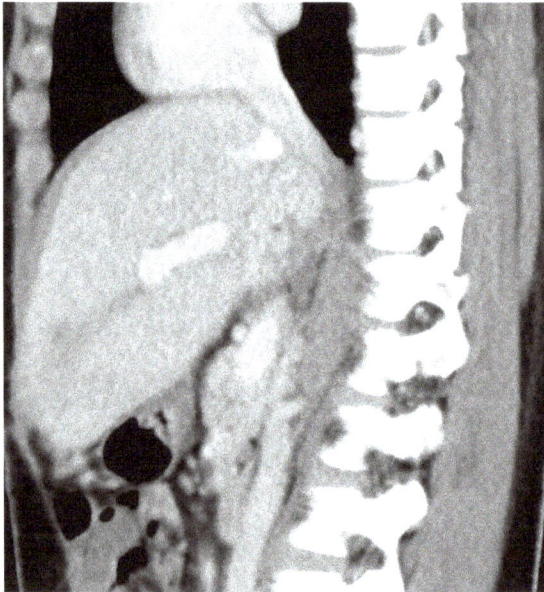

Figure 11. Grade 2 liver injury

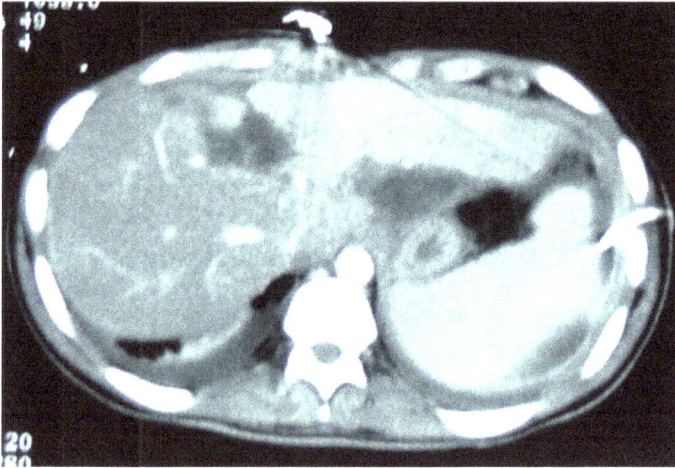

Figure 12. Grade 3 liver injury that was treated non surgically

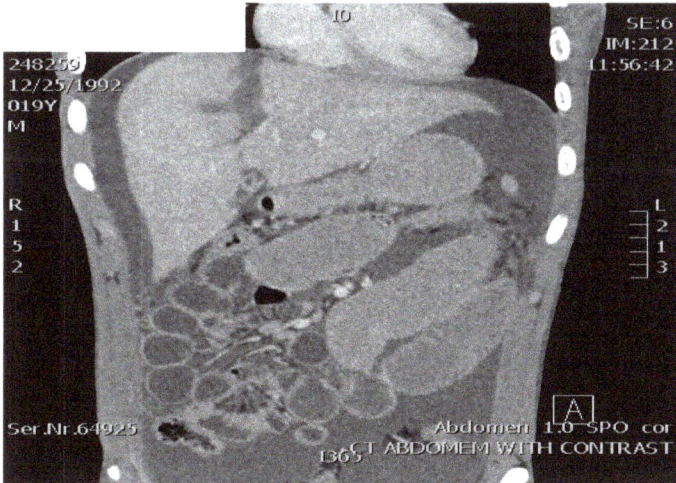

Figure 13. Grade 4 liver injury that was treated non surgically

6. Management

6.1. Non operative

The countercurrent argument was that nonoperative treatment (NOM) was associated with virtually a 100% mortality rate, so all patients with suspected or diagnosed liver injuries must have an operation. Improved mortality rates during and after World War II assured the primacy of operative treatment [64].

Three observations prompted the move towards nonoperative treatment. First, the practice of nonoperative treatment was initially advocated for splenic injuries and then extended to the liver. The success in children led to attempts of nonoperative treatment in adults [65]-[66] Second, the high rate of nontherapeutic operations in many patients with blunt hepatic injuries was not in patients' best interest. Third, the advent of CT scanning greatly facilitated both diagnosis and grading of injuries and gave some reassurance that the intestinal injuries had not occurred.

There has been several reports started since 1985, were Trunkey *etal* [67], defined the criteria for NOM:

- haemodynamic stability
- absence of peritoneal sign
- Availability of CT
- Monitor in ICU
- Facility of immediate surgery
- Absence of other organ injuries

These criteria has become more and more less strict, were multiple reports are trending more to NOM [3]. There is no time limit for NOM, continues monitoring is the only key to take the patient to the operating room [68]. Other reports even went to the extreme as if the patient had risk factors by the injury severity score (ISS) [69] and all patients should be treated first by NOM regardless of their trauma [70]. However, all of these reports mentioned that this is possible with the addition of angiography and embolization that made the NOM more feasible and more successful.

The success rate of nonoperative treatment has been remarkably high. The necessity for operations for ongoing hemorrhage has been reported to be from 5% to 15%. There remains a concern over missed bowel injuries that have been reported from 1% to 3%.[71]-[75].

Nonoperative treatment of abdominal stab wounds has been practiced successfully in numerous centers and is on the rise. NOM of gunshot wounds has been more controversial, however, many reports are calling to add these group of patients to the NOM group [76]-[79] Demetriades and colleagues(2006) reported 152 patients with penetrating solid organ injuries. 28.4% of all liver injuries were successfully managed nonoperatively [80]. However, in the last few years NOM has emerged a huge mile stone. Appropriately selected patients with liver gunshot injuries deemed feasible, safe, and effective, regardless of the liver injury severity [77]. However, they all mentioned that CT scan was mandatory before adopting the NOM. Another report stated that regardless of the grade of liver trauma, NOM is safe and effective in appropriately selected patients with liver gun shoot injuries treated in centers with suitable facilities [79].

6.2. Operative

6.2.1. Damage control surgery

As the first intention when taking the patient to the operating room is to do damage control surgery (DCS). This usually implies saving the patient's life and stopping the bleeding. This will make the patient more stable and in a better physiologically and hemodynamically state to be able to have the definitive treatment.

Skin preparation should allow for extension of a midline abdominal incision to a median sternotomy or right thoracotomy, if necessary, for adequate exposure of posterior liver injuries [81]-[82]. If the indication for surgery is an obvious penetrating through-and-through liver injury, or the patient failed the NOM and is clear liver injury only a bilateral subcostal incision is a useful alternative and has been adopted by some to have better liver exposure (fig 14).

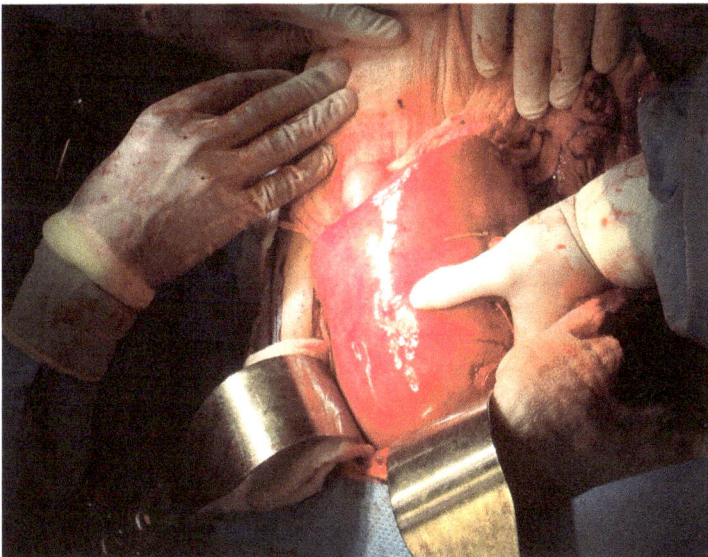

Figure 14. Mobilization of the right hemi-liver to achieve excellent exposure of the injury

DCS includes perihepatic packing and partial abdominal closure or Bogota bag. Usually an average of six laparotomy pads can be packed to get the tamponade effect between the liver and the abdominal wall. The timing of re-exploration is controversy but usually 12-24 hours is safe time for re-exploration were the patients condition permits (fig 15).

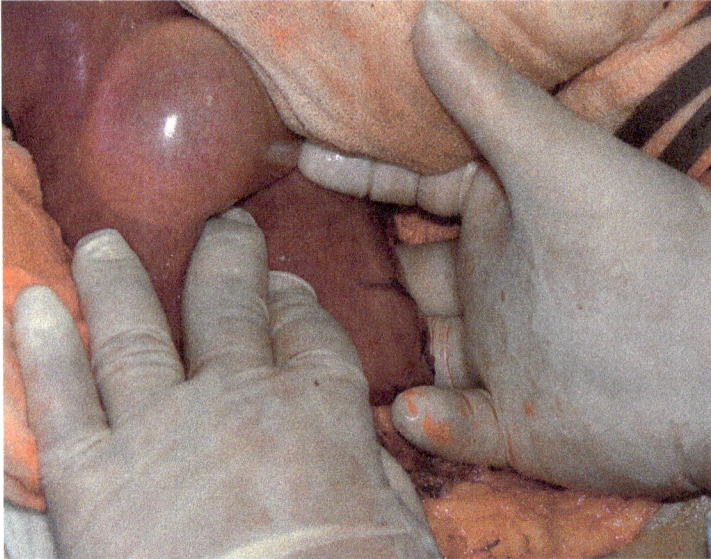

Figure 15. Packs as it was done in the first DCS were the bleeding stopped, fingers demonstrating the liver laceration

Even 30 years after the resurrection of packing as a treatment alternative, it remains an important part of the armamentarium of surgeons in managing difficult hepatic injuries. It is always better to have a patient with packs to come and deal with on another day, than trying to stop the bleeding with no success, especially if the surgeon has limited experience, which usually happens in the first operation. As many hospitals have a general surgeon on-call with limited liver or trauma experience.

If a major liver injury is encountered, initial control of bleeding can be achieved with temporary tamponade of the right upper quadrant using packs, portal triad occlusion (Pringle manoeuvre) (Fig 16a &b), bimanual compression of the liver or even manual compression of the abdominal aorta above the coeliac trunk [83]-[84]. Attempts to evaluate the liver injury before adequate resuscitation may result in further blood loss and worsening hypotension.

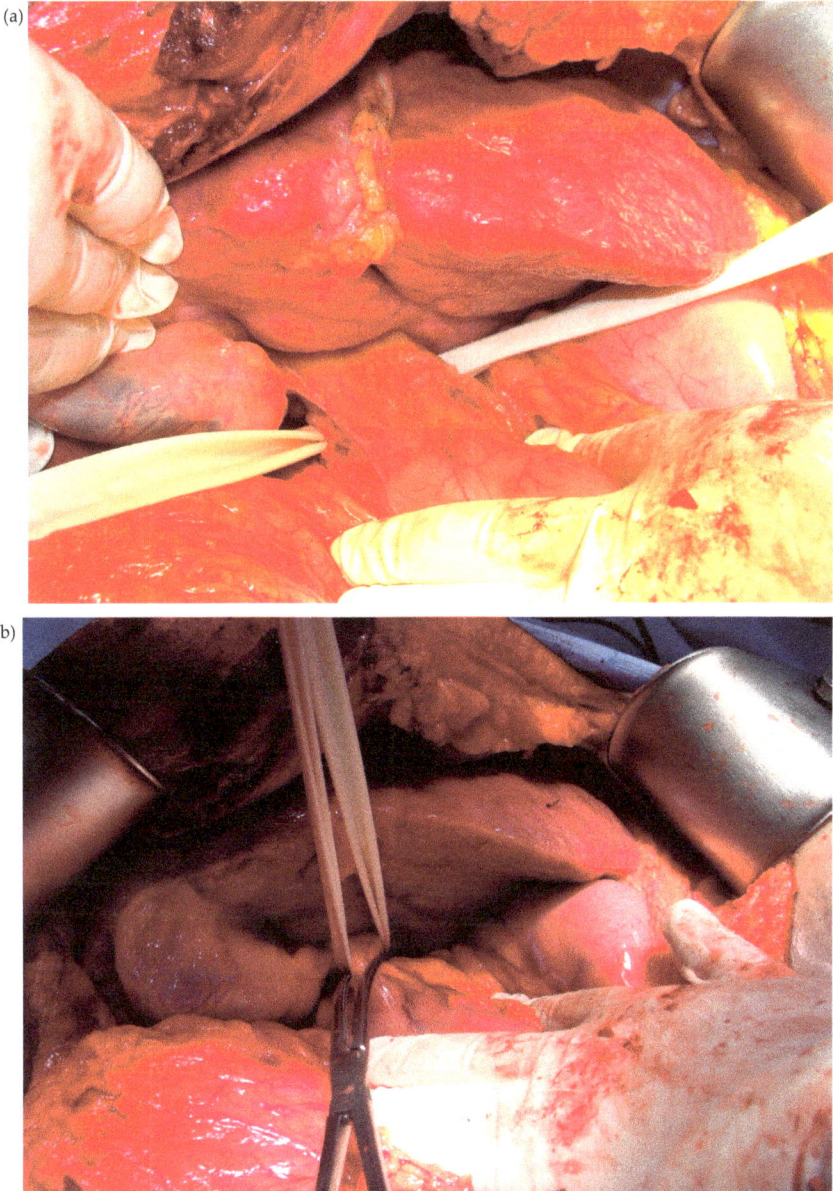

Figure 16. a. Tape inserted around the portal triad. b. Pringles manouver were the clamp is gently applied to occlude the portal triad

Digital compression of the portal triad (Pringle manoeuvre) can be used diagnostically and compression can be maintained with an atraumatic vascular clamp if haemorrhage decreases [85]. The clamp should be occluded only to the degree necessary to compress the blood vessels in order not to injure the common bile duct. If haemorrhage is unaffected by portal triad occlusion, major vena cava injury or atypical vascular anatomy should be suspected 86-87 Although the permitted occlusion time of the portal triad is controversial, most authors now agree that clamping of the hepatic pedicle for up to 1h is well tolerated with no adverse effects on liver function [81],[88]

After initial intraoperative resuscitation, the liver must be mobilized adequately to allow a thorough examination of the damaged area, unless the injury is already accessible through the incision [81,84,89] The liver is mobilized by dividing the falciform, triangular and coronary ligaments, and by placing abdominal packs posteriorly to maintain this position [90]. This manoeuvre allows the surgeon to determine the nature and severity of the injury and to decide on the necessary surgical technique. Care should be taken to avoid impairing venous return, by either excessive lifting and/or rotation of the mobilized liver, or excessive packing causing caval compression [90].

There are several tricks to stop the bleeding other than the one mentioned before, however we advise that most of these should be done by experienced surgeons in a stable patient or if the patient is still bleeding after trying the previous methods mentioned. Several specific modalities began to be used more often to treat arterial bleeding. Hepatorrhaphy was used with increased frequency. When the arterial bleeding occurred deep within the hepatic parenchyma, a tractotomy was advocated to expose and suture ligate the arterial flow. But control of deep arterial bleeding was often technically difficult to accomplish.[91]-[93]

In response to futile attempts to directly suture ligate arterial bleeding, Dr Aaron's group performed ligation of the hepatic artery.[94] Initially performed at the Louisville General Hospital to control arterial hemorrhage from a ruptured hepatic adenoma, Mays found this technique useful to control arterial bleeding in trauma patients. A literal explosion in its use occurred in Louisville, and surgeons there proposed it to prevent rebleeding.[95]-[96] A high rate of infection led to reconsideration of its use, and it was subsequently used less frequently [103], although it remained an operation that could occasionally be life-saving.97-98

Major venous bleeding was recognized as a major source of mortality, particularly in patients who had been in high-speed motor vehicle crashes. The nearly uniform lethality of retrohepatic vena caval injuries with attempt at direct repair led to the development of the atriocaval shunt. This technique, developed by Schrock and associates, [99] theoretically bypassed the caval injury and allowed direct suture repair of the cava itself and main hepatic veins. The operation required opening the chest to expose the atria. This bicavitary exposure accelerated hypothermia and coagulopathy in many patients. Consequently, the mortality rate remained high, but the concept of direct repair of this deadly injury was very important.

Both previously mentioned bleeding problems often were treated initially with temporary inflow occlusion by clamping the portal triad. The concept of inflow occlusion actually pre-dated Pringle, [85] but his work published in 1908 was rediscovered and popularized in the 1960s after rarely being mentioned in the literature for more than 50 years.

Diffuse bleeding from damaged or devitalized liver increasingly required surgical treat-ment. Reports on civilian liver injuries from the 1950s generally cautioned against debride-ment of damaged liver for fear it would worsen preexisting hemorrhage. Absorbable gauze packing and drainage were mostly used for this problem. As the forces of injury increased, other techniques were required.

Resectioned debridement was increasingly used. There was a brief flurry of activity with use of major anatomic resections, but the high mortality rate of this procedure led to discontinu-ing its use in most centers.[100]-[101] The omental pedicle described for liver injury in 1910 and mentioned occasionally through the years was reintroduced by Stone and Lamb[102] and gained widespread popularity.

In summary; as a general surgeon facing a major hepatic injury in the middle of the night think of NOM and try not to rush to the operating room unless clearly indicated. However, if you were forced to the operating room do the minimal to stop the bleeding (DCS). If major procedure is required, the decision must be made early in the operation were technical /clin-ical expertise and speed are critical. Plan definitive surgeries in a stable patient were optimal condition ably.

6.2.2. Definitive surgery

This is usually carried out in a stable patient by an experienced surgeon at a second stage to deal with a certain problem (Fig 17). One of the commonest problem is bile leak and collec-tion with an incidence of 6-20 %. This is usually after the patient recovered, were they devel-op an intra-abdominal collection that is best treated by a radiological applied drain. Then it can be investigated by MRCP or ERCP. The MRCP is non invasive, however with the collec-tion it can have very little input. ERCP is advocated by some to be much better were the leak is identified and can be treated by sphinctrotomy and a stent [104] with very high success rate [105]. However, some of these patients fail and require surgical ligation of the leak which is much easier when the location is identified pre-operatively and a stent is in place to increase the success rate.

Another reason to go to the operating room is liver necrosis and abscess formation that occurs when bleeding stoops and demarcation of the live is obvious. Liver necrosis might increase with attempts to stop the bleeding with angioembolization in NOM or by arterial ligation and packing in DCS.The best option will be to drain the abscess radio-logically were this might be sufficient. However, if not we advise operative drainage and an anatomical liver resection to maintain adequate live tissue and maintain a good vas-cular supply. This should be carried out by an experienced liver surgeon to get the best result (Fig 18).

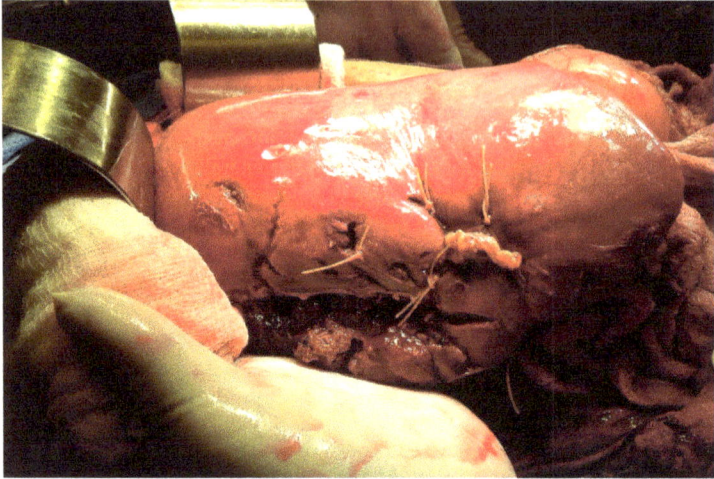

Figure 17. Full mobilization in a second look operation to stop the bleeding and to do definitive surgery.

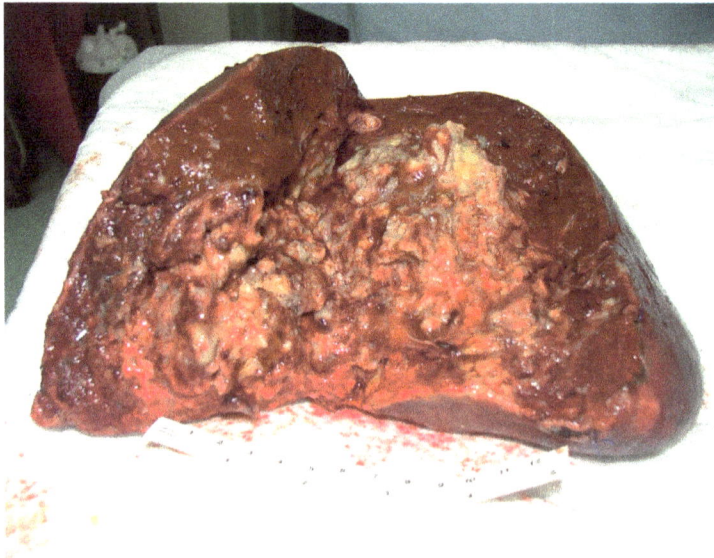

Figure 18. Liver necrosis following embolization with NOM for bleeding. The patient was treated by right hemi hepatectomy because the necrosis could not be drained radiologically.

Liver resection might be necessary with reported frequency of 2% to 5% in most series, with an overall mortality of 17.8% and morbidity around 30%.[106-108] (Fig 19).

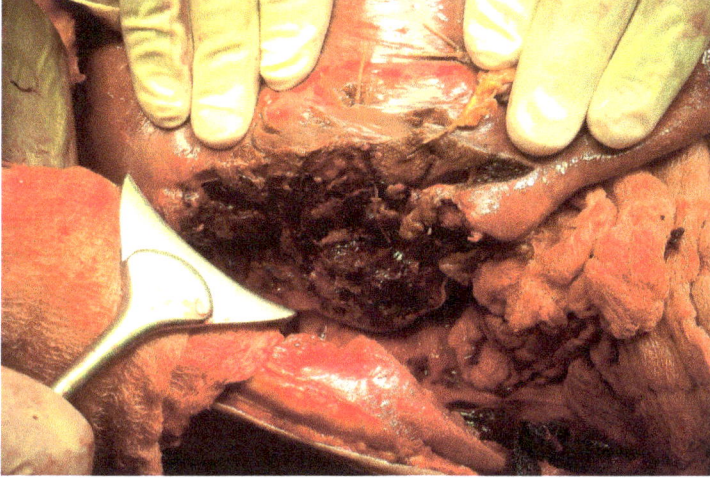

Figure 19. Liver trauma which was treated with a right posterior sectionectomy (seg 6&7)

Liver transplantation has been reported in the literature as an extreme intervention in cases of severe and complicated hepatic trauma. The main indications for liver transplant in such cases were uncontrollable bleeding and postoperative hepatic insufficiency. Liver transplant for trauma is a rare condition with 20 cases described in the literature [109]. Esquivel *et al.* first reported the use of liver transplantation in two patients with progressive hepatic failure and uncontrollable bleeding. [110]. The transplant decision is difficult because usual criteria are not validated, liver's potential recovery is difficult to evaluate and sepsis and head injuries often associated, complicating the decision because of their own prognosis. [111].

7. Complications

7.1. Non operative

The most common complication of NOM is failure, ending with the patient in the operating room. This is even more serious, because the patient most of the time is in a worse state than what he was and bleeding (the leading cause) is still ongoing. This also is more profound if it occurs in the middle of the night or with a surgeon of limited liver expertise. It should be borne in mind that this most common complication usually arises as a result of inappropriate selection of a patient for conservative management [23]. The failure rate ranges from 6-10% [68, 112] especially when it was combined with arterial emobolization, however, the incidence of liver necrosis was higher [113] (Fig 20a &b).

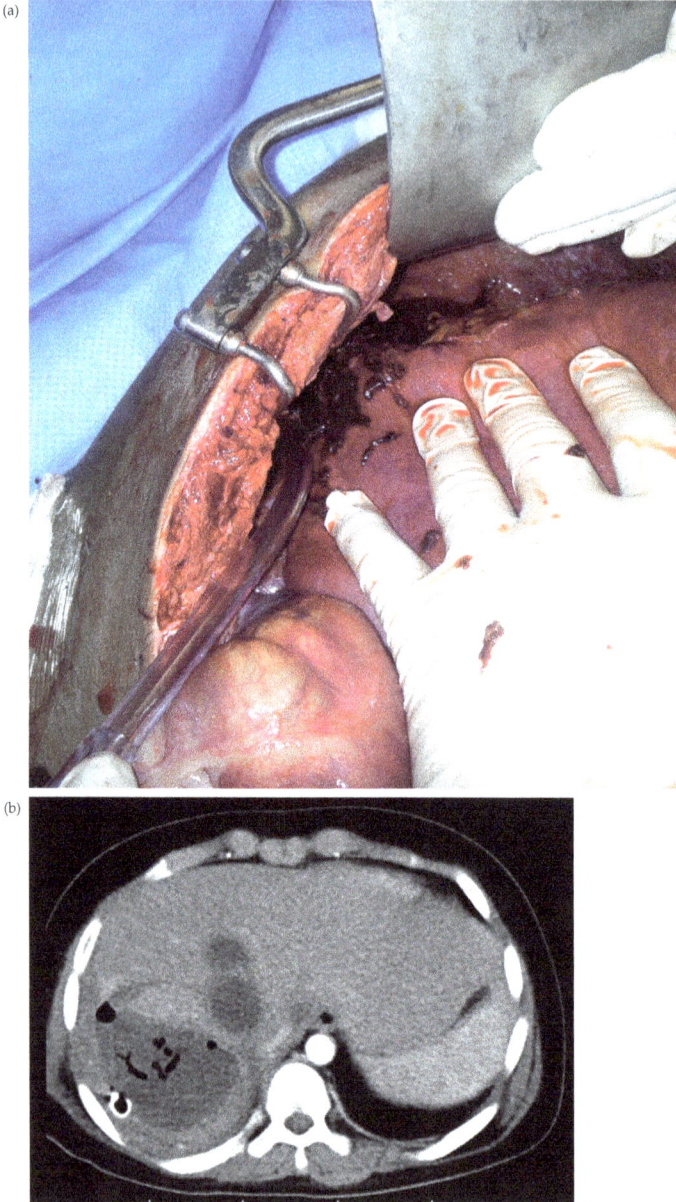

Figure 20. a. Failed NOM showing the bleeding from the liver dome. b. Same patient with grade 4 liver injury that failed NOM, drain left in place.

Complications can arise from injuries that have not been recognized at the time of initial presentation or /and become apparent after initial delay. Associated injuries seem to be the most important factors predisposing to postoperative problems [114]-[117].

In a recent multicenter study, hepatic complications developed in 5% (13 of 264) of patients with grade 3 injuries, 22% (36 of 166) of patients with grade 4 injuries, and 52% (12 of 23) of patients with grade 5 injuries. Univariate analysis revealed 24-hour crystalloid, total and first 24-hour packed red blood cells, fresh frozen plasma, platelet, and cryoprecipitate requirements and liver injury grade to be significant, but only liver injury grade and 24-hour transfusion requirement predicted complications by multivariable analysis. They came out with the Conclusion that NOM of high-grade liver injuries is associated with significant morbidity and correlates with grade of liver injury. Screening patients with transfusion requirements and high-grade injuries may result in earlier diagnosis and treatment of hepatic-related complications [118]. We have discussed in the previous section the management of each of these complications as a part of the operative management to liver trauma.

7.2. Operative

Rebleeding in the postoperative period is a challenging problem. Delayed haemorrhage is the most common complication of the non-operative management of hepatic injuries and is the usual indication for a delayed operation [119]. Coagulopathy, inadequate initial surgical repair and missed retrohepatic venous injury may result in further haemorrhage. Confirmed coagulation defects should be corrected as rapidly as possible with fresh frozen plasma and platelet transfusions.

Some authors recommend reoperation after transfusion of 10 units of blood in 24 h [120], however the limit of 6 units in the first 12 h seems to be more reasonable [121]-[122]. In cases with slow rebleeding when the limit of 6 units has not been exceeded, embolization of the bleeding vessels may be helpful [122]. Multiple bleeding vessels is usually the cause of failure because the vascular lesions distal to the area of embolization with rich collateral circulation, or bleeding from the portal or hepatic veins [123]-[125]

Late complications like sepsis, bile leak and liver failure occur at a later stage. Intra-abdominal sepsis in the postoperative period occurs in approximately 7-12 per cent of patients 126 Predisposing factors include the presence of shock and increased transfusion requirements, increased severity of liver injury, associated injuries such as small bowel or colonic perforation, the use of perihepatic packs, superficial suturing of deep lacerations with intrahepatic haematoma formation, and the presence of devitalized parenchyma. Adequate initial surgical management in an effort to reduce transfusion requirements, with debridement of all devitalized tissue and early removal of perihepatic packs, has been recommended to reduce the incidence of septic complications [81],.

Arteriovenous fistula is not an uncommon complication with an incidence of less than 3%. It can manifest after liver injury as an arterioportal fistula that can result in portal hypaertension and is usually treated by embolization [127].

8. Outcome

The mortality rate from liver trauma has fallen from 66 per cent in World War I, to 27 per cent in World War II, to current levels of 10-15 per cent [8],[10],[12],[128]-[129]. Better knowledge of liver pathophysiology and anatomy, and enhanced resuscitation, anaesthesia and intensive care, have contributed to this improvement. Schweizer et al,(1993) compared outcome to grade of injury. The overall mortality was 12% [9], specially with the livers excellent regeneration capability (Fig 21).

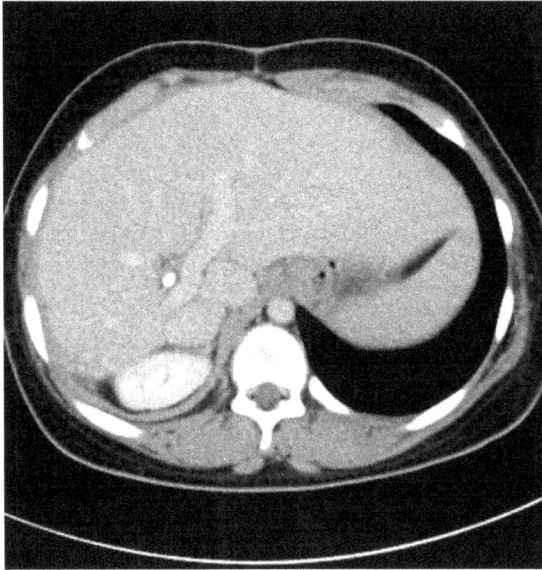

Figure 21. Liver regeneration post resection of the right liver

The mechanism of injury has an important bearing on mortality rate with blunt trauma carrying a higher mortality rate (10-30 per cent)[130]. than penetrating liver trauma (0-10 per cent)[10-11].

While most early deaths in patients with liver trauma seem to be due to uncontrolled haemorrhage and associated injuries, most late deaths result from head injuries and sepsis with multiple organ failure [131].

Author details

Bilal O. Al-Jiffry[1,2] and Owaid AlMalki[1]

1 Surgery, Taif University, Taif, Saudi Arabia

2 Surgery, AlHada Military Hospital, Taif, Saudi Arabia

References

[1] Wachtel T. Critical care concepts in the management of abdominal trauma. Crit Care Nurs Q. 1994;17(2):34-50.

[2] Feliciano DV. Surgery for liver trauma. Surg Clin North Am 1989; 69: 273-84.

[3] Cox EF. Blunt abdominal trauma. A five 5-year analysis of 870 patients requiring celiotomy. Ann Surg 1984; 199: 467-74.

[4] Clemente N, Di Saverio S, Giorgini E, Biscardi A, Villani S, Senatore G, Filicori F, Antonacci N, Baldoni F, Tugnoli G. Management and outcome of 308 cases of liver trauma in Bologna Trauma Center in 10 years. Ann Ital Chir. 2011 Sep-Oct;82(5):351-9

[5] Li Petri S, Gruttadauria S, Pagano D, Echeverri GJ, Di Francesco F, Cintorino D, Spada M, Gridelli B. Surgical management of complex liver trauma: a single liver transplant center experience. Am Surg. 2012 Jan;78(1):20-5

[6] A. Nawaz Khan H. Vadeyar Liver Trauma emedicine September 2005

[7] Matsch T, Begquist D, Hedelin M, Findblack B. Leberverletzungen nachstumpfem Bauchtrauma. Unfallchirurgie 1982; 85: 524-8.

[8] Schweizer W, Tanner S, Baer HU, Huber A, Berchtold R, Blumgart LH. Diagnostik und Therapie von Leberverletzungen beim polytraumatisierten Patienten. Helv Chir Acta 1989; 55: 597-612.

[9] Schweizer W, Tanner S, Baer HU, Lerut J, Huber A, Gertsch P et al. Management of traumatic liver injuries. Br J Surg 1993; 80: 86-8.

[10] Krige JE, Bornman PC, Terblanche J. Liver trauma in 446 patients. South Afr J Surg 1997; 35: 10-15.

[11] Feliciano DV, Mattox KL, Jordan GL Jr, Burch JM, Bitando CG, Cruse PA. Management of 1000 consecutive cases of hepatic trauma (1979-1984). Ann Surg 1986; 204: 438-45.

[12] Cogbill TH, Moore EE, Jurkovich GJ, Feliciano DV, Morris JA, Mucha P. Severe hepatic trauma: a multi-center experience with 1335 liver injuries. J Trauma 1988; 28: 1433-8.

[13] Park RW, Chrysos E, Diamond T, Management of liver trauma. Br J Surg 1999;86:1121-35.

[14] Parray FQ, Wani ML, Malik AA, Thakur N, Wani RA, Naqash SH, Chowdri NA, Wani KA, Bijli AH, Irshad I, Nayeem-Ul-Hassan. Evaluating a conservative approach to managing liver injuries in Kashmir, India. J Emerg Trauma Shock. 2011 Oct;4(4):483-7

[15] Liver resection and liver transplantation: the anatomy of the liver and associated structures. Jamieson Glyn, Launois B. In: The Anatomy of General Surgical Operation, Ed. Jamieson GG. Elsevier Churchill Livingstone, Edinburgh 2nd Ed. 2006. Chapter2, pp 8-23

[16] Gray`s anatomy of the human body, twentieth edition, Philadelphia , 2000.

[17] Peng SY. Isolated caudate lobe resection. In: Hepatocellular Carcinoma, Ed. Law WY, world Scientific Singapore2008. Chapter 26, pp 465-489

[18] Kawarada Y, Das BC, Taoka H. Anatomy of the hepatic hilar area: the plate system. Journal of HBP surgery 2000; 7: 580-586.

[19] Scheuerlein H, Kockerling F. The anatomy of the liver. In: liver surgery, Operative techniques and Avoidance of Complications. J.A. Barth, Heidelberg.2001, pp 9-38.

[20] Sherlock DJ, Bismuth H. Secondary surgery for liver trauma. Br J Surg 1991; 78: 1313-17.

[21] Arrillo EH, Wohltmann C, Evolution in the treatment of complex blunt liver injuries. Curr Probl Surg 2,001 Jan; 38(1): 1-60.

[22] Paterson-Brown, Core topics in general and emergency surgery; third edition 2005. Elsevier 239-257

[23] Garden, hepatobiliary and pancreatic surgery; third edition 2003. Elsevier 331-347

[24] . Bain IM, Kirby RM, Tiwary P, et al. Survey of abdominal ultrasound and diagnostic peritoneal lavage for suspected intra-abdominal injury following blunt trauma. Injury. 1999;29:65–71.

[25] Bode PJ, Edwards MJR, Kruit MC, van Vugt AB. Sonography in a clinical algorithm for early evaluation of 1671 patients with blunt abdominal trauma. Am J Radiol. 1999;172:905–911.

[26] Kimura A, Otsuka T. Emergency center ultrasonography in the evaluation of hemoperitoneum: a prospective study. J Trauma 1991; 31: 20-3.

[27] Hoffmann R, Nerlich M, Muggia-Sullam M, Pohlemann T, Wippermann B, Regel G et al. Blunt abdominal trauma in cases of multiple trauma evaluated by ultrasonography: a prospective analysis of 291 patients. J Trauma 1992; 32: 452-8.

[28] Pachter HL, Feliciano DV. Complex hepatic injuries. Surg Clin North Am 1996; 76: 763-82.

[29] Carrillo EH, Platz A, Miller FB, Richardson JD, Polk HC Jr. Non-operative management of blunt hepatic trauma. Br J Surg 1998; 85: 461-8.

[30] Goletti O, Ghiselli G, Lippolis PV, Chiarugi M, Braccini G, Macaluso C et al. The role of ultrasonography in blunt abdominal trauma: results in 250 consecutive cases. J Trauma 1994; 36: 178-81.

[31] Rozycki GS, Ochsner MG, Schmidt JA, Frankel HL, Davis TP, Wang D et al. A prospective study of surgeon-performed ultrasound as the primary adjuvant modality for injured patient assessment. J Trauma 1995; 39: 492-500.

[32] McKenney MG, Martin L, Lentz K, Lopez C, Sleeman D, Aristide G et al. 1000 consecutive ultrasounds for blunt abdominal trauma. J Trauma 1996; 40: 607-12.

[33] Richards JR, McGahan JP, Pali MJ, Bohnen PA. (1999) Sonographic detection of blunt hepatic trauma: hemoperitoneum and parencymal patterns of injury. J Trauma. 1999;47:1092–1097.

[34] Soto JA, Morales C, Murena F, Sanabria A, Guevara JM, Suarez T. Penetrating stab wounds to the abdomen: use of serial US and contrast enhanced CT in stable patients. Radiology. 2001;220:365–371.

[35] Hochmuth A, Fleck M, Hauff P, et al. First experience in using a new ultrasound mode and ultrasound contrast agent in the diagnosis of blunt renal trauma: a feasibility study in an animal model. [Preliminary report]. Invest Radiol. 2000;35:205–211.

[36] Adam A, Roddie ME. CT of the liver and biliary tract. In:Blumgart LH (ed.) surgery of the liver and the biliary tract, 2nd edn. Edinburgh: Churchill Livingstone, 1994;pp 243-70.

[37] Safi F, Weiner S, Poch B et al. surgical management of liver rupture. : Chirurgie 1999,70:253-8.

[38] Cachecho R, Clas D, Gersin K et al. Evolution in the management of the complex liver injury at a level 1 trauma center. J Trauma 1998; 45:79-82.

[39] Strong RW. The management of blunt liver injuries. Aust NZ J Surg 1999; 69:609-16.

[40] Toombs BD, Sandler CM, Rauschkolb EN, Strax R, Harle TS. Assessment of hepatic injuries with computed tomography. J Comput Assist Tomogr 1982; 6: 72-5.

[41] Carrillo EH, Wohltmann C, Evolution in the treatment of complex blunt liver injuries. Curr Probl Surg 2001 Jan; 38(1): 1-60.

[42] Casillas VJ, Amendola MA, et al, Imaging of nontraumatic hemorrhagic hepatic lesions. Radiographics 2000 Mar-Apr; 20(2): 367-78.

[43] Fang JF, Chen RJ, Wong YC, et al: Classification and treatment of pooling of contrast material on computed tomographic scan of blunt hepatic trauma. J Trauma 2000 Dec; 49(6): 1083-8.

[44] Meredith JW, Trunkey DD. CT scanning in acute abdominal injuries. Surg Clin North Am. 1988;68:255–268.

[45] Federle MP, Jeffrey RB. Hemoperitoneum studied by computed tomography. Radiology. 1983;148:187–192.

[46] Federle MP, Goldberg HI, Kaiser JA, et al.. Evaluation of abdominal trauma by computed tomography. Radiology. 1981;138:637–644.

[47] Toombs BD, Lester RC, Ben-Menachem Y, et al.. Computed tomography in blunt trauma. Rad Clin North Am. 1981;19:17–35.

[48] McGehee M, Kier R, Cohn SM, McCarthy SM: Comparison of MRI with postcontrast CT for the evaluation of acute abdominal trauma. J Comput Assist Tomogr 1993 May-Jun; 17(3): 410-3.

[49] Shuman WP. CT of blunt abdominal trauma in adults. Radiology 1997; 205: 297-306.

[50] Vock P, MRI. In: Blumgart LH (ed.) Surgery of the liver and biliary tract, 2nd edn. Edinburgh: Churchill Livingstone, 1994; pp271-82.

[51] Poletti PA, Mirvis SE, Shanmuganathan K, et al: CT criteria for management of blunt liver trauma: correlation with angiographic and surgical findings. Radiology 2000 Aug; 216(2): 418-27

[52] Hagiwara A, Yukioka T, Ohta S et al. non-surgical management of patients with blunt hepatic injury; efficacy of transcatheter arterial embolization. Am J Roentgenol 1997; 169:1151-6.

[53] Carrillo EH, Spain DA, Wohltmann CD et al.Interventional techniques are useful adjuncts in the non-operative management of hepatic injuries. J Trauma 1999;46:619-22.

[54] Sugimoto K, Asari Y, Sakaguchi T et al. ERCP in the non-surgical management o blunt liver trauma. J Trauma 1993;35:192-9.

[55] Sosa JL, Markley M, Sleeman D, Puente I, Carrillo E. Laparoscopy in abdominal gunshot wounds. Surg Laparosc Endosc 1993; 3: 417-19.

[56] Sosa JL, Arrillaga A, Puente I, Sleeman D, Ginzburg E, Martin L. Laparoscopy in 121 consecutive patients with abdominal gunshot wounds. J Trauma 1995; 39: 501-6.

[57] Ditmars ML, Bongard F. Laparoscopy for triage of penetrating trauma: the decision to explore. J Laparoendosc Surg 1996; 6: 285-91

[58] Hallfeld KK, Trupka AW, Erhard J et al. Emergency laparoscopy for abdominal stab wounds. Surg Endosco 1998; 12:907-10.

[59] Chen RJ, Fang JF,Lin BC et al. selective application of laparoscopy and fibrin glue in the failure of non-operative management of blunt hepatic trauma. J Trauma1998;44:691-5.

[60] Pilcher CJ, Wesolowski MS, Jawad MA. Laparoscopic applications for abdominal trauma injuries. AORN J 1996; 64: 366-75.

[61] Raphael T, Villavicencio , John A.Aucar. Analysis of laparoscopy in trauma. JACS 1999;189:pp11-20.

[62] Moore EE, Shackford SR, Pachter HL, McAninch JW, Browner BD, Champion HR et al. Organ injury scaling: spleen, liver and kidney. J Trauma 1989; 29: 1664-6.

[63] 14 Ochsner MG, Jaffin JH, Golocovsky M, Jones RC. Major hepatic trauma. Surg Clin North Am 1993; 73: 337-52.

[64] David Richardson, changes in the management of injuries to the liver and spleen. JACS May 2005 pages 648-669

[65] Richie JP, Fonkalsrud EN. Subcapsular hematoma of the liver. Arch Surg. 1972;104:781–784

[66] Karp MP, Cooney DR, Pros GA, et al.. The non-operative management of pediatric hepatic trauma. J Pediatr Surg. 1983;18:512–518.

[67] Meyers AA, Crass RA, Lim RA, et al.. Selective non-operative management of blunt liver injury using computed tomography. Arch Surg. 1985;120:550–554

[68] Parks NA, Davis JW, Forman D, Lemaster D. Observation for nonoperative management of blunt liver injuries: how long is long enough? J Trauma. 2011 Mar;70(3):626-9

[69] Norrman G, Tingstedt B, Ekelund M, Andersson R. Non-operative management of blunt liver trauma: feasible and safe also in centres with a low trauma incidence. HPB (Oxford). 2009 Feb;11(1):50-6

[70] Letoublon C, Chen Y, Arvieux C, Voirin D, Morra I, Broux C, Risse O. Delayed celiotomy or laparoscopy as part of the nonoperative management of blunt hepatic trauma. World J Surg. 2008 Jun;32(6):1189-93

[71] Marx JA, Moore EE, Jordan RC, et al.. Limitations of computed tomography in the evaluation of acute abdominal trauma—prospective randomized study. J Trauma. 1985;25:933–938.

[72] Buckman RF, Piano G, Dunham CM, et al.. Major bowel and diaphragmatic injuries associated with blunt spleen or liver rupture. J Trauma. 1988;28:1317–1321.

[73] Fischer RP, Miller-Crotchet P, Reed RL. The hazards of non-operative management of adults with blunt abdominal injury. J Trauma. 1988;28:1445–1449.

[74] Kemmeter PR, Hoedema RE, Foote JA, et al. Concomitant blunt enteric injuries with injuries of the liver and spleen (a dilemma for trauma surgeons). Am Surg. 2001;267:221–226.

[75] Sherk JP, Oakes DD. Intestinal injuries missed by computed tomography. J Trauma. 1990;30:1–7.

[76] Schnüriger B, Talving P, Barbarino R, Barmparas G, Inaba K, Demetriades D. Current practice and the role of the CT in the management of penetrating liver injuries at a Level I trauma center. J Emerg Trauma Shock. 2011 Jan;4(1):53-7

[77] Navsaria PH, Nicol AJ, Krige JE, Edu S. Selective nonoperative management of liver gunshot injuries. Ann Surg. 2009 Apr;249(4):653-6

[78] Velmahos GC, Constantinou C, Tillou A, Brown CV, Salim A, Demetriades D. Abdominal computed tomographic scan for patients with gunshot wounds to the abdomen selected for nonoperative management. J Trauma. 2005 Nov;59(5):1155-60; discussion 1160-1

[79] Omoshoro-Jones JA, Nicol AJ, Navsaria PH, Zellweger R, Krige JE, Kahn DH. Selective non-operative management of liver gunshot injuries. Br J Surg. 2005 Jul;92(7): 890-5

[80] Demetriades,Demetrios, Selective nonoperative management of penetrating abdominal solid organ injuries. Ann. Surg 2006;244:pp620-28

[81] Wilson RH, Moorehead RJ. Hepatic traumaand its management. Injury 1991;22:439-45.

[82] Stain SC, Yellin AE, Donovan AJ. Hepatic trauma. Arch Surg 1988; 123: 1251-5.

[83] Feliciano DV, Pachter HL. Hepatic trauma revisited. Curr Probl Surg 1989; 26: 453-524

[84] Canizaro PC, Pessa ME. Management of massive hemorrhage associated with abdominal trauma. Surg Clin North Am 1990; 70: 621-34.

[85] Pringle JH. Notes on the arrest of hemorrhage due to trauma. Ann Surg. 1908;48:546–566.

[86] Moore EE, Edgar J. Poth Lecture. Critical decisions in the management of hepatic trauma. Am J Surg 1984; 148: 712-16.

[87] Walt AJ, Bender JS. Injuries of the liver. In: Schwartz SI, Ellis H, eds. Maingot's Abdominal Operations. Vol. 2. Norwalk, Connecticut: Appleton-Century-Crofts, 1985: 1577-90.

[88] Shuman WP. CT of blunt abdominal trauma in adult . radiology 1997; 205: 297-306.

[89] Smadja C, Traynor O, Blumgart LH. Delayed hepatic resection for major liver injury. Br J Surg 1982; 69: 361-4.

[90] Ochsner MG, Jaffain JH, Golocovsky M. Jones RC. Major hepatic trauma. Surg clin north am 1993;73:337-52.

[91] Lucas CE, Ledgerwood AM. Prospective evaluation of hemostatic techniques for liver injuries. J Trauma. 1976;16:442–451.

[92] Feliciano DV, Mattox KL, Jordan GL, et al.. The management of 1000 consecutive cases of hepatic trauma. Ann Surg. 1988;204:438–495.

[93] Trunkey DD, Shires GT, McClellan R. Management of liver trauma in 811 consecutive patients. Ann Surg. 1974;179:722–728.

[94] Morris JA, Eddy VA, Blinman TA, et al.. The staged celiotomy for trauma (issues in unpacking and reconstruction). Ann Surg. 1993;217:576–586.

[95] Aaron WS, Fulton RL, Mays ET. Selective ligation of the hepatic artery for trauma of the liver. Surg Gynecol Obstet. 1975;141:187–189.

[96] Mays ET, Conti S, Fallahzadkh H, et al.. Hepatic artery ligation. Surgery. 1979;86:536–543

[97] Mays ET. Hepatic trauma. Curr Prob Surg. 1976;13:1–86.

[98] Flint LM, Polk HC. Selective hepatic artery ligation (limitations and failures). J Trauma. 1979;19:319–323.

[99] Schrock T, Blaisdell FW, Mathewson C, et al.. Management of blunt trauma to the liver and hepatic veins. Arch Surg. 1968;96:698–704.

[100] FA, Moore EE, Seagraves A. Non-resectional management of major hepatic trauma. Amer J Surg. 1985;150:725–729.

[101] Walt AJ. The mythology of hepatic trauma or babel revisited. Amer J Surg. 1978;135:1218.

[102] Stone HH, Lamb JM. Use of pedicled omentum as an autogenous pack for control of hemorrhage in major injuries of the liver. Surg Gynecol Obstet. 1975;141:92–94.

[103] Carmona RH, Peck D, Lim RC. The role of packing and re-operation in severe hepatic trauma. J Trauma. 1984;24:779–784.

[104] Wahl WL, Brandt MM, Hemmila MR, Arbabi S. Diagnosis and management of bile leaks after blunt liver injury. Surgery. 2005 Oct;138(4):742-7; discussion 747-8

[105] Sugimoto K, Asari Y, Sakaguchi T et al. ERCP in the non-surgical management o blunt liver trauma. J Trauma 1993;35:192-9.

[106] Pachter HL, Spencer FC, Hofstetter SR, et al. Significant trends in the treatment of hepatic injuries. Experience with 411 injuries. Ann Surg 1992;215:492–500.

[107] Polanco P, Leon S, Pineda J, et al. Hepatic resection in the management of complex injury to the liver. J Trauma 2008;65(6):1264–9 [discussion: 1269–70].

[108] Richardson JD, Franklin GA, Lukan JK, et al. Evolution in the management of hepatic trauma: a 25-year perspective. Ann Surg 2000;232:324–30.

[109] Honore C, et al. Liver transplantation for hepatic trauma: Discussion about a case and its management. J Emerg Trauma Shock. 2011 Jan;4(1):137-9.

[110] Liver replacement after massive hepatic trauma. Esquivel CO, Bernardos A, Makowka L, Iwatsuki S, Gordon RD, Starzl TE. J Trauma. 1987 Jul;27(7):800-2

[111] Delis SG, Bakoyiannis A, Selvaggi G, Weppler D, Levi D, Tzakis AG. Liver transplantation for severe hepatic trauma: experience from a single center. World J Gastroenterol 2009;15:1641-4.

[112] Clemente N, Di Saverio S, Giorgini E, Biscardi A, Villani S, Senatore G, Filicori F, Antonacci N, Baldoni F, Tugnoli G. Management and outcome of 308 cases of liver trauma in Bologna Trauma Center in 10 years. Ann Ital Chir. 2011 Sep-Oct;82(5):351-9

[113] Beuran M, Nego I, Ispas AT, Păun S, Runcanu A, Lupu G, Venter D. Nonoperative management of high degree hepatic trauma in the patient with risk factors for failure: have we gone too far? J Med Life. 2010 Jul-Sep;3(3):289-96

[114] Fabian TC, Croce MA, Stanford GG, Payne LW, Mangiante EC, Voeller GR et al. Factors affecting morbidity following hepatic trauma. A prospective analysis of 482 injuries. Ann Surg 1991; 213: 540-8.

[115] 126 Flint LM, Mays ET, Aaron WS, Fulton RL, Polk HC. Selectivity in the management of hepatic trauma. Ann Surg 1977; 185: 613-18.

[116] Bender JS, Geller ER, Wilson RF. Intra-abdominal sepsis following liver trauma. J Trauma 1989; 29: 1140-5.

[117] Menegaux F, Langlois P, Chigot JP. Severe blunt trauma of the liver: study of mortality factors. J Trauma 1993; 35: 865-9.

[118] Rosemary A. Kozar, Frederick A. Moore, C. Clay Cothren, ; Risk Factors for Hepatic Morbidity Following Nonoperative Management Multicenter Study Arch Surg. 2006;141:451-459.

[119] Carrillo EH, Platz A, Miller FB, Richardson JD, Polk HC Jr. Non-operative management of blunt hepatic trauma. Br J Surg 1998; 85: 461-8.

[120] Cue JI, Cryer HG, Miller FB, Richardson JD, Polk HC Jr. Packing and planned reexploration for hepatic and retroperitoneal hemorrhage: critical refinements of a useful technique. J Trauma 1990; 30: 1007-13

[121] Beal SL. Fatal hepatic hemorrhage: an unresolved problem in the management of complex liver injuries. J Trauma 1990; 30: 163-9.

[122] De Toma G, Mingoli A, Modini C, Cavallaro A, Stipa S. The value of angiography and selective hepatic artery embolization for continuous bleeding after surgery in liver trauma: case reports. J Trauma 1994; 37: 508-11.

[123] Brick SH, Taylor GA, Potter BM, Eichelberger MR. Hepatic and splenic injury in children: role of CT in the decision for laparotomy. Radiology 1987; 165: 643-6.

[124] Krige JEJ, Bornman PC, Terblanche J. Therapeutic perihepatic packing in complex liver trauma. Br J Surg 1992; 79: 43-6.

[125] Tisnado J, Beachley MC, Cho SR. Control of intrahepatic bleeding by superselective embolization of the middle hepatic artery. South Med J 1982; 75: 70-1.

[126] Morimoto RY, Birolini D, Junqueira AR Jr, Poggetti R, Horita LT. Balloon tamponade for transfixing lesions of the liver. Surg Gynecol Obstet 1987; 164: 87-8.

[127] Oishi AJ, Nagorney DM Portl hypertension, variceal bleeding and high output cardiac failure secondary to an intrahepatic arterioportal fistula. HPB surg 1993;7:53-9.

[128] Pachter HL, Liang HG, Hofstetter SR. Liver and biliary tract trauma. In: Moore EE, Mattox KL, Feliciano DV, eds. Trauma. 2nd ed. Norwalk, Connecticut: Appleton and Lange, 1991: 441-63.

[129] Helling TS, Morse G, McNabney WK, Beggs CW, Behrends SH et al. Treatment of liver injuries at level I and level II centres in a multi-institutional metropolitan trauma system. The Midwest Trauma Society Liver Trauma Study Group. J Trauma 1997; 42: 1091-6.

[130] Sherman HF,Savage BA, Jones LM et al. non-operative management of blunt hepatic injuries: safe at any grade? J Trauma 1994; 37:616-21.

[131] Cox EF, Flancbaum L, Dauterive AH, Paulson RL. Blunt trauma to the liver. Analysis of management and mortality in 323 consecutive patients. Ann Surg 1988; 207: 126-34

Permissions

The contributors of this book come from diverse backgrounds, making this book a truly international effort. This book will bring forth new frontiers with its revolutionizing research information and detailed analysis of the nascent developments around the world.

We would like to thank Hesham Abdeldayem, MD, for lending his expertise to make the book truly unique. He has played a crucial role in the development of this book. Without his invaluable contribution this book wouldn't have been possible. He has made vital efforts to compile up to date information on the varied aspects of this subject to make this book a valuable addition to the collection of many professionals and students.

This book was conceptualized with the vision of imparting up-to-date information and advanced data in this field. To ensure the same, a matchless editorial board was set up. Every individual on the board went through rigorous rounds of assessment to prove their worth. After which they invested a large part of their time researching and compiling the most relevant data for our readers. Conferences and sessions were held from time to time between the editorial board and the contributing authors to present the data in the most comprehensible form. The editorial team has worked tirelessly to provide valuable and valid information to help people across the globe.

Every chapter published in this book has been scrutinized by our experts. Their significance has been extensively debated. The topics covered herein carry significant findings which will fuel the growth of the discipline. They may even be implemented as practical applications or may be referred to as a beginning point for another development. Chapters in this book were first published by InTech; hereby published with permission under the Creative Commons Attribution License or equivalent.

The editorial board has been involved in producing this book since its inception. They have spent rigorous hours researching and exploring the diverse topics which have resulted in the successful publishing of this book. They have passed on their knowledge of decades through this book. To expedite this challenging task, the publisher supported the team at every step. A small team of assistant editors was also appointed to further simplify the editing procedure and attain best results for the readers.

Our editorial team has been hand-picked from every corner of the world. Their multi-ethnicity adds dynamic inputs to the discussions which result in innovative outcomes. These outcomes are then further discussed with the researchers and contributors who give their valuable feedback and opinion regarding the same. The feedback is then collaborated with the researches and they are edited in a comprehensive manner to aid the understanding of the subject.

Apart from the editorial board, the designing team has also invested a significant amount of their time in understanding the subject and creating the most relevant covers. They scrutinized every image to scout for the most suitable representation of the subject and create an appropriate cover for the book.

The publishing team has been involved in this book since its early stages. They were actively engaged in every process, be it collecting the data, connecting with the contributors or procuring relevant information. The team has been an ardent support to the editorial, designing and production team. Their endless efforts to recruit the best for this project, has resulted in the accomplishment of this book. They are a veteran in the field of academics and their pool of knowledge is as vast as their experience in printing. Their expertise and guidance has proved useful at every step. Their uncompromising quality standards have made this book an exceptional effort. Their encouragement from time to time has been an inspiration for everyone.

The publisher and the editorial board hope that this book will prove to be a valuable piece of knowledge for researchers, students, practitioners and scholars across the globe.

List of Contributors

Hesham Abdeldayem, Amr Helmy, Hisham Gad, Essam Salah, Amr Sadek, Tarek Ibrahim, Elsayed Soliman, Khaled Abuelella, Maher Osman, Amr Aziz, Hosam Soliman, Sherif Saleh, Osama Hegazy, Hany Shoreem, Taha Yasen, Emad Salem, Mohamed Taha, Hazem Zakaria, Islam Ayoub and Ahmed Sherif
Department of Surgery, National Liver Institute, Egypt

Ahmad Madkhali
Department of surgery, College of Medicine, King Saud University, Riyadh, Saudi Arabia

Murad Aljiffry
Department of surgery, College of Medicine, King Abdulaziz University, Jeddah, Saudi Arabia

Mazen Hassanain
Department of surgery, College of Medicine, King Saud University, Riyadh, Saudi Arabia College of Medicine, Liver Disease Research Centre, King Saud University, Riyadh, Saudi Arabia

S. M. Robinson
Institute of Cellular Medicine, Newcastle University, Framlington Place, Newcastle upon Tyne, UK

J. Scott
Department of Radiology, Freeman Hospital, Newcastle upon Tyne, UK

D. M. Manas and S. A. White
Department of HPB Surgery, Freeman Hospital, Newcastle upon Tyne, UK

Julio C. Wiederkehr, Izabel M. Coelho and Sylvio G. Avilla
Federal University of Paraná, Curitiba, Brazil
Hospital Pequeno Príncipe, Curitiba, Brazil

Barbara A. Wiederkehr and Henrique A. Wiederkehr
Hospital Pequeno Príncipe, Curitiba, Brazil

Chunbao Guo and Mingman Zhang
Dept. of hepatobiliary Surgery, Children's Hospital, Chongqing Medical University, Chongqing P. R. China, P. R. China

Hiroshi Yoshida
Department of Surgery, Nippon Medical School Tama Nagayama Hospital, Japan
Department of Surgery, Nippon Medical School, Japan

Yasuhiro Mamada, Nobuhiko Taniai, Takashi Tajiri and Eiji Uchida
Department of Surgery, Nippon Medical School, Japan

Hao Lu, Guoqiang Li, Ling Lu, Ye Fan, Xiaofeng Qian, Ke Wang and Feng Zhang
Liver Transplantation Center, First Affiliated Hospital of Nanjing Medical Univerisity, Nanjing, China

Mirela Patricia Sîrb Boeti and Irinel Popescu
University of Medicine and Pharmacy "Carol Davila", Bucharest, Romania

Răzvan Grigorie
Fundeni Clinical Institute, Department of General Surgery and Liver Transplantation, Buchares, Romania

Elsayed Ibrahim Salama
Pediatric Department, National, Menoufia University, Egypt

Rajan Jagad, Ashok Thorat and Wei-Chen Lee
Division of Liver and Transplantation Surgery, Department of General Surgery, Chang-Gung Memorial Hospital at Linkou, Chang-Gung University College of Medicine, Taiwan

Ahmad Mohamed Sira and Mostafa Mohamed Sira
Department of Pediatric Hepatology, National Liver Institute, Menofiya University, Egypt

Bilal O. Al-Jiffry
Surgery, Taif University, Taif, Saudi Arabia
Surgery, Al Hada Military Hospital, Taif, Saudi Arabia

Owaid AlMalki
Surgery, Taif University, Taif, Saudi Arabia

www.ingramcontent.com/pod-product-compliance
Lightning Source LLC
Chambersburg PA
CBHW070738190326
41458CB00004B/1219